THIRD EDITION

SERIOUS STRENGTH TRAINING

Contents

THIRD EDITION

SERIOUS STRENGTH TRAINING

Tudor O. Bompa, PhD

Mauro Di Pasquale, MD

Lorenzo J. Cornacchia

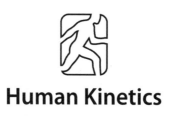

Human Kinetics

Library of Congress Cataloging-in-Publication Data

Bompa, Tudor O.
    Serious strength training / Tudor O. Bompa, Mauro Di Pasquale, Lorenzo J. Cornacchia. -- 3rd ed.
        p. cm.
    Includes bibliographical references and index.
    1. Weight training. 2. Bodybuilding. 3. Muscle strength. I. Di Pasquale, Mauro G. II. Cornacchia, Lorenzo, 1968-
III. Title.
    GV546.B55 2012
    613.7'1--dc23
                                    2012022403
ISBN-10: 1-4504-2244-6 (print)
ISBN-13: 978-1-4504-2244-4 (print)

This publication is written and published to provide accurate and authoritative information relevant to the subject matter presented. It is published and sold with the understanding that the author and publisher are not engaged in rendering legal, medical, or other professional services by reason of their authorship or publication of this work. If medical or other expert assistance is required, the services of a competent professional person should be sought.

Permission notices for material reprinted in this book from other sources can be found on page xi.

The web addresses cited in this text were current as of September 2012, unless otherwise noted.

Acquisitions Editor: Justin Klug; **Developmental Editor:** Heather Healy; **Assistant Editor:** Claire Marty; **Copyeditor:** Patricia MacDonald; **Indexer:** Nan N. Badgett; **Permissions Manager:** Martha Gullo; **Graphic Designer:** Fred Starbird; **Cover Designer:** Keith Blomberg; **Photograph (cover):** Milos Markovic/istockphoto; **Photo Production Manager:** Jason Allen; **Art Manager:** Kelly Hendren; **Associate Art Manager:** Alan L. Wilborn; **Illustrations:** © Human Kinetics, unless otherwise noted; **Printer:** United Graphics

Human Kinetics books are available at special discounts for bulk purchase. Special editions or book excerpts can also be created to specification. For details, contact the Special Sales Manager at Human Kinetics.

Printed in the United States of America   10 9 8 7 6 5 4 3 2 1

The paper in this book is certified under a sustainable forestry program.

Human Kinetics
Website: www.HumanKinetics.com

United States: Human Kinetics
P.O. Box 5076
Champaign, IL 61825-5076
800-747-4457
e-mail: humank@hkusa.com

Canada: Human Kinetics
475 Devonshire Road Unit 100
Windsor, ON N8Y 2L5
800-465-7301 (in Canada only)
e-mail: info@hkcanada.com

Europe: Human Kinetics
107 Bradford Road
Stanningley
Leeds LS28 6AT, United Kingdom
+44 (0) 113 255 5665
e-mail: hk@hkeurope.com

Australia: Human Kinetics
57A Price Avenue
Lower Mitcham, South Australia 5062
08 8372 0999
e-mail: info@hkaustralia.com

New Zealand: Human Kinetics
P.O. Box 80
Torrens Park, South Australia 5062
0800 222 062
e-mail: info@hknewzealand.com

E5632

Preface

If you are reading this book, you clearly have an interest in bodybuilding and strength training, but do not allow the title or photos to mislead you into thinking *Serious Strength Training* can benefit only professional bodybuilders and strength trainers; this is not true. This book can also benefit beginner and recreational athletes. We included photos that are aesthetically pleasing, that provide a "wow" factor and accentuate the specific muscle groups highlighted within chapters, but you may not want to look like a professional bodybuilder or become bulky like a strength athlete. The choice is yours, and the level of bodybuilding and strength training you choose to undertake is entirely up to you.

Strength training is the only sport dedicated solely to the aesthetics of the human body. The roots of strength training and bodybuilding lie in Roman and Greek antiquity. These civilizations used physical activity as a means of striving for a perfect balance between body and mind. Sculptures from these ancient societies reflect their perceptions of the perfect human form—large, strong, well-defined muscles, all in perfect proportion, or balance.

Today, however, some bodybuilders and athletes have abandoned the idea of the perfect human body for the novelty of a freaky body part. They seem to favor mass over symmetry, bulk over chiseled lines, bloat over definition, and quantity over quality. Although mass is important, we must realize that its value does not exceed the value of symmetrical lines, well-proportioned limbs, and deeply striated muscles. To attain the ultimate body, one must never lose sight of the balance that shapes the perfect form. To achieve this level of development requires dedication, patience, and—most important—a solid understanding of the body, training principles, exercise prescription, nutrition, and planning. This book introduces a revolutionary approach to strength training and bodybuilding that will bring the body to its perfect state, naturally, with *periodization*. Read on to see how this book can help you build the ultimate physique!

GET BIGGER AND STRONGER!

Dr. Tudor O. Bompa developed periodization in Romania in 1963. The Eastern Bloc countries used his unique system for years as they achieved virtual domination of the athletic world. The system has also been published worldwide in many journals and magazines. Bompa is the author of several books, including *Theory and Methodology of Training: The Key to Athletic Performance* (1963, 1985, 1990, and 1994) and *Periodization of Strength: The New Wave in Strength Training* (1993). In 1988, he applied his concept of periodization to the sport of bodybuilding, and his periodization of bodybuilding system has been published in *Iron Man Magazine* as the Iron Man Training System since 1991. In 1996, Dr. Bompa worked with Lorenzo Cornacchia to write a monthly column called EMG Analysis (Iron Man Publication). Since then, Dr. Bompa has published *Periodization Training for Sports, Second Edition* (2005), and *The Theory and Methodology of Training, Fifth Edition* (2009).

Periodization for serious strength training and bodybuilding is a method of organizing training to achieve optimal gains in mass, strength, and definition, without encountering the pitfalls of overtraining, stagnation, and injury. Different training phases such as *anatomical adaptation, hypertrophy, maximum strength, muscle definition,* and *transition* are manipulated according to individual training goals. This approach ensures that an athlete will peak at appropriate times and can build or maintain a splendid physique year-round. Whether you are just beginning to train or are a seasoned pro, this book has the training plan you need, complete with detailed daily training programs.

GET MASSIVE AND RIPPED!

Serious Strength Training includes a nutrition and supplement program to correspond with each phase of training. The body's needs change as training changes, so we must take nutrition and supplementation into account and not leave it to chance. The metabolic diet, coupled with the periodization of supplementation, gives athletes the tools needed to reach optimal levels of strength, mass, and definition. Dr. Mauro Di Pasquale spends a substantial amount of time researching supplementation formulas to work in conjunction with the metabolic diet.

Dr. Di Pasquale was a world-class athlete for more than 15 years, winning the world championship in powerlifting in 1976 and the World Games in 1981. Today he balances a busy career as a licensed physician in Ontario, Canada, with his demanding schedule as a consultant and researcher. Dr. Di Pasquale's licensed profession and research have contributed to his experience and vast knowledge in periodization of training, dieting, and supplementation.

GET SMART!

Cutting-edge research, directed by kinesiologist and former NWA (National Wrestling Alliance) light-heavyweight wrestler Lorenzo Cornacchia, gives you the last word on the best exercises for strength, mass, and shape. Scientific studies, using state-of-the-art EMG (electromyography) equipment, identify the exercises that produce the greatest amount of electrical muscular activation. Part III, Maximum Stimulation Exercises, ranks exercises in order of their effectiveness and provides pictures for each movement to ensure proper execution.

GET STARTED!

For those who have been using the periodization training system over the past few years, it has meant better results—increased muscle size, tone, and definition—without the ever-present pain, strain, and exhaustion typical of other programs. For those about to begin using these techniques, don't look back. Training will never be the same again!

Acknowledgments

We would like to dedicate this book to Paul Ricciardi, who lost his fight with Hodgkin's lymphoma in October 2010 at the young age of 36. His strength and fight were something to be admired.

We would like to thank Leanna Taggio for her hard work and dedicated research in helping to edit and organize *Serious Strength Training, Third Edition*.

We would also like to thank Christina Sangalli for the initial stages of manuscript preparation.

We are grateful to the following people for their expert contributions to the completion of this book.

Lenny Visconti, BPHE, BSc (PT), CAFC

Jacquie Laframboise, PhD

Cassandra Volpe, PhD

Louis Melow, PhD

Shiraz Kapadia, BSc (PT)

Marni Pepper, BSc (PT)

Teddy Temertzoglou, BPHE

We are equally indebted to York University for the use of their EMG research facilities and equipment.

We express our appreciation to the friends and close associates who have contributed either directly or indirectly to the completion of this book:

Bernadette Taggio

Kelly Gallacher

Bonnie Hicks

John Poptsis

Laura Binetti

Michael Berger

Mike Cotic

Carmela Caggianiello

Patricia Gallacher

Trevor Butler

Frank Covelli

Special thanks to our partners Mike Cotic and Trevor Butler for the coordination and scheduling of the Fitness Fanatix Gym Facility.

We thank Terry Park for his high professionalism in the many hours necessary to take and edit the required photographs. Special thanks to Sammy Wong and Peter Robinson for their photographs and hard work.

Special thanks to all the bodybuilders and fitness models who posed for photographs.

Special thanks to Stephen Holman, editor in chief of *Iron Man Magazine*; Tom Deters, DC, associate publisher of *Flex* (Weider Publications); and Mark Casselman, science editor of *Muscle & Fitness*.

Finally, we would like to thank the professionals at Human Kinetics for their contributions. We are indebted to Justin Klug and Heather Healy, who helped make this project a great success.

Credits

Figures 1.5, 3.1, 3.2, 3.3, 3.4, 3.5, 3.6, 3.7, 3.8, 3.9, 3.10, 12.1, tables 3.1, 3.3, 4.2, 12.1, appendix C and D tables: Reprinted from T.O. Bompa, 1996, *Periodization of strength*, 4th ed. (Toronto: Veritas).

Figure 3.11 Reprinted from T.O. Bompa, 1983, *Theory and methodology of training: The key to athletic performance*, 3rd ed. (Dubuque: Kendall Hunt). Modified from N. Yakovlev, 1967, *Sports biochemistry* (Leipzig: Deutsche Hochschule für Körperkultur).

Figures 3.12 and 3.13 Reprinted, by permission, from T.O. Bompa, 1983, *Theory and methodology of training: The key to athletic performance*, 3rd ed. (Dubuque: Kendall Hunt).

Figures 5.3, 5.4, 5.5, 5.6, text on page 96: Adapted from M. Di Pasquale, 2002, *The anabolic solution for recreational and competitive bodybuilders*, 3rd ed. [Online]. Available: www.metabolicdiet.com/books/as_bb.pdf [April 25, 2012].

Figures 6.1, 6.2, 6.3, 6.4, 7.1, table 6.1: Reprinted from M. Di Pasquale, 2002, *The anabolic solution for recreational and competitive bodybuilders*, 3rd ed. [Online]. Available: www.metabolicdiet.com/books/as_bb.pdf [April 25, 2012].

PART ONE

SCIENCE of STRENGTH TRAINING

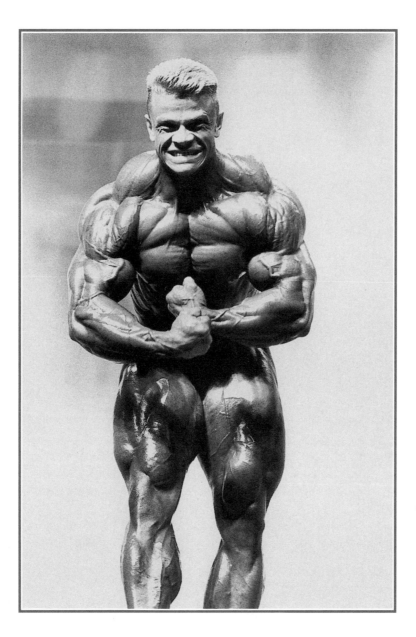

Adapting to the Training Stimulus

Understanding certain theoretical principles and fundamental concepts in strength training and bodybuilding, as well as having general overall knowledge, allows athletes, at any level, to create training programs that will help them achieve their goals and meet their specific training needs. To effectively utilize the information in this book, you must understand muscle contraction and how muscles produce work.

MUSCLES AND MUSCLE CONTRACTION

Three separate layers of connective tissue surround skeletal muscle (see figure 1.1). The outmost layer is the epimysium. The middle connective tissue, the perimysium, surrounds the individual bundles of muscle fibers, called the fasciculi (singular = fasciculus). Each muscle fiber within a fasciculus is surrounded by a connective tissue called the endomysium. The membrane surrounding the muscle fiber cell is referred to as the sarcolemma. Satellite cells located above the sarcolemma play a key role in muscle growth and repair (Wozniak et al. 2005).

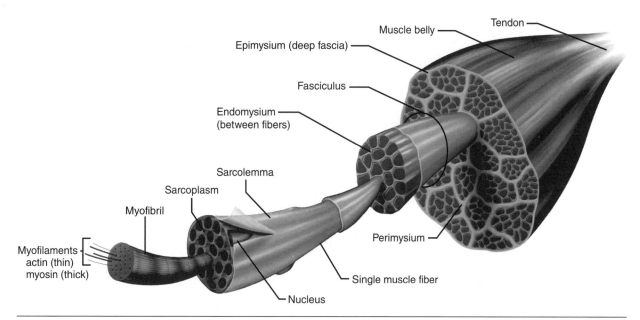

FIGURE 1.1 The three layers of connective tissue in skeletal muscle: epimysium (outer layer), perimysium (middle layer that surrounds fasciculi), and endomysium (surrounds individual muscle fibers).

Each muscle fiber has threadlike protein strands called myofibrils that contain the contractile proteins myosin (thick filaments) and actin (thin filaments), whose actions are very important in muscle contraction (figure 1.2). The ability of a muscle to contract and exert force is determined by its design, the cross-sectional area, the fiber length, and the number of fibers within the muscle. Dedicated training increases the thickness of muscle filaments, thereby increasing both muscle size and force of the contraction.

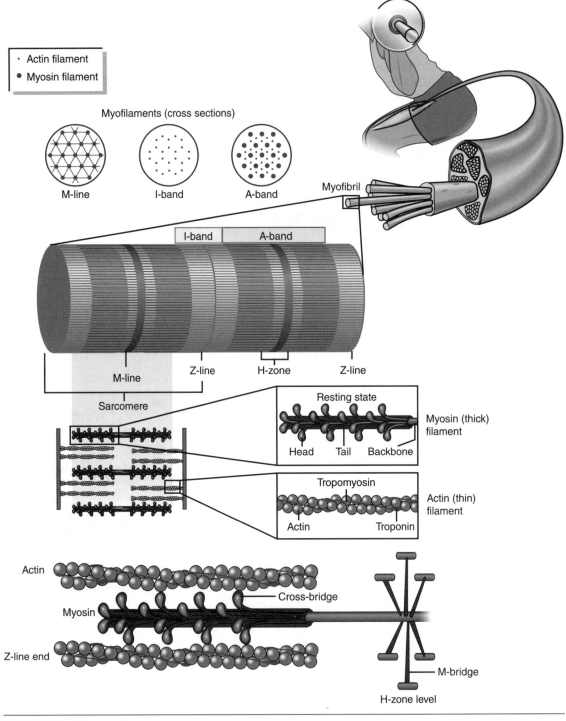

FIGURE 1.2 Muscle cell.

MECHANISM OF MUSCLE CONTRACTION: SLIDING FILAMENT THEORY

According to the sliding filament theory of contraction, muscle contraction involves the two contractile proteins (actin and myosin) in a series of mechanical events. Each myosin filament is surrounded by six actin filaments. The myosin filaments contain crossbridges, which are tiny extensions that reach toward the actin filaments. When the impulse from a motor nerve reaches a muscle cell, it stimulates the entire fiber, creating chemical changes that allow the actin filaments to join with the myosin crossbridges. The binding of myosin to actin via crossbridges releases energy that causes the crossbridges to swivel, pulling or sliding the myosin filament over the actin filament. This sliding motion causes the muscle to shorten (contract), producing force (figure 1.3). Once the stimulation ceases, the actin and myosin filaments separate, returning the muscle to its resting length. This crossbridge activity explains why the force a muscle generates depends on its initial length before contraction. The optimal length before muscle contraction is resting length (or slightly greater) because all the crossbridges can connect with the actin filaments, slowing development of maximal tension.

The highest force output occurs when contraction begins at a joint angle of approximately 110 to 120 degrees. Contractile force diminishes if the muscle length before contraction is either shorter or longer than resting length. When the length is significantly shorter than resting length (i.e., already partially contracted), the actin and myosin filaments already overlap, leaving fewer crossbridges open to "pull" on the actin filaments. When a muscle is significantly beyond resting length before contraction, the force potential is small because the actin filaments are too far away from the crossbridges to be able to join and shorten the muscle.

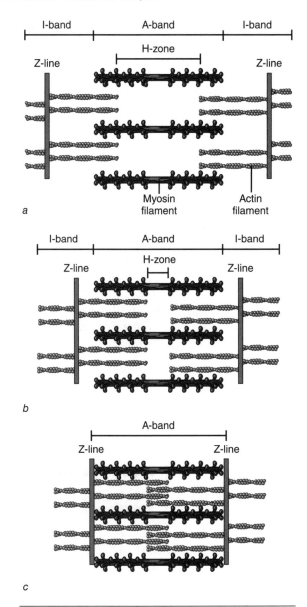

FIGURE 1.3 Contraction while muscle is shortened.

The Motor Unit

Skeletal muscle cells are connected to nerve cells, called motor neurons, that extend outward from the spinal cord. The motor unit consists of the motor neurons and all the muscle fibers it innervates (figure 1.4). The contraction process in muscles is stimulated from the motor neurons. The site where the motor neurons and muscle cells connect is called the neuromuscular junction. This junction is where the sarcolemma forms a pocket referred to as the motor end plate.

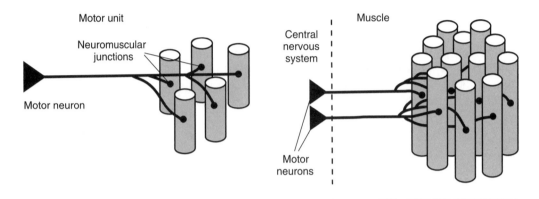

FIGURE 1.4 Motor unit.

Reprinted, by permission, from A.J. Vander, J.H. Sherman, and D.S. Luciano, 1990, *Human physiology: The mechanisms of body function*, 5th ed. (New York: McGraw-Hill), 296. © The McGraw-Hill Companies, Inc.

It is essential to understand that the motor neuron does not physically make contact with the muscle fiber but is separated by a short gap called the neuromuscular cleft. When a nerve impulse reaches the end of the motor nerve, the neurotransmitter acetylcholine is released. Acetylcholine diffuses across the synaptic cleft to complete the task of binding with receptor sites on the motor end plate. This key process allows the sarcolemma to increase permeability to sodium, resulting in a depolarization (a change in the cell's membrane potential, making it more positive or less negative) called the end-plate potential (EPP). If the threshold potential is reached, an action potential occurs, an impulse travels along the muscle cell membrane, and the muscle contracts (Ruegg 1992).

Muscle Fiber Types

Muscle fibers differ in their biochemical (metabolic) functions. Three individual muscle fiber types exist in human skeletal muscle: slow twitch fibers, referred to as Type I, and fast twitch fibers, identified as Type IIa and Type IIx. Type I fibers contain high numbers of oxidative enzymes (high mitochondrial volume). The fibers are surrounded by a greater amount of capillaries (blood vessels) and have higher concentrations of myoglobin (a red protein containing heme that carries and stores oxygen in muscle cells) than any other fibers. These key components provide Type I fibers with a large capacity for aerobic metabolism and a high resistance to fatigue.

Type IIa fibers are referred to as intermediate fibers or fast oxidative glycolytic fibers. This type of fiber contains biochemical and fatigue characteristics that are between Type I and Type IIx. Type IIa fibers are extremely adaptable. In respect to endurance training, they can increase their oxidative capacity to identical levels as Type I (Booth and Thomason 1991). Type IIx fibers are referred to as fast twitch fibers or fast glycolytic fibers and have a relatively small mitochondrial volume. Since they are rich in glycolytic enzymes, Type IIx fibers have a limited capacity for aerobic metabolism and a low resistance to fatigue (Powers and Howley 2009).

Slow twitch and fast twitch fibers exist in relatively equal proportions within the body—proportions not thought to be greatly affected by strength training and bodybuilding. The distribution of fiber types can vary, both within the same muscle and between different muscles. The arms tend to have a higher percentage of fast twitch fibers than the legs; the biceps averages about 55 percent fast twitch and the triceps 60 percent, whereas the soleus muscle (in the calf) averages around 24 percent fast twitch (Fox, Bowes, and Foss 1989). The proportion of fast twitch fibers within a muscle plays an important role in strength training and bodybuilding. Muscles containing a higher percentage of fast twitch fibers are capable of quicker and more powerful contractions, while those with more slow twitch fibers resist fatigue and are useful for endurance activities.

The recruitment of muscle fibers is load dependent. During moderate- and low-intensity activity, slow twitch fibers are recruited as workhorses. As the load increases, a greater number of fast twitch fibers are activated during contractions.

There are no clear differences in muscle fiber distribution between female and male athletes. People with an inherited predisposition for a greater number of fast twitch fibers are more genetically suited to strength training and bodybuilding than are people who inherit a predisposition for a greater number of slow twitch fibers. Yet while genetics is an important factor in determining success, it is not the only one. Regardless of genetic makeup, every person, through intensive training and proper nutrition, can improve muscle size, tone, and definition.

HOW MUSCLES WORK

The musculoskeletal frame of the body is an arrangement of bones attached to one another by a series of ligaments at structures called joints. The muscles crossing these joints provide the force necessary for body movements. Skeletal muscles do not contract independently of one another; movements about a joint involve several muscles, each with a different role.

Agonists and synergists are muscles that work together as a team, cooperating to perform a movement. The agonists are the prime movers, while the synergists provide assistance. Antagonists act in opposition to agonists during movement. The interaction between agonist and antagonist muscle groups directly influences athletic movements. In most cases, especially for skilled and experienced athletes, the antagonist muscles are relaxed, allowing motions to be performed with ease. A motion that looks jerky, or is performed rigidly, may result from improper interaction between the two groups. Only by relaxing the antagonists can an athlete improve the flow and smoothness of a muscle contraction.

Prime movers are the muscles primarily responsible for producing a comprehensive strength movement. During a biceps curl, for example, the prime mover is the biceps muscle, while the triceps acts as an antagonist and needs to be relaxed in order to facilitate smooth flexion.

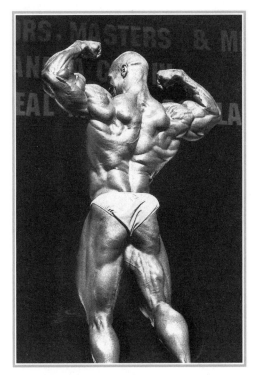

Mr. Olympia Ronnie Coleman's muscular physique.

The line of pull for strength training and bodybuilding is an imaginary line that crosses the muscle longitudinally, connecting the two extreme heads of the muscle. A muscle contraction achieves its highest physiological and mechanical efficiency when performed along the line of pull. Here's an example: You can flex your elbow with your palm held in several different positions. With the palm turned upward, the line of pull is direct, creating the highest efficiency. With the palm facing down, efficiency of contraction decreases because the tendon of the biceps muscle wraps around the radius bone. In this case, the line of pull is indirect, which wastes a large portion of the contractile force. For maximum strength gains and optimal muscle efficiency, perform strength exercises along the line of pull.

Stabilizers (or fixators) are usually smaller muscles that contract isometrically to anchor, or steady, a bone so that prime movers have a firm base to pull on. A stabilizer may be another muscle in the same limb, but muscles of other parts of the body may also act as stabilizers so that a limb can perform a motion. For example, in preacher curls (elbow flexion, with the upper arms rested on a firm support), the shoulders, upper arms, and abdominal muscles are contracted isometrically to stabilize the shoulders so the biceps have a stable base to pull.

Types of Muscle Contraction

Skeletal muscles are responsible for both contraction and relaxation. A muscle contracts when it is stimulated, and when the contraction stops the muscle relaxes. Bodybuilders and strength athletes use various types of contractions depending on the scope of their training phase and the equipment being used. There are three types of contractions—isotonic, isometric, and isokinetic.

Isotonic   Isotonic (dynamic), from the Greek *isos* + *tonikos* (equal tension), is the most familiar type of muscle contraction. As the term implies, during an isotonic contraction the tension is constant throughout the entire range of motion. There are two types of isotonic contractions: concentric and eccentric.

- In concentric, from the Latin *com* + *centrum* (having a common center), the muscle shortens in length. Concentric contractions are possible only when the resistance (i.e., weight load) is less than the athlete's maximum potential. Examples of concentric contractions include the curling action of a biceps curl and the extending motion of a leg extension.

- Eccentric, or negative, contractions reverse the process of a concentric action—that is, eccentric contractions return muscles to their starting point. During a biceps curl, the eccentric component occurs when the arm extends to the starting point after the curl. During a leg extension, eccentric work is being done when the legs bend at the knee toward the starting position. During an eccentric contraction, the muscles are yielding either to the force of gravity (as in free weights) or to the force of a machine's pull. Under such conditions, the muscle lengthens as the joint angle increases, thus releasing a controlled tension.

Isometric   In isometric (static) contractions—from the Greek *isos + metrikos* (equal in measurement)—the muscle develops tension without changing length. During an isometric contraction, the application of force against an immovable object forces the muscle to develop high tension without altering its length. For example, if you push against a wall, tension is created in your muscles although they remain the same length. The tension developed from this type of contraction is often higher than that developed during an isotonic contraction.

Isokinetic   Isokinetic, from the Greek *isos + kineticos* (equal motion), describes a contraction with constant velocity over the full range of motion. Isokinetic work needs special equipment designed to allow a constant velocity of contraction regardless of the load. During the movement, an athlete performs both concentric and eccentric contractions while the machine provides a resistance that is equal to the force generated by the athlete. The benefit of this type of training is that it allows the muscle to work maximally throughout the entire movement. It eliminates the "sticking point," or weak spot, that is present in every exercise motion.

Types of Strength and Their Significance in Training

Various types of strength training are needed to build and sculpt the most muscular, defined, and symmetrical yet injury-free physique possible.

General strength is the foundation of the entire strength and bodybuilding program. It must be the sole focus of training during the early training phase of an experienced lifter; for entry-level strength trainers or bodybuilders, it must be the sole focus for the first few years. A low level of general strength can limit overall progress, leaving the body susceptible to injury and with diminished ability to build muscle strength and size.

Maximum strength refers to the highest force that can be performed by the neuromuscular system during a maximum contraction. It reflects the heaviest load an athlete can lift in one attempt, expressed as 100 percent of maximum, or one-repetition maximum (1RM). For training purposes, it is crucial to know one's maximum strength for each exercise, since it is the basis for calculating loads for every strength phase. (See appendix C for frequently used percentages of a range of 1RMs. See appendix D for an alternative way to find 1RM.)

Muscle endurance is the muscle's ability to sustain work for a prolonged period. It is used largely in endurance training and also plays a crucial role in bodybuilding and strength training programs. This type of endurance is used extensively during the muscle definition (or "cuts") phase of training.

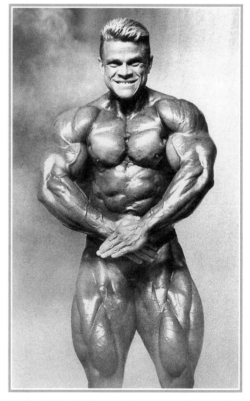

Roland Cziurlok's amazing size and strength are the results of employing maximum strength training.

PRINCIPLES OF STRENGTH TRAINING AND BODYBUILDING

Training is a complex activity governed by principles and methodological guidelines designed to help athletes achieve the greatest possible muscle size and definition. The principles of training explained in this section are very important training guidelines that must be considered at the start of an organized training program.

Principle 1: Vary Your Training

Bodybuilding and strength training are highly demanding activities that require hour after hour of dedicated training. The pressure of continually increasing training volume and intensity, along with the repetitive nature of weightlifting, can easily lead to boredom, which may become an obstacle to motivation and success.

The best medicine for monotonous training is variety. To add variety, you must be familiar with training methods and periodization planning (see part IV) and be comfortable with a multitude of different exercises for each muscle group (see part III). Variety in training improves psychological well-being as well as training response. The following suggestions will help you add variety to your training.

- Choose different exercises for each specific body part instead of doing your favorite exercises each time. Change the order in which you perform certain exercises. Remember, both your mind and your body become bored; they both need variety.
- Incorporate variety into your loading system as suggested by the step-loading principle (discussed under principle 3).
- Vary the type of muscle contractions done in your workouts (i.e., include both concentric and eccentric work).
- Vary the speed of contraction (slow, medium, and fast).
- Vary equipment so you go from free weights to machine weights to isokinetics and so on.

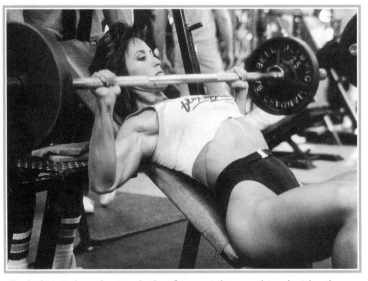

Rachel McLish understands that free weights combined with other equipment provide variety in her training.

Principle 2: Observe Individual Differences

Rarely do two people come to training with exactly the same history and agenda. Everyone is different in genetics, athletic background, eating habits, metabolism, training desire, and adaptation potential. Strength athletes and bodybuilders, regardless of their level of development, must have individualized training programs. Too often, entry-level athletes are seduced into following the training programs of advanced athletes. Advice given by these seasoned athletes is inappropriate for novices, no matter how well intentioned. Beginners, whose muscles, ligaments, and tendons are unaccustomed to the stresses of serious weight training, require a longer period of adjustment, or adaptation, in order to avoid injury.

Often the following factors influence a person's work capacity:

- Training background. The work demand should be proportional to your experience, background, and age.

- Individual work capacity. Not all athletes who are similar in structure and appearance have the same work tolerance. Individual work abilities must be assessed before determining the volume and intensity of work. This will increase the odds of becoming successful and remaining injury free.

- Training load and rate of recovery. When planning and evaluating the training load, consider the factors outside training that place high demands on you. For example, you must consider time commitments for school, work, or family, and even the distance traveled to the gym, because these factors can affect the rate of recovery between training sessions. You should also consider that any destructive or negative lifestyle habits will affect your rate of recovery.

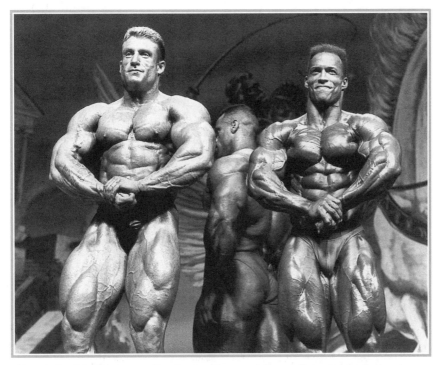

No two bodybuilders are alike. Dorian Yates and Shawn Ray—both gloriously big and symmetrical—each have their own individual look, style, and training needs.

Principle 3: Employ Step-Type Loading

The theory of progressive load increments in strength training has been known and employed since ancient times. According to Greek mythology, the first person to apply the theory was Milo of Croton, who was a pupil of the famous mathematician Pythagoras (c. 580-500 BC) and an Olympic wrestling champion. In his teen years, Milo decided to become the strongest man in the world and embarked on this mission by lifting and carrying a calf every day. As the calf grew and became heavier, Milo became stronger. Finally, when the calf had developed into a full-grown bull, Milo, thanks to a long-term progression, was able to lift the bull and was indeed the strongest man on earth. Improvements in muscle size, tone, and definition are a direct result of the amount and quality of training performed over a long period of time. From the entry level right up to the Mr. or Ms. Olympia level, the training workload must increase gradually, in accordance with each person's physiological and psychological abilities, if gains in muscle size, tone, and definition are to continue.

The most effective technique for load patterning is the step-loading principle because it fulfills the physiological and psychological requirements that increased training load must be followed by a period of unloading. The unloading phase is a key element that allows the body to adapt to the new, more intense stressors and regenerate itself in preparation for yet another load increase. Since everyone responds differently to stress, each athlete must plan a loading schedule that fits her specific needs and rate of adaptation. For instance, if the load is increased too abruptly it may exceed the body's adaptation capacity, disrupting the physiological balance of the overload-to-adaptation cycle. Once this disruption occurs, adaptation will be less than optimal, and injuries might occur.

The step-type approach involves the repetition of a microcycle, or a week of training, in which the resistance is increased over several steps, followed by an unloading step to ensure recuperation (figure 1.5).

Note that each step represents more than one single workout, which means the workload is not increased at every training session. One workout provides insufficient stimulus to produce marked changes in the body. Such adaptation occurs only after repeated exposure to the same training loads. In figure 1.5, each step represents 1 week, each vertical line indicates a change in load, and each horizontal line represents the week over which you use and adapt to that load. The percentages indicated above each step are the suggested percentages of maximum.

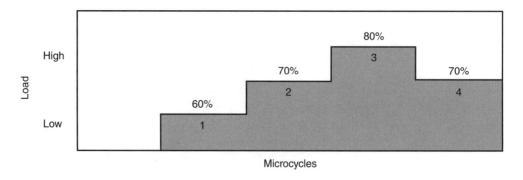

FIGURE 1.5   The step-type method of increasing training load.

Reprinted from Bompa 1996.

You can see the progression for the first 3 weeks, as well as the decrease for the unloading phase in the 4th week.

Let's look at how your body responds to the step-loading approach. On Monday, for example, you begin a microcycle (a new step) by increasing the workload. After Monday's workout your body is in a state of fatigue—a physiological crisis—because it is unaccustomed to such stress. When the same level continues, your body will probably be comfortable with the load by Wednesday and adapt to it in the following 2 days. By Friday, you should feel really good and capable of lifting even heavier loads. After the crisis of fatigue comes a phase of adaptation, which in turn is followed by a physiological rebound, or improvement. By the next Monday, you should feel physically and mentally comfortable, which indicates that it is time to challenge the level of adaptation once more.

Each step of the microcycle brings improvements until you reach the unloading (regeneration) phase (step 4). This phase gives your body the time it needs to replenish its energy stores, restore a psychological balance, and rid itself of the fatigue that has accumulated over the preceding 3 weeks. The fourth step in this example becomes the new lowest step for another phase of load increments. Figure 1.6 illustrates how microcycles (steps) fit into the context of a longer training cycle, where the goal is to build muscle size.

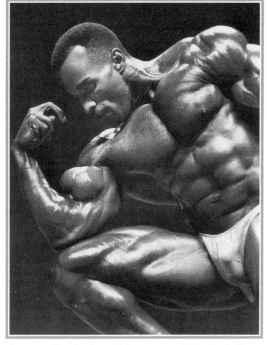

Darrem Charles hits a biceps pose. This kind of muscle development occurs only with carefully planned training.

Although the load increments may seem small, remember that because you are getting stronger your maximum weight values are increasing, which means your percentages of maximum are increasing as well. For example, the first time you reached the high step of 80 percent, your 80-percent-of-maximum weight for a specific exercise may have been 120 pounds (55 kg). Three weeks later, because of your adaptation and strength gains, your 80 percent may have increased to 130 pounds (60 kg). Consequently, you use progressively heavier loads over the long term, despite the fact that your percentages of maximum remain the same.

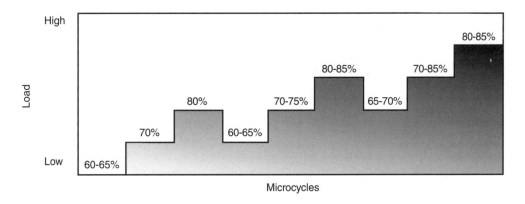

FIGURE 1.6   An example of how to structure training loads over a longer period of time.

THREE BASIC LAWS OF STRENGTH TRAINING AND BODYBUILDING

The training principles just discussed provide a loose guideline for general training. There are also three laws of strength training that must be adhered to if an athlete is to proceed injury free to a more comprehensive, rigorous training program. Entry-level bodybuilders and strength athletes often begin training programs without being aware of the strain they will encounter and without understanding the progression or training methodology behind the program. These are usually the people who tend to seek advice from seasoned athletes (who may not be qualified to give it) and who, consequently, find themselves out of their league and on a collision course with injury. Adherence to the following training laws will ensure the proper anatomical adaptation of a young or untrained body before subjecting it to the rigors of strength training.

Law 1: Before Developing Muscle Strength, Develop Joint Flexibility

Most strength training exercises, especially those employing free weights, use the whole range of motion around major joints. In some exercises, the weight of the barbell compresses the joints to such a degree that, if the person does not have good flexibility, strain and pain can result.

Consider deep squats: During a deep squat, compression of the knee joints may cause an inflexible athlete a lot of pain or even injury. Also, in the deep-squat position, a lack of good ankle flexibility forces the person to stay on the balls of the feet and toes, rather than on the flat of the foot where a good base of support and balance is ensured. Development of ankle flexibility (i.e., dorsiflexion, or bringing the toes toward the shin) is essential for all strength trainers but especially for entry-level athletes (Bompa, Di Pasquale, and Cornacchia 2003).

Good flexibility can greatly reduce or eliminate the incidence of injuries (Fredrick and Fredrick 2006). Flexibility aids in the elasticity of the muscles and provides a wider range of motion in the joints. Unfortunately, research on this subject has produced mixed reviews, causing athletes at all levels to neglect stretching programs. Regular stretching creates several essential training benefits, such as improved flexibility, reduced muscle soreness, good muscular and joint mobility, and greater efficiency in muscular movements and fluidity of motion (Nelson and Kokkonen 2007).

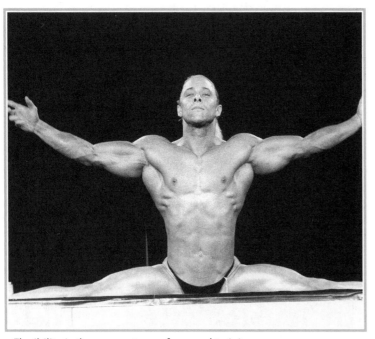

Flexibility is the cornerstone of a sound training program.

Law 2: Before Developing Muscle Strength, Develop the Tendons

The rate of gain in muscle strength always has the potential to exceed the rate at which tendons and ligaments can adapt to higher tensions. It is crucial that the tendons and ligaments have time to adapt, but because many people lack a long-term vision, they prematurely use heavy loads to develop specific muscle groups without strengthening the support systems of those muscles. It's like building a house on the sand—it may look good for a little while, but at high tide the whole thing is destroyed. Build your body on a rock-solid foundation, and this will not happen to you.

Tendons and ligaments are trainable and can actually increase in diameter as a result of proper anatomical adaptation training (see chapter 12), which increases their ability to withstand tension and wear. This training is accomplished via a low-load program for the first 1 to 2 years of training. Shortcuts are not the answer to achieving a well-developed, injury-free body. Patience will ultimately pay off.

Law 3: Before Developing the Limbs, Develop the Body's Core

It is true that big arms, shoulders, and legs are impressive, and a lot of training must be dedicated to these areas. Yet the trunk is the link between these areas, and the limbs can only be as strong as the trunk. The trunk has an abundance of abdominal and back muscles: Bundles that run in different directions surround the core of the body with a tight and powerful support system. A poorly developed trunk represents a weak support system for the hard-working arms and legs. So in spite of temptations in this direction, an entry-level training program must not revolve around the legs, arms, and shoulders. The focus must first be on strengthening the core area of the body—the muscles of the abdomen, lower back, and spinal column.

Back muscles consist of long and short muscles that run along the vertebral column. They work together as a unit, with the rotators and diagonal muscles, to perform many movements. Abdominal muscles run lengthwise (rectus abdominis), crosswise (transversus abdominis), and diagonally (abdominal obliques), enabling the trunk to bend forward and sideways, to rotate, and to twist. Since the abdominal muscles play important roles in many exercises, weakness in this area can severely limit the effectiveness of many strength actions.

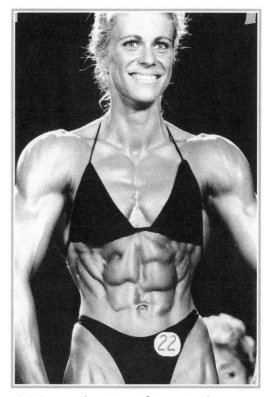

Anja Langer, the picture of symmetry, knows the importance of building a strong foundation.

Understanding the Periodization System

The field of strength training, especially that of bodybuilding, is saturated with methods and programs that are unproven and often lack logic. Scientific research cannot support the novel systems that pop up in magazines and on the Internet at an astounding rate. You will do well to ignore fads and follow well-tested approaches validated both by research and in competition. The following discussion about periodization training will help you comprehend and apply the periodized training programs and nutrition plans suggested in parts II and III.

THE PERIODIZATION SYSTEM

Although Tudor Bompa's *Periodization of Bodybuilding* was copyrighted in May 1988 (as an adaptation for bodybuilding of the earlier-developed *Periodization of Strength*), many people—athletes and authors alike—still do not fully understand this very successful training system. Some authors describe periodization as "the science behind reps and sets" or the principle of "progression of the training load per week," while others characterize it as a "philosophy." Others have simply decided, without research, understanding, or testing, that periodization doesn't work. In fairness to the periodization system of training, we urge you to try it first and then draw your own conclusions.

One of the major goals of this book is to help all athletes learn to plan their own training programs and eventually to help more bodybuilders and strength trainers properly

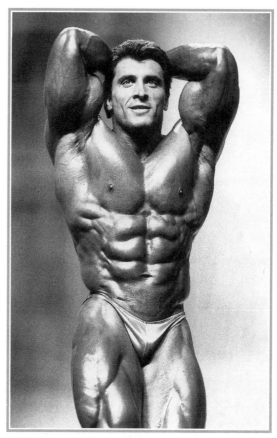

Milo Sarcev understands that in training, nothing happens by accident; progress happens by design.

use the periodization system. Periodization is the most effective way to organize a training program. This organization refers to two major elements:

1. How to structure a longer period of time, such as a year of training, into smaller and more manageable phases.

2. How to structure the program into specific training phases, such as the following:

   - **Anatomical adaptation (AA)**—the beginning and progressive training performed after a break or an extended absence from the sport
   - **Hypertrophy (H)**—a training phase in which the objective is to increase muscle size
   - **Mixed training (M)**—the progressive transition from the H phase to the MxS phase; accomplished by utilizing both phases during mixed training programs
   - **Maximum strength (MxS)**—a training phase in which the objective is to increase muscle tone and density
   - **Muscle definition (MD)**—a training phase using specific training methods, where the objective is to burn fat and in the process further improve muscle striation and vascularization
   - **Transition (T)**—where the objective is recovery and regeneration before beginning another phase

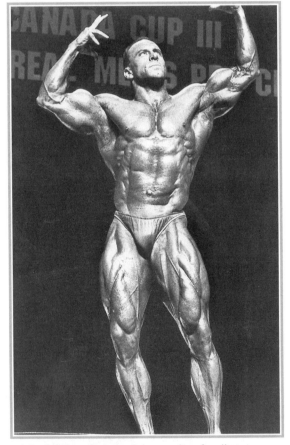

John McGough reaped the results of well-structured training phases.

The preceding sequence of training phases is essential because it outlines an entire training cycle. First, it facilitates the development of muscle size via the hypertrophy phase. It then improves muscle tone and muscle separation during a maximum strength phase. Once muscle size and tone reach the level you want, training focuses on the development of muscle definition, where muscle striation is enhanced.

Periodization is not a rigid system in which only the basic model is the legitimate one. On the contrary—since there are several variations of the basic model, you can choose the one that best suits your own training goals. The chapters in part IV provide suggested phase-specific training and nutrition programs that will facilitate your ability to plan a true periodization program according to your specific needs. In addition to presenting highly organized and phase-specific training programs, periodization provides a variety of year-round training methods as well as phase-specific training loads that employ different variations of both muscle stimulation and contraction for optimal muscle growth and strength.

Very few strength trainers and bodybuilders follow a well-adjusted and carefully designed plan. Through periodization we intend to promote a new type of athlete—one who is in control of his body and whose training leads to complete body development. The new athlete will have impressive muscular development and will cultivate muscle density, tone, definition, symmetry, and strength superior to that of traditional bodybuilders who use antiquated training philosophies. Regardless of whether you are training just to look attractive or to compete professionally, the ideal for every athlete is to acquire the desired amount of muscle mass without sacrificing physical appearance.

The basic model of periodization presented in figure 2.1 illustrates the proper sequence of training phases and may be adapted to address the specific needs of individual athletes. Many variations of this plan are possible to meet the different needs of each bodybuilder and strength trainer. This particular plan uses September as the starting point, although you can use any month of the year when developing your own plan.

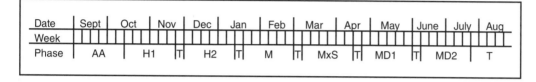

Date	Sept	Oct	Nov	Dec	Jan	Feb	Mar	Apr	May	June	July	Aug
Week												
Phase	AA	H1	T	H2	T	M	T	MxS	T	MD1	T	MD2	T

FIGURE 2.1   The basic model of the annual plan for periodization of bodybuilding and strength training. AA is anatomical adaptation, H is hypertrophy, M is mixed training, MxS is maximum strength, MD is muscle definition, and T is transition.

The small blocks beneath each month represent the weeks, or microcycles. You must plan in advance how many weeks are appropriate for each phase. The bottom row of the chart divides the year into training phases. Organize these phases in a way that ensures you meet your goals at the appropriate time. For example, a competitive athlete might design an annual plan to peak for major shows. Recreational bodybuilders and strength trainers more concerned with aesthetics might wish to plan for vacations and other activities.

PERIODIZATION OF TRAINING FOR INCREASED SIZE

Periodization is not a rigid concept. Figure 2.1 is a basic structure that will not apply to every bodybuilder and strength trainer. Each athlete has different personal and professional commitments, so we offer different variations of training plans. Please keep in mind that the suggested variations do not exhaust all the possible options. You should construct an individualized periodization plan according to your unique set of needs and obligations. The options presented here are intended to help implement the concept of periodization according to individual needs.

Double periodization is an option for people who cannot commit themselves to the year-round training program recommended in figure 2.1. It is also an option for people with better training backgrounds or for those seeking more variety in training.

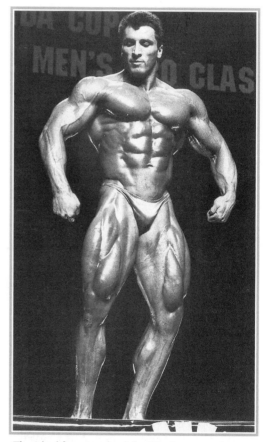

The ideal for every bodybuilder is to acquire the desired amount of muscle mass without sacrificing physical appearance.

In the double-periodization model (figure 2.2), the months of the year are numbered rather than named to let you commence training at any time throughout the year. The phases in this model follow the same sequence as those in the basic model (figure 2.1), except the annual plan is divided into two halves and the sequence is repeated. Additionally, for each training phase in figure 2.2, the number in the upper right corner of the boxes in the bottom row indicates the number of weeks for each phase.

1	2	3	4	5	6	7	8	9	10	11	12
4	6		6		6	2	4		6		6	6	4
AA	H	T	MxS	MD	T	AA	H	T	MxS	MD	T

FIGURE 2.2 A double-periodization model.

Double Periodization for Athletes With Family Obligations
Figure 2.3 presents another variation of the basic model that revolves around the busiest times of the year for someone with a family. During Christmas and summer vacation periods, training is often disorganized and interrupted because of family commitments. To prevent the frustration that accompanies periods of fragmented training, it is better to actually structure an annual plan around the main holidays of the year. Again, the number in the upper right corner indicates the number of weeks for each phase.

Sept	Oct	Nov	Dec	Jan	Feb	Mar	Apr	May	June	July	Aug
4	6		6	2	4		6		6		6		6	4
AA	H	MxS	T	AA	H1	T	H2	MxS	T	MD	T

FIGURE 2.3 A double-periodization model revolving around the holidays of the year.

As figure 2.3 indicates, minitransition phases are planned during holiday times. The plan prescribes two hypertrophy phases in which the purpose of training is to increase muscle size. Certainly, other variations of the basic structure are possible. For instance,

- H2 could be replaced by a mixed program of H and MxS in proportions decided by the athlete;
- H2 could be replaced by MxS, if the development of this strength quality is the goal; or
- H2 could be divided into 3 weeks of MxS followed by 3 weeks of H.

Periodization Program for Entry-Level Bodybuilders Entry-level bodybuilders and strength trainers should create their own programs or follow the model in figure 2.4. This figure presents months by number—month 1 represents the first month of training with a new program. Resist the temptation to copy the programs of experienced bodybuilders. Entry-level athletes have fragile bodies that are not ready for the challenge designed for experienced athletes. Beginners must be extra careful to progressively increase the training load by performing a lower number of training sessions and hours per week, planning longer AA phases, and confronting the body with less overall stress in training.

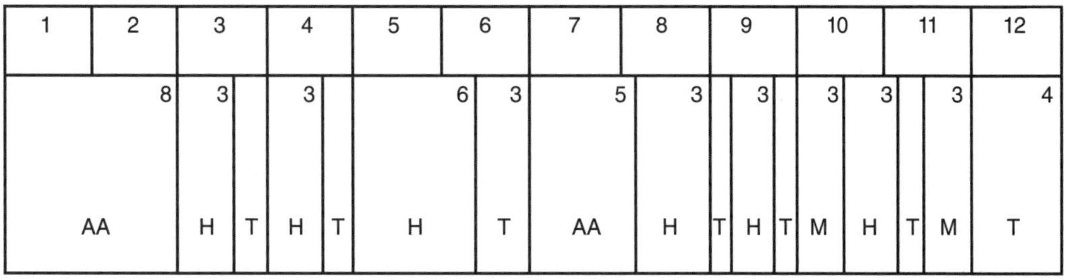

1	2	3	4	5	6	7	8	9	10	11	12
	8	3	3		6	3	5	3	3	3	3	3	4
AA	H	T	H	T	H	T	AA	H	T H	T M	H	T M	T

FIGURE 2.4 A periodization program for entry-level bodybuilders and strength trainers.

In this entry-level program, AA is 8 weeks long, giving the muscle tissues, ligaments, and tendons adequate time to prepare for the phases to come. To make adaptation to hypertrophy a careful and gradual process, the first two H phases are only 3 weeks long, separated by a 1-week regeneration T phase. After 4 months, the anatomy of an entry-level athlete should have progressively adapted to training, permitting longer H phases. The first half of the program ends with a 3-week T phase, giving the body a long period of regeneration before a new and slightly more difficult program begins.

Periodization Program for Recreational Bodybuilders Those who have completed 1 to 2 years of bodybuilding or strength training could follow an annual plan such as figure 2.5 presents. T phases occur during the Christmas and summer holidays to allow recreational bodybuilders time to enjoy other activities. Note that, except for the first AA and H phases, a T phase of 1 to 2 weeks is planned throughout to avoid high levels of fatigue and overtraining. As with the other figures, the numbers in the top row refer to months, and the numbers in the upper right corner of the boxes in the bottom row indicate the number of weeks to devote to the phase.

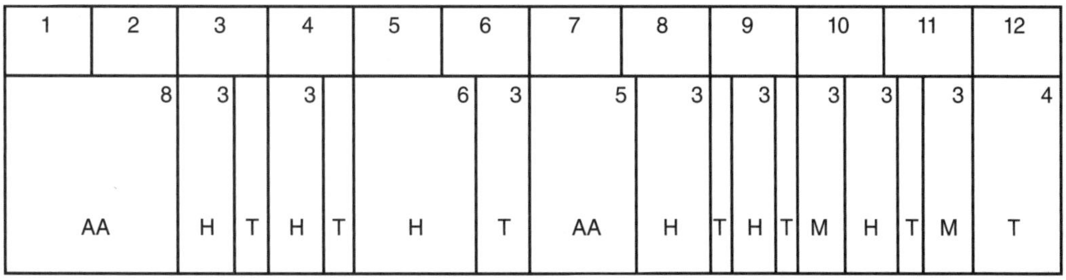

1	2	3	4	5	6	7	8	9	10	11	12
	8	3	3		6	3	5	3	3	3	3	3	4
AA	H	T	H	T	H	T	AA	H	T H	T M	H	T M	T

FIGURE 2.5 A periodization program for recreational bodybuilders and strength trainers.

Nonbulk Program for Female Athletes   Figure 2.6 describes a program for athletes who want more variety in training. This high-variety program has many alternations of training phases. It was created for bodybuilders and strength trainers (especially female athletes) who want to sculpt a toned, muscular, and symmetrical body without packing on bulky muscles.

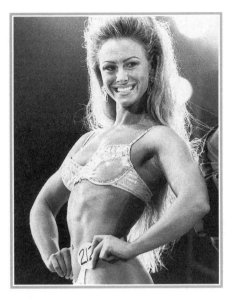

A toned and symmetrical physique.

Sept	Oct		Nov	Dec		Jan	Feb	Mar		Apr	May		June		July	Aug
3	3	3	3	3	3	4	3	3	3	3	3	3	3	4	4	
AA	H	MxS T	M	MD	T	AA	H	M	T	MD	MxS T	MD	M	T	MD	T

FIGURE 2.6   A periodization program for female bodybuilders and strength trainers or those who do not want to train for bulk.

TRIPLE-PERIODIZATION PLAN: DESIGN AND DURATION

The triple-periodization plan is suitable for recreational bodybuilders and strength trainers or for busy professionals who cannot easily commit themselves to a year-long plan such as the basic model or even to a double-periodization plan. Shorter modules, such as the one in figure 2.7, help these athletes achieve the basic goals of well-developed bodies and good fitness, while taking into account their social needs during the main holidays of the year.

Sept	Oct	Nov	Dec		Jan	Feb	Mar		Apr		May	June	July	Aug
7	3	3	2		3	6	3		3	2	3	3	3 3	5
AA	H	T	M	T	AA	H	T	M	MD	T	AA	H T	MxS MD	T

FIGURE 2.7   Triple periodization: a recommended program for recreational or busy professional bodybuilders and strength trainers.

HYPERTROPHY (MASS) PROGRAM

An athlete whose primary training objective is building muscle size could use the program outlined in figure 2.8. It follows a double-periodization plan, whereby most of the training program is dedicated to developing muscle hypertrophy. Longer H phases, alternated with M training toward the end of each segment, will stimulate the highest possible development of muscle size. Our periodized approach to mass training differs from traditional programs in that the M phases, which mix hypertrophy with maximum strength training, have the important merit of developing short-term and, more significantly, chronic hypertrophy.

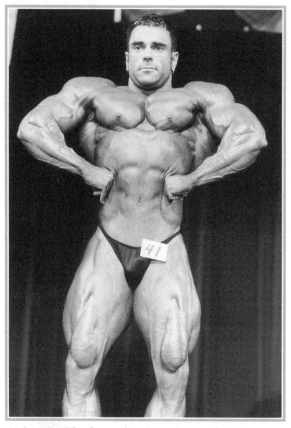

Nelson Da Silva knows how to gain muscle mass.

1	2	3	4	5	6	7	8	9	10	11	12
3	6		6	3	3	3	2	3	6	3	3	4	4
AA	H	T	H	T	M	H	M	T	AA	H	T	M	H	M	T

FIGURE 2.8 A hypertrophy (mass) training program.

PERIODIZATION PLAN STRESSING MAXIMUM STRENGTH

Many bodybuilders would like to develop large muscles and, more important, muscle tone, high muscle density, and certainly stronger muscles. Increased chronic hypertrophy results from following a training program such as that in figure 2.9. As figure 2.9 illustrates, the program to maximize strength follows a double-periodization plan. The fact that MxS dominates this program means the training recruits more fast twitch muscle fibers—resulting in chronic hypertrophy and muscles that are well defined and visibly striated. As before, the numbers in the top row refer to months, and the numbers in the upper right corner of the boxes in the bottom row indicate the number of weeks for each phase.

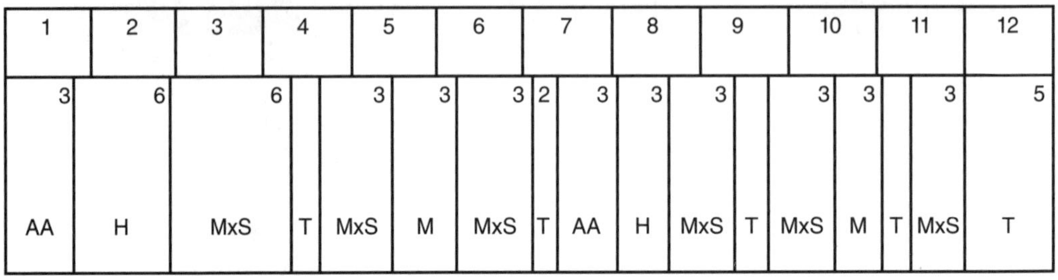

1	2	3	4	5	6	7	8	9	10	11	12
3	6	6		3	3	3	2	3	3	3		3	3		3	5
AA	H	MxS	T	MxS	M	MxS	T	AA	H	MxS	T	MxS	M	T	MxS	T

FIGURE 2.9 A periodization plan stressing maximum strength.

PERIODIZATION PLAN STRESSING MUSCLE DEFINITION

Some athletes have already reached their desired level of muscle hypertrophy; they now want to improve muscle definition in order to achieve total body development. People who have already tested our program (especially women) have reported incredible changes in their bodies. The majority drastically trimmed their waists while at the same time significantly increasing muscle definition in the upper body, buttocks, and legs. Some have even reported gains in strength. In one of our female groups, 68 percent lost substantial weight and changed their overall body shapes so much they had to change their wardrobes. They achieved this weight loss by natural means and not as a result of some diet gimmick—just natural, honest, and dedicated training. This is the healthy way.

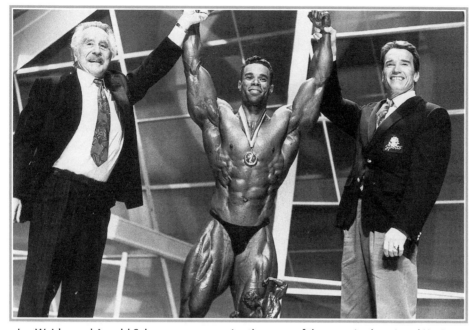

Joe Weider and Arnold Schwarzenegger raise the arms of the amazingly striated Kevin Levrone.

This plan, shown in figure 2.10, is a double-periodization program that focuses on burning subcutaneous fat, thus allowing for better-striated and more visible muscles. The purpose of periodized bodybuilding training is to sequence specific types of strength training in order to obtain maximum gains. These phases can be combined to create a certain type of adaptation, allowing bodybuilders to model their bodies to reach maximum hypertrophy, muscle tone, or muscle definition. After the first year of using periodized training plans, bodybuilders become better accustomed to creating models of training that fit their own needs.

1	2	3	4	5	6	7	8	9	10	11	12
3	6	3	4		6	2	3	6	3	4	3	4
AA	H	MxS	T	MD	T	MD	T	AA	H	MxS	T	MD	MD	T

FIGURE 2.10 A periodization plan stressing muscle definition.

Designing the Perfect Program

To obtain both continual improvement and the necessary balance between work and regeneration, athletes must pay constant attention to the amounts of work (volume) and the loads (intensity) they use in training. They must continuously monitor the load, number of exercises, number of sets, rest intervals, and types of split routines they employ. Athletes who wish to design their own training programs need to understand all these training elements and combine them effectively for their own bodies.

A well-structured periodized training program is essential for success. Traditional bodybuilding programs, where the highly regarded "no pain, no gain" theory is the norm, consistently result in overtraining. Strategies such as low-intensity days and supercompensation can help prevent overtraining. Use these days to enjoy a different type of bodybuilding training.

VOLUME AND INTENSITY

Training volume is the quantity of work performed. It incorporates the following integral parts:

- The duration of training (in hours)
- The cumulative amount of weight lifted per training session or phase
- The number of exercises per training session
- The number of sets and repetitions per exercise or training session

Bodybuilders should maintain training logs in order to correctly monitor the total volume of work performed and to help plan the total volume of training for future weeks and months. Training volume varies among people according to their training background, work tolerance, and biological makeup. Mature athletes with a solid background in strength training will always be able to tolerate higher volumes of training. Regardless of a person's experience, however, any dramatic or abrupt increase in training volume can be detrimental. Such increases can result in high levels of fatigue, inefficient muscular work, and greater risk of injury. This is why a well-designed, progressive plan, along with an appropriate method of monitoring load increments, is crucial to your well-being and training success.

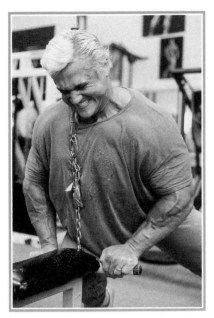

Now there's intensity: Tom Platz gives it his grunting, vein-bulging, teeth-gnashing best.

Training volume also changes with the type of strength training performed. For instance, high-volume training is planned during the muscle definition phase in order to burn more fat and, consequently, develop better muscle striations. Medium-volume training, on the other hand, is typical for maximum strength or power training. Muscle size and definition improve only as a result of careful and constant physiological adaptation, which depends on the proper manipulation of the quantity, or volume, of training.

One adaptation that occurs as a result of progressively higher volumes of training is a more efficient and faster recovery time between sets and between training sessions. Faster recovery permits more work per training session and per week, encouraging even further increases in training volume.

In strength training, intensity—expressed as a percentage of 1RM—is a function of the power of the nervous stimuli employed in training. The strength of a stimulus depends on the load, the speed at which a movement is performed, the variation of rest intervals between repetitions and sets, and the psychological strain that accompanies an exercise. Thus, the intensity is determined by the muscular effort involved and the energy spent by the central nervous system (CNS) during strength training. Table 3.1 gives the intensities and loads employed in strength training.

A supermaximum load exceeds one's maximum strength. In most cases, loads between 100 and 125 percent of 1RM are used by applying eccentric force, or by resisting the force of gravity. When using supermaximum loads you should have two spotters, one at each end of the barbell, to assist you and protect you from accident or injury; if you use the eccentric method in a bench press without spotters, the barbell could fall on your chest because the weight is actually heavier than you can lift.

During the maximum strength phase, only bodybuilders with a strong background or base in strength training can use supermaximum loads. Most other athletes should restrict themselves to a load of up to 100 percent, or 1RM. The load, however, should also relate to the type of strength being developed, as scheduled in the periodization plan.

TABLE 3.1   **Intensity Values (Loads) Used in Strength and Bodybuilding Training**

Intensity value	Load	Percentage of 1RM	Type of contraction
1	Supermaximum	101-105	Eccentric, isometric
2	Maximum	90-100	Concentric
3	Heavy	80-89	Concentric
4	Medium	50-79	Concentric
5	Low	30-49	Concentric

Reprinted from Bompa 1996.

NUMBER OF EXERCISES

One of the keys of an effective training program is to have an adequate repertoire of exercises from which to choose. Athletes should build their repertoire of exercises to meet several key characteristics for their training programs.

Exercises That Stimulate the Greatest Amount of Electrical Activity   The greater the electrical activity, the more muscle fibers are recruited, resulting in greater gains in muscle strength and size (see chapter 9). To maximize this effect, it is critical to know which loading pattern to use, how that pattern should vary in a given training phase, which lifting technique to use, and how the load increments can vary in order to induce supercompensation.

Level of Development   One of the main objectives of an entry-level bodybuilding program is the development of a strong anatomical and physiological foundation. Without such a base, consistent improvement will be unlikely. Entry-level strength trainers and bodybuilders need a number of exercises (about 12 to 15) that collectively address the major muscle groups of the body. The duration of this type of training may be from 1 to 3 years, depending on the person's background (and level of patience). Training programs for advanced bodybuilders follow a completely different approach. The main training objective for these athletes is to increase muscle size, density, tone, and definition to the highest possible levels.

Individual Needs   As training progresses over the years, some bodybuilders develop imbalances between different parts of the body. When this occurs, they should adapt their programs by giving priority to exercises that stress the underdeveloped parts of the body.

Training Phase   As outlined by the periodization concept, the number of exercises varies according to the phase of training (see chapters 12 through 17 in part IV). The order of exercises in bodybuilding must be phase specific, taking into account the scope of training for each particular phase. Just as the rest interval, volume of training, exercises, and so on vary according to the different kinds of strength being developed, so must the order of performing exercises.

For example, in the maximum strength training phase, exercises are cycled in vertical sequence as they appear on the daily program sheet. The athlete performs one set of each exercise, starting from the top and moving down, and repeats the cycle as often as prescribed. The advantage of this method is that it allows for better recovery of each muscle group. By the time exercise 1 is repeated, enough time has elapsed to promote almost full recovery. When you are lifting 90 to 105 percent 1RM, this much rest is necessary if training is to remain at a high intensity throughout the session.

If, however, the phase of training is hypertrophy, then all the sets for exercise 1 are performed before moving on to the next exercise—this is a horizontal sequence. This sequence exhausts the muscle group much faster, leading to greater increases in muscle size. Local muscle exhaustion is the main training focus of the hypertrophy phase.

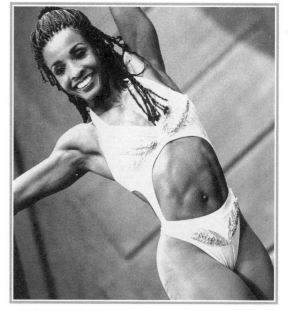

Madonna Grimes achieved her superfit body through proper exercise selection.

TECHNIQUE FOR LIFTING AND RANGE OF MOTION

Correct form and good technique increase the effectiveness of targeting a given muscle group. Good technique also ensures that muscle contraction occurs along the line of pull. Any contraction that is performed along the line of pull increases the mechanical effectiveness of that particular exercise. For instance, a squat performed with the feet wider than shoulder-width apart and the toes pointed diagonally (often done in powerlifting) is not mechanically effective since the quadriceps muscles are not contracting along the line of pull. Placing the feet at shoulder width and with toes pointed forward and slightly to the side is more effective since the contraction of the muscles is along the line of pull. Similarly, arm curls intending to target the biceps muscle are performed along the line of pull only when the palm is facing up (supination), as in preacher curls.

For an exercise to be effective and have good fluidity, it must be performed throughout the entire range of motion (ROM). Using the full range of motion ensures maximum motor unit activation. In addition, bodybuilders should always stretch at the end of the warm-up to maintain a good range of motion and excellent flexibility, during the rest interval between sets and as part of the cool-down. Good stretching practice keeps the muscle elongated and speeds the rate of recovery between workouts. Stretching also helps the overlapped myosin and actin return to their normal anatomical states, where biochemical exchanges are optimized.

LOADING PATTERNS

A serious training program follows a number of variations of distinct loading patterns that pertain to the pyramid loading formation. These variations include the pyramid loading pattern as well as the double-, skewed-, and flat-pyramid loading patterns.

Pyramid The pyramid is one of the most popular loading patterns in bodybuilding (figure 3.1). Notice that as the load progressively increases to maximum, the number of sets decreases proportionately. The physiological advantage of using the pyramid is that it ensures the activation or recruitment of most, if not all, of the motor units.

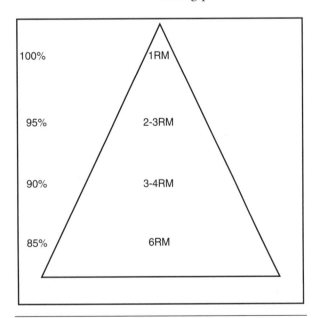

FIGURE 3.1 An example of the pyramid loading pattern. The number of repetitions (inside the pyramid) refers to their number per training session.

Reprinted from Bompa 1996.

Double Pyramid   The double pyramid is two pyramids, one mirroring the other (figure 3.2). In this loading pattern, beginning at the bottom, the load increases progressively up to 95 percent 1RM and then decreases again for the last sets. Note that as the load increases the number of repetitions, shown inside the pyramid, decreases and vice versa.

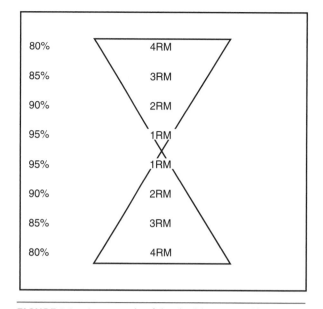

FIGURE 3.2 An example of the double-pyramid loading pattern.

Reprinted from Bompa 1996.

Skewed Pyramid   The skewed pyramid (figure 3.3) is an improved variant of the double pyramid. In this pattern, the load constantly increases throughout the session, except during the last set when it is lowered. The purpose of this last set is to provide variation and motivation, since the athlete must perform the set as quickly as possible.

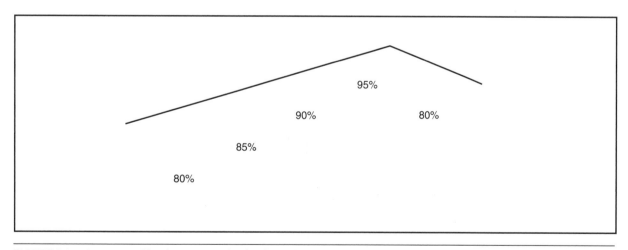

FIGURE 3.3   A suggested loading pattern for the skewed pyramid.

Reprinted from Bompa 1996.

Flat Pyramid The flat-pyramid loading pattern (Bompa 1999) can provide maximum training benefits (figure 3.4). A comparison between the traditional pyramids and the flat pyramid explains why this is the most effective loading pattern. In the traditional pyramids the load varies too much, often ranging between 60 percent to more than 100 percent of 1RM. Load variations of such magnitude cross over three intensity (load) borders—medium, heavy, and maximum.

To produce hypertrophy, the load must range between 60 and 80 percent 1RM, whereas for maximum strength the load must be 80 to 100-plus percent 1RM. The flat pyramid gives the physiological advantage of providing the best neuro-muscular adaptation for a given type of strength training because it keeps the load within one intensity level. This prevents the body from becoming confused by several different intensities.

The flat pyramid begins with a warm-up set (60 percent 1RM), and then the load stabilizes for the entire exercise at 70 percent 1RM. Another set at 60 percent 1RM may be performed at the end of each exercise for variety. Variations of the flat pyramid are possible depending on the phase and scope of training, as long as the load stays within the boundaries of the required intensity for a given phase:

70% - 80% - 80% - 80% - 80% - 70%

80% - 90% - 90% - 90% - 90% - 80%

85% - 95% - 95% - 95% - 95% - 85%

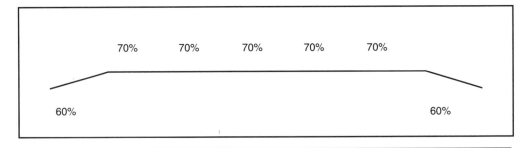

FIGURE 3.4 An example of the flat-pyramid loading pattern.

Reprinted from Bompa 1996.

REPETITIONS PER SET

Strength trainers and bodybuilders who follow traditional methods regarding the number of repetitions performed per set—that is, those who go to the gym every day and always perform 8 to 12 sets—will be shocked by the numbers recommended in table 3.2. Very few people have thought of performing 150-rep sets. High repetitions of this nature should be performed during the MD phase when you are trying to increase lean muscle mass to be show or contest ready. Remember, each training phase is different and requires a separate approach to loading rest intervals, number of reps, and exercise order.

TABLE 3.2	**Number of Repetitions Appropriate for Each Training Phase**	

Training phase	Training purpose	Number of repetitions
Maximum strength	Increase muscle strength and tone	1-7
Hypertrophy	Increase muscle size	6-12
Muscular endurance	Increase definition	30-150

LIFTING SPEED

The speed of lifting is an important component of strength and bodybuilding training. For the best results, some types of work must be executed quickly, while others must be performed at a medium pace. The speed with which you intend to lift, however, is not necessarily reflected in the appearance of the lift. For example, when you lift a heavy load that is 90 percent of 1RM, the performed motion might look slow; however, the force against the resistance must be applied as quickly as possible. Only under this condition will you be able to synchronize and recruit all the motor units necessary to defeat the resistance.

The fast twitch muscle fibers are recruited for action only when the application of force is fast and vigorous. You can usually maintain optimal speed throughout the first half of a set. Once fatigue sets in, speed often declines and a great deal of mental concentration is required to complete the intended number of repetitions.

NUMBER OF SETS

A set represents the number of exercise repetitions followed by a rest interval. The number of sets prescribed per exercise and workout depends on several factors, including how many exercises you perform in a training session, the phase of training, how many muscle groups you want to train, and how experienced you are.

Exercises in a Training Session As the number of exercises increases, the number of sets per exercise declines—for as energy and work potential decrease, the ability to perform numerous exercises and repetitions for a very high number of sets declines. As work potential improves, however, the number of sets per workout that you can tolerate will improve.

Training Phase As explained in chapter 2, an athlete goes through several training phases during a year of training. Each phase has a specific objective related to creating the best possible body shape. In the adaptation phase, where the scope of training is just overall adaptation, the number of sets per exercise is not high (two or three). In the hypertrophy phase, however, where the objective is to increase muscle size, it is necessary to perform the highest number of sets you can tolerate.

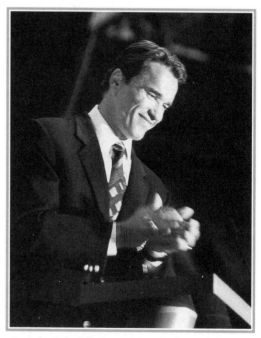

From bodybuilder to movie star, former governor of California Arnold Schwarzenegger finds time to keep in shape and motivate others.

Muscle Groups Trained per Session If training only one or two muscle groups in a given session, you can perform more sets per muscle group than if you are training three or four muscle groups. But when selecting the muscle groups per training session, you must consider how many training sessions are planned per week and how much time you can dedicate per workout. The more training sessions you have each week, the fewer the muscle groups you need to focus on in each session. If there is a shortage of time, use multijoint (compound) exercises.

Bodybuilder's Experience The classification of the bodybuilder (i.e., entry level, recreational, advanced) also plays a part in determining the number of sets included in the training session. As you become more experienced and achieve a high state of adaptation to weight training, you can perform more sets per body part per workout. For example, while an advanced bodybuilder might prepare for a contest by performing 20 or 30 sets for two or three muscle groups, a recreational athlete might train the same muscle groups with only 15 or 20 sets.

Rest Interval Energy is a crucial commodity in bodybuilding. The type of energy system used during a given workout depends on the phase of training (e.g., hypertrophy vs. muscle definition), the load employed, and the duration of the activity. High-intensity training can completely deplete your energy stores. To complete the workout, you must take a rest interval (RI) between each set in order to replenish the depleted fuel stores before you perform the next set.

Bodybuilders must realize that the RI and restoration of energy between sets and training sessions are as important as the training itself. The amount of time allowed between sets determines, to a high degree, the extent to which the energy source will be replenished before the next set. Careful planning of the RI is crucial if you are to avoid needless physiological and psychological stress during training.

STEPS FOR DESIGNING A TRAINING PROGRAM

Bodybuilders and strength trainers should understand the goals they are trying to accomplish. You can design an effective training program by using the following steps.

1. Select the Type of Strength Sought Strength training should be phase specific and designed to meet the needs of the person. Decide on the appropriate percentage of 1RM to be used and the number of reps and sets based on the type of strength sought. The strength training gains that bodybuilders and different athletes try to achieve can be sport specific or concentrated on overall body strength to transition into increased muscular gains during the hypertrophy phase. Details on training methods and progression are provided in part IV.

2. Select the Exercises Identify the prime movers, and then select the exercises that can best stimulate these muscles to meet your individual needs. These needs might depend on your background or foundation, your individual strengths and weaknesses, or the disproportionate development among your muscle groups and body parts. For example, if you have the capacity to develop massive legs quickly but your upper body takes longer to grow, then select exercises to compensate the weaker part to encourage growth and restore symmetry.

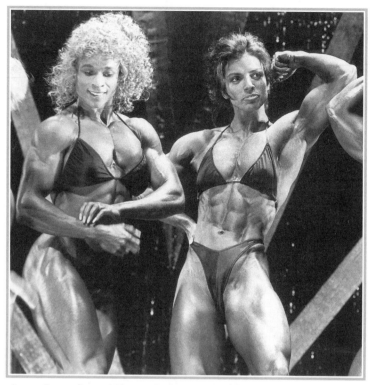

Laura Creavalle and Sharon Bruneau strut their stuff.

Selection of exercises is also phase specific. For example, during the anatomical adaptation phase, most muscle groups are worked in order to develop a better overall foundation, whereas in the muscle definition phase, training becomes more specific and exercises are selected to target the prime movers.

3. Test Maximum Strength   Knowing your 1RM for each exercise is crucial for the concept of periodization, as each workout is planned using percentages of 1RM. If for some reason you are unable to test 1RM for each exercise, try to test 1RM for at least the dominant exercise within the training program. Often strength trainers randomly choose the load and number of repetitions, or they follow the programs of others instead of using their own specific data, which is 1RM for each exercise. Because continual improvement in maximum strength, recovery ability, lifting techniques, and other factors occurs from phase to phase, any data other than 1RM for each exercise are valid for only a short time.

Among some members of the bodybuilding world, an unfounded belief exists that testing for 1RM is dangerous. Some trainers maintain that injury will result if a lifter puts forth a maximal effort; however, an adequately trained athlete can lift 100 percent once in a 4-week period without danger. Keep in mind, though, that a very thorough and progressive warm-up must precede any test for 1RM. If an athlete is still reluctant to test for 100 percent, another option is to test for a 3RM or 5RM (i.e., maximum weight that can be lifted three or five times before exhaustion) and then conclude what the 1RM would be. (See appendix C for a chart that gives the estimated 1RM for submaximal values.)

4. Develop the Actual Training Program   The fourth step is to develop the actual training program. By this point, you know which exercises are to be performed, the 1RM for each exercise, and the type of strength to be developed. With this information, you can select the number of exercises, the percentage of 1RM, the number of reps, and the number of sets.

This program cannot be the same, however, for each training phase. The training demand must be progressively increased so you are forced to adapt to increasing workloads—such adaptation is required in order to increase muscle size, tone, and strength. You can increase the training demand by any of the following means: Increase the load, decrease the rest interval, increase the number of repetitions, or increase the number of sets.

Table 3.3 illustrates a hypothetical program to demonstrate how to set up your own program. Before looking at the chart, be sure you understand the notation used to express the load, number of reps, and number of sets. For example, the following description

$$80/10 \times 4$$

represents the load and the number of reps and sets. The number 80 represents the load as a percentage of 1RM, so the lifter is using a load that is 80 percent of 1RM. The number 10 represents the number of repetitions per set, and the number 4 represents the number of sets.

Although many books and articles on this subject actually take the liberty of prescribing the load in pounds or kilograms to be used, please notice that we do not. There is little basis on which someone could legitimately suggest the weight an athlete should use without knowing anything about the athlete! The load must be suggested as a percentage of 1RM. This allows strength trainers and bodybuilders to specifically calculate the load for each exercise according to their individual potential, within the requirements of a given training phase.

TABLE 3.3	Hypothetical Training Program to Illustrate Format Design		
Ex no.	**Exercise**	**Load/# reps × sets**	**RI (min)**
1	Leg press	80/6 × 4	3
2	Flat bench press	75/8 × 4	3
3	Leg curl	60/10 × 4	2
4	Half squat	80/8 × 4	3
5	Abdominal curl	15 × 4	2
6	Deadlift	60/8 × 3	2

Reprinted from Bompa 1996.

The first column of table 3.3 lists the exercises by number, or the order in which they are performed during the training session. The second column lists the exercises. The third column shows the load, number of reps, and number of sets. The last column gives the RI required after each set.

5. Test to Recalculate 1RM   Finally, test to recalculate 1RM. Another test for 1RM is needed before the beginning of each new phase to ensure that progress is acknowledged and new loads are based on the new gains made in strength.

TRAINING CYCLES

A good bodybuilding program improves muscle size, tone, density, and definition. A training program is successful only when it has these characteristics:

- It is a part of a longer plan.
- It is based on the scientific knowledge available in the field.
- It uses periodization as a guideline for planning training throughout the year.

The program must have short-term goals and long-term goals that are phase specific. Each training phase has its own objectives, so it is necessary to design the daily and weekly programs to meet these objectives, while coinciding with the overall plan.

The development of a plan with both short- and long-term goals must take into account a person's background, physical potential, and rate of adaptation to the physiological challenges imposed by training. In chapters 12 through 17, we introduce you to several types of plans; and since planning theory is very complex, we discuss annual planning only as it pertains to bodybuilding.

Training Session

The training session, or daily program, includes a warm-up, the main workout, and a cool-down. Each of these three parts of the training session has its own goals. The first part prepares you for the training planned that day; the work is done in the second, or main, part of the workout; and the third part cools you down and speeds up your recovery before the next training session.

Warm-Up   The purpose of the warm-up is to prepare you for the program to follow. During the warm-up your body temperature rises, enhancing oxygen transport and preventing, or at least reducing, ligament sprains and muscle and tendon strains. It also stimulates central nervous system activity, which coordinates all the systems of the body, speeds up motor reactions through faster transmission of nerve impulses, and improves coordination. For the purpose of strength and bodybuilding training, the warm-up consists of two parts:

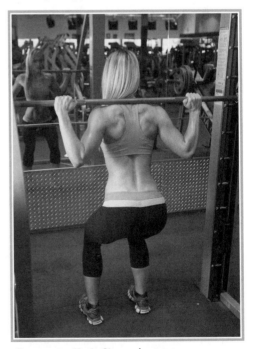

1. **General warm-up (10 to 12 minutes).** This part consists of light jogging, cycling, or stair climbing, followed by stretching exercises. This ritual prepares the muscles and tendons for the workout by increasing blood flow and body temperature. During this time, you can mentally prepare for the main part of the training session by visualizing the exercises to be performed and motivating yourself for the eventual strain of training.

2. **Specific warm-up (3 to 5 minutes).** This part is a short transition period that consists of performing a few repetitions of each planned exercise using significantly lighter loads. This prepares your body for the specific work to be done during the main part of the workout.

Fitness star Kasia Sitarz always warms up before an intensive training session.

Main Workout This part of the training session is dedicated to performing the actual bodybuilding exercises. For the best results, make up the daily program well in advance of the workout, and write it down on paper or, better yet, in a logbook. To know the program in advance is of psychological benefit because it enables you to better motivate yourself and focus more clearly on the task at hand.

The duration of a training session depends on the type of strength being developed and the specific training phase of your model of periodization. For example, the longest workouts are needed for the hypertrophy phase because there are many sets to perform. As a result, a hypertrophy workout may be as long as 2 hours, especially if there are a large number of exercises. Multijoint exercises are beneficial in a hypertrophy workout because they save you time.

The recommended duration of a workout, both in specific sports as well as in bodybuilding, has shifted dramatically over the years. From the 1960s to the early 1970s, the duration of suggested workouts was often 2.5 to 3 hours. The results from numerous scientific investigations have had a dramatic influence on the recommended duration of a workout, demonstrating that you may improve more over the course of three 1-hour workouts than during a single 3-hour workout. In the case of strength training and bodybuilding, longer workouts result in a hormonal shift. Specifically, testosterone levels decrease, promoting breakdown (catabolism) of protein, which has a negative effect on muscle building.

The type of strength or bodybuilding training dictates, to a very high degree, the duration of a workout. It is also important to realize that the rest intervals employed greatly influence the duration of a training session. The following durations are suggested for each type of strength training session:

- 1 to 1.25 hours for anatomical adaptation and general conditioning
- 1 to 2 hours for hypertrophy training
- 1 to 1.5 hours for maximum strength training
- 1.5 hours for muscle definition training

Cool-Down Just as the warm-up is a transition period to take the body from its normal biological state to a state of high stimulation, the cool-down is a transition period that produces the opposite effect. The job of the cool-down is to progressively bring the body back to its normal state of functioning.

A cool-down of 10 to 25 minutes consists of activities that facilitate faster recovery and regeneration. After a tough workout, the muscles are exhausted, tense, and rigid. To overcome this, you must allow for muscle recovery (see chapter 4). Hitting the showers immediately after the last exercise, though tempting, is not the best course of action.

Removal of lactic acid from the blood and muscles is necessary if the effects of fatigue are to be eliminated quickly. The best way to achieve this is by performing 10 to 25 minutes of light, continuous aerobic activity, such as jogging, cycling, or rowing, which will cause the body to continue perspiring. This will remove about half the lactic acid from the system and help you recover more quickly between training sessions. Remember, the faster you recover, the greater the amount of work you can perform in the next training session.

Microcycle

The microcycle is the weekly training program and is probably the most important tool in planning. Throughout the annual plan, the nature and dynamics of the microcycles change according to the phase of training, the training objectives, and the physiological and psychological demands of training. Well-organized bodybuilders should also seriously consider load variations. The work, or the total stress per microcycle, is increased mainly by increasing the number of training days per week. The total work per week follows the principle of step-type loading.

Loading Patterns   Because of unscientific theories—such as "no pain, no gain" and overloading—that have dominated the sports of bodybuilding and strength training, most athletes believe in training hard day in and day out regardless of the season. It is not surprising that most of them constantly feel exhausted and frustrated because they do not achieve expected gains, and many quit because they stop enjoying their sport. To avoid such undesirable outcomes, athletes need to follow the step-type loading pattern and alternate intensities inside each microcycle. Figures 3.5 through 3.7 illustrate low-, medium-, and high-intensity variations. (These three microcycles also represent the first three microcycles of each of the macrocycles shown in figures 3.9 and 3.10. See the upcoming macrocycle section.) Other variations are possible, depending on individual circumstances.

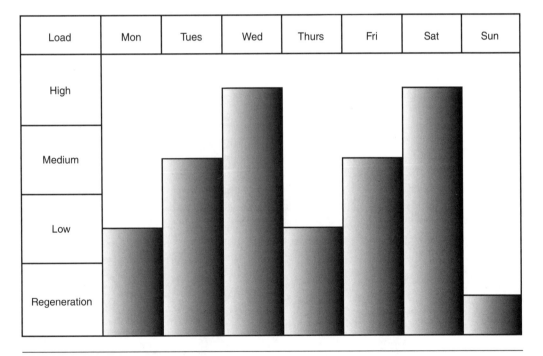

FIGURE 3.5   A low-intensity microcycle.

Reprinted from Bompa 1996.

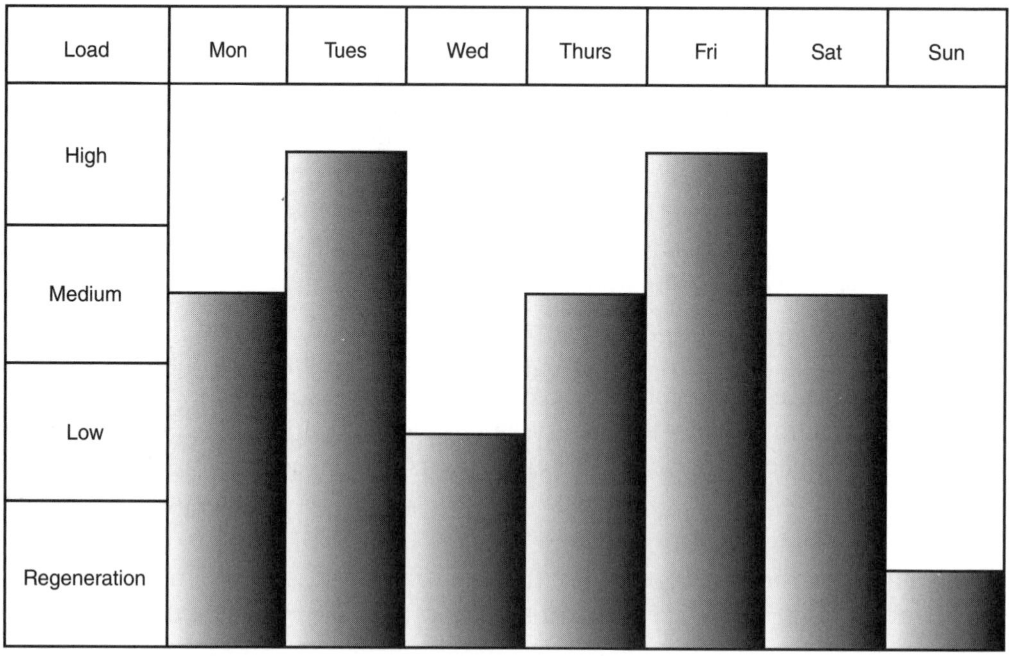

Load	Mon	Tues	Wed	Thurs	Fri	Sat	Sun
High							
Medium							
Low							
Regeneration							

FIGURE 3.6 A medium-intensity microcycle.

Reprinted from Bompa 1996.

Load	Mon	Tues	Wed	Thurs	Fri	Sat	Sun
High							
Medium							
Low							
Regeneration							

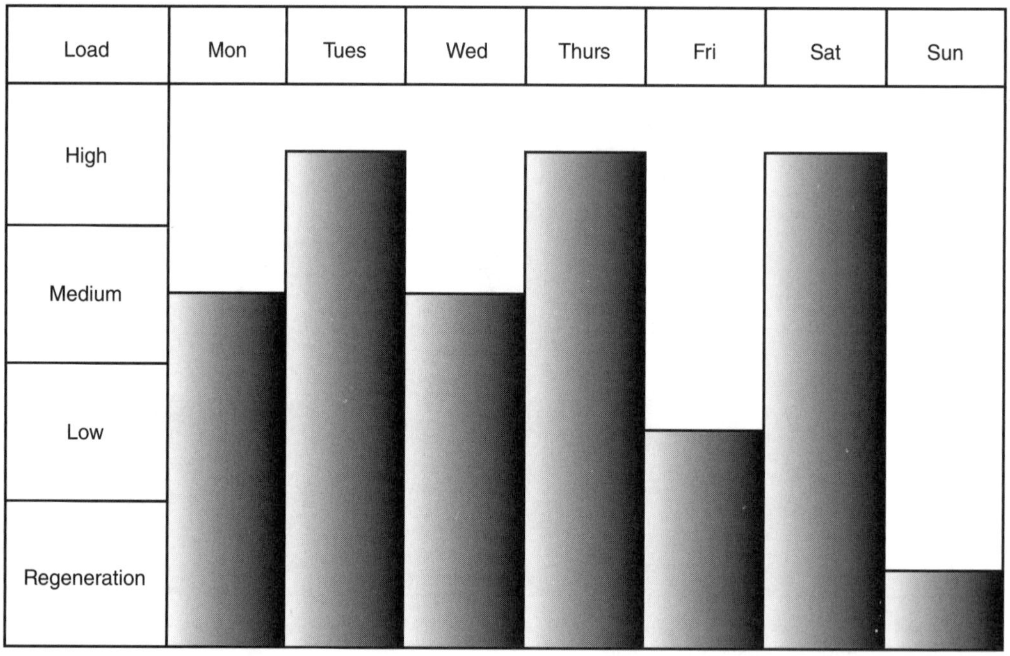

FIGURE 3.7 A high-intensity microcycle.

Reprinted from Bompa 1996.

Any microcycle variation includes low-intensity days, and these days represent a crucial concept in training—one that not only aids in reaching recovery and supercompensation (see the Supercompensation section later in this chapter) but also helps prevent overtraining, which is so common among bodybuilders who follow the traditional "no pain, no gain" philosophy. Athletes might legitimately question the role of low-intensity days, but they serve a valuable purpose. The body uses the fuels adenosine triphosphate (ATP) and phosphocreatine (PC), which are replenished from protein and fat (gluconeogenesis). For high-intensity workouts that consist of low-rep sets and rest intervals of 2-3 minutes, which are typical of maximum strength training, the ATP-PC system provides the energy. Under these conditions, energy stores can be replenished in about 24 hours, which means the next day's workout can also be of high intensity.

Every high-intensity workout session, however, creates physiological strain and mental or psychological stress, caused by the intense concentration that is necessary to tackle the challenging loads. Consequently, after such a workout the athletes must be concerned with two things: (1) whether their energy stores will be replenished before the next workout and (2) whether they will be mentally ready for the next session. These factors make it necessary to plan in advance for low-intensity days after 1 or 2 days of hard training, such as the low-intensity days shown in figures 3.5 through 3.7.

Figure 3.8 gives another option for planning a microcycle, in which two challenging days are planned back to back. Please note that this type of microcycle is only for highly trained strength trainers and bodybuilders who have a high adaptive response and are capable of tolerating intense physiological and psychological strain.

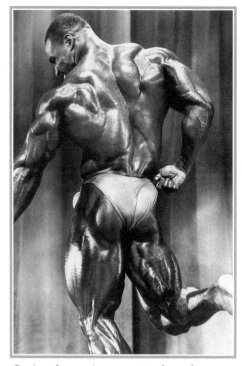

During the maximum strength workouts that are necessary to create a body this massive, the energy system taxed (ATP-PC) can be replenished in approximately 24 hours.

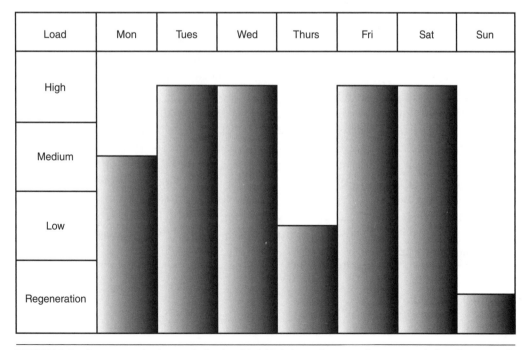

FIGURE 3.8   A suggested microcycle for the third, high-intensity step of a macrocycle for elite strength trainers and bodybuilders.

Reprinted from Bompa 1996.

If, however, the session consists of high-rep sets, as proposed for the muscle definition ("cuts") phase, or if the workout is especially long (2 to 3 hours), the breakdown and oxidation of body fat supplies a large proportion of the fuel. After these long and exhausting workouts, the complete restoration of glycogen often takes 48 hours. The same duration of time is necessary for protein synthesis, implying that only after 48 hours is the same muscle group ready for another workout. Figure 3.7 suggests an appropriate microcycle structure for this type of training.

Training Frequency   The frequency of training sessions depends on the athlete's classification, training phase, and training background. Recreational bodybuilders must progressively introduce training. At first they can plan 2 relatively short strength training sessions per microcycle. Once this training regimen is handled easily, the frequency can gradually be increased to 3 or 4 sessions per microcycle. Higher-level athletes who are taking part in shows can plan 6 to 10 training sessions per microcycle.

As you will learn in part III, the number of training sessions also depends on the phase of training: 3 to 5 for anatomical adaptation, 4 to 6 or even higher for professional bodybuilders and strength trainers, and 6 to 10 during the maximum strength and hypertrophy phases.

An athlete's training background and resulting work tolerance are important factors in determining the frequency of training sessions per microcycle. Obviously well-trained athletes with 2 to 3 years of experience can train with ease at least four times per microcycle, which translates into visible improvements in size and muscle tone. These athletes can tolerate more work than novices.

Macrocycle

To plan a program, you must understand how the microcycle fits into a longer training phase—namely, the macrocycle, or 4 weeks of training—and how to plan the load of training per microcycle. Load increments within the macrocycle must follow a step-type progression. Figure 3.9 illustrates the standard approach for load increments for the microcycles within a macrocycle. With regard to intensity, macrocycles follow the principle of step-type loading. The load progressively increases over three microcycles (weeks), and then declines for a regeneration cycle to facilitate recuperation and replenishment of energy before another macrocycle begins. (Figures 3.5, 3.6, and 3.7 provide appropriate examples of how to plan the first three microcycles in figure 3.9.)

Based on the model shown in figure 3.9, figure 3.10 gives a practical example suggesting load increments and using the notation explained in this chapter. This figure illustrates that the work, or the total stress in training, increases in steps, with the highest point being in step 3. (Figures 3.5, 3.6, and 3.7 provide appropriate examples of how to plan the first three microcycles in figure 3.10.) Step 4 is a regeneration cycle in which the load and number of sets are lowered. This lessens the fatigue that has developed during the first three steps and allows the body to replenish its energy stores. Step 4 also allows the athlete to psychologically relax.

To increase the work from step 1 to step 3, there are two options: (1) increase the load (the highest one being in step 3) or (2) increase the number of sets (from five total sets in step 1 to seven total sets in step 3). In this example, both options are used at the same time—an appropriate approach for athletes with a solid background in training. Other options will suit the needs of different classifications. Entry-level athletes, for example, have difficulty tolerating higher loads and an increased number of sets, so it is more important for them to increase the number of exercises. This approach will develop their entire muscular system and help the ligaments and tendons adapt to strength training.

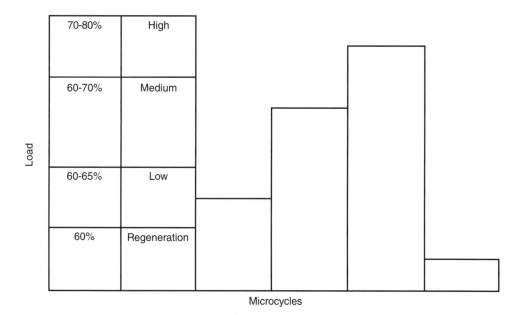

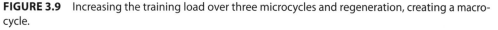

FIGURE 3.9 Increasing the training load over three microcycles and regeneration, creating a macrocycle.

Reprinted from Bompa 1996

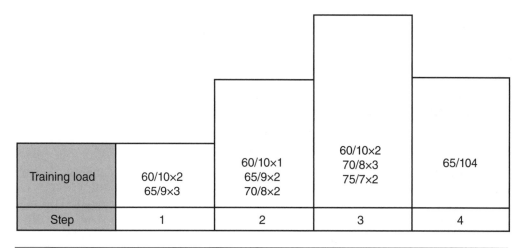

FIGURE 3.10 A practical example of load increments over a macrocycle.

Reprinted from Bompa 1996.

SUPERCOMPENSATION

Supercompensation is the state of physiological and psychological arousal that ideally occurs before a day of high-intensity training. Supercompensation can only be achieved, however, if work and regeneration are timed perfectly. Mistakes in timing are what turn supercharged workouts into daily-grind sessions. Figure 3.11 illustrates the supercompensation cycle of a training session.

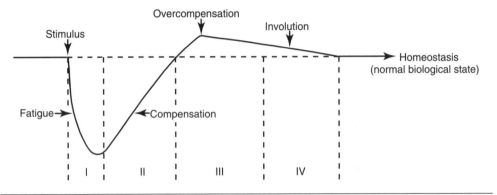

FIGURE 3.11 The supercompensation cycle of a training session.

Reprinted from Bompa 1983.

Under normal conditions of rest and proper diet, a person is in a balanced state (homeostasis). As figure 3.11 illustrates, a certain level of fatigue is reached, both during and at the end of a training session. This fatigue is caused by the depletion of fuel stores, lactic acid accumulation in the working muscles, and psychological stress. The abrupt drop of the homeostasis curve illustrates the reduction of functional capacity to perform high-quality work, the depletion of free fatty acids, and the fact that the muscles are in a state of catabolism, or a posttraining state of protein degradation. Levels of insulin, which increases the rate of glucose transport to the working muscles, decline in the blood.

The time between the end of one session and the beginning of another is the phase of compensation during which the biochemical sources of energy are replenished. The return of the curve toward the normal biological state, or homeostasis, is slow and progressive, indicating that the replenishment of lost energy stores requires several hours. If the rest interval between two high-intensity training sessions is planned correctly, the energy sources (ATP-PC) are fully replaced, and the body also acquires some fuel reserves. This energy rebound puts athletes into a state of supercompensation and gives them the energy needed to train even harder. Furthermore, the state of compensation represents the beginning of the anabolic state of the muscles, when protein is resynthesized and blood insulin levels return to normal. This compensation phase is essential for adaptation to training and, consequently, for improving muscle size, tone, and definition.

If the time between two workouts is too long, the supercompensation will fade away (involution), resulting in little, if any, improvement in work capacity. The optimal recovery period needed for supercompensation varies according to the type and intensity of training as shown in table 3.4.

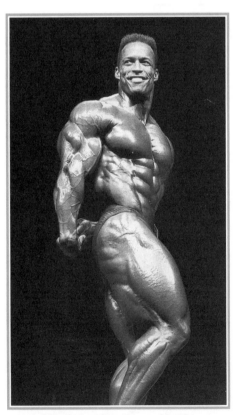

A well-fueled and well-rested body can be pushed to the limits to achieve maximum results.

TABLE 3.4	Time Needed for Supercompensation to Occur After Different Types of Training	
Type of training	**Energy system**	**Time needed for super-compensation (hours)**
Aerobic (cardiorespiratory)	Glycogen, fats	6-8
Maximum strength	ATP-PC	24
Hypertrophy, muscle definition	Glycogen	36

The way loads are planned directly affects how the body responds to training. For example, if an athlete follows the philosophy of lifting as heavy a load as possible day in and day out, and the intensity of training per microcycle does not vary, then the supercompensation curve changes drastically. Under these conditions the body never has time to replenish its energy stores and comes closer to exhaustion with every workout. Figure 3.12 illustrates what happens to the body and to training potential when continuous exhaustive training is employed over a prolonged period of time.

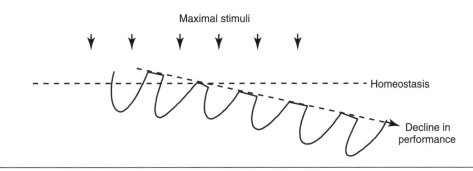

FIGURE 3.12   The effect of continuous overload training on one's body and working capacity.
Reprinted from Bompa 1983.

As we can see from figure 3.12, it is still possible to reach supercompensation during the first 2 or 3 days of constant overloading because fatigue has not yet affected the body's overall potential. As constant overload training continues, however, fatigue increases, taking the body further away from its balanced state (homeostasis). After about 3 or 4 days, every workout begins in a state of residual fatigue. At this stage supercompensation is never reached, and the bodybuilder's training capacity and growth potential are inhibited. Eventually the athlete reaches a very high level of exhaustion and a very low level of motivation. From this point, overtraining and breakdown are only steps away.

In comparison, when you alternate heavy training days with light training days, as suggested in figures 3.5 through 3.7 (pages 39 and 40), and follow the step-loading principle, the supercompensation curve forms a wave-like pattern, as shown in figure 3.13, that hovers around and above the body's homeostasis level. Energy stores are continuously replenished, and the body is not striving to operate in a state of exhaustion or fatigue. When the body is rested and full of fuel, it can be pushed to heights never dreamed of before. By training this way, you can expect supercompensation to occur every 2 to 4 days.

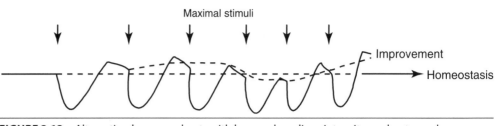

Maximal stimuli

Improvement

Homeostasis

FIGURE 3.13 Alternating heavy workouts with low- and medium-intensity workouts produces a wavelike curve of improvement.

Reprinted from Bompa 1983.

Improvements in your working potential and feelings of overall well-being occur mostly on the days when you experience supercompensation. This is also the time when growth and muscle size increase. Since every bodybuilder and strength trainer wants these positive outcomes, you should carefully plan your training program so that heavy and intense training is followed by an easy day that encourages supercompensation.

SPLIT ROUTINES

Although split routines are a necessity for seriously committed bodybuilders, they are not necessarily appropriate for recreational athletes whose goals are to look fit, strong, and toned. These recreational bodybuilders will probably get the best results from training three times a week with a total-body routine.

Most serious bodybuilders train very frequently, from four to six times a week. But it is difficult to challenge the same muscles in consecutive training sessions. Split routines allow these athletes to train the various muscle groups every second

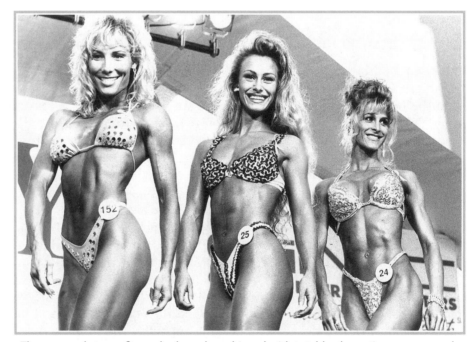

The sexy and strong fitness look can be achieved with total-body routines as opposed to the split routines favored by many hard-core bodybuilders.

day or so in order to achieve better recovery between workouts. Table 3.5 is a classic example of a 6-day split routine. Many athletes believe that a program such as the classic split routine, which trains each muscle group twice per week, is sufficient to stimulate an optimal adaptive response to training. Others believe that training a muscle group to exhaustion only once a week is sufficient stimulus to make the desired gains in muscle size, tone, and definition.

We seriously question both these modes of thinking: Twice a week is not enough. For continual improvements, workouts must *constantly challenge* your present state of adaptation. To provoke a new adaptive response, you should progressively increase your training load using the step-type loading method. Depending on the load used, this approach will stimulate an increase in muscle size or an increase in tone and strength. Competitive bodybuilders should work some muscle groups three times a week during certain training phases. (Please note that this is feasible only if you decrease the number of sets and exercises per muscle group to the lowest level realistically possible, to ensure that your energy is spent most effectively.) Table 3.6 suggests the number of sets for each muscle or muscle group per workout. These suggestions apply to recreational bodybuilders with 2 to 3 years' experience and to advanced and professional bodybuilders and strength trainers.

TABLE 3.5	Classic 6-Day Split
Day	**Body part**
1	Legs, calves, and shoulders
2	Chest and biceps
3	Back and triceps
4	Legs, calves, and shoulders
5	Chest and biceps
6	Back and triceps
7	Rest

TABLE 3.6	Suggested Sets Per Workout
Muscle	**Number of sets per workout**
Chest	8
Back	10
Quadriceps	6
Hamstrings	4-6
Calves	6-8
Biceps	6
Triceps	6
Shoulders	10-12
Abdominals	6

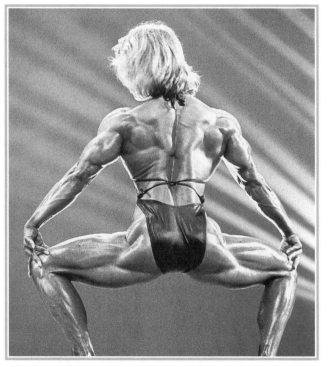

The beautifully sculpted physique of Laura Creavalle is attributed to her well-structured periodized training program.

TABLE 3.7	**High-Adaptive-Response 6-Day Spilt**

Day	Body part
1	Chest, back, and arms
2	Legs, calves, shoulders, and abdominals
3	Chest, back, and arms
4	Legs, calves, shoulders, and abdominals
5	Chest, back, and arms
6	Legs, calves, shoulders, and abdominals
7	Rest

TABLE 3.8	**High-Adaptive-Response 6-Day Double Split**

Day	Time	Body part
1	a.m.	Legs and calves
	p.m.	Chest and biceps
2	a.m.	Shoulders and triceps
	p.m.	Back and abdominals
3	a.m.	Legs and calves
	p.m.	Chest and biceps
4	a.m.	Shoulders and triceps
	p.m.	Back and abdominals
5	a.m.	Legs and calves
	p.m.	Chest and biceps
6	a.m.	Shoulders and triceps
	p.m.	Back and abdominals
7		Rest

The high-adaptive-response 6-day split outlined in table 3.7 trains each body part three times per week and allows each muscle group 48 hours of recovery before it is trained again. The same approach can be used on a double-split routine. Table 3.8 shows one of many possible combinations.

Although most bodybuilders believe the split routine allows sufficient recovery between training sessions, this belief does not accord with the reality of the energy systems' requirements. Although a split routine helps eliminate local muscle fatigue (the fatigue acquired by a group of muscles worked to exhaustion), it does little to facilitate overall replenishment of the body's energy stores. If athletes perform exhaustive workouts every day, their glycogen stores become depleted regardless of whether they use a split routine. Remember, exhaustive workouts use glycogen as the main fuel source, taking it from the working muscles as well as from the liver. The body needs 48 hours to fully restore glycogen levels and synthesize protein and cannot operate optimally if a person trains to exhaustion every 24 hours.

Accelerating Muscle Recovery

R ecovery is one of the most important elements of successful training. Athletes who understand the concept avoid critical fatigue and overtraining. Strength athletes are constantly exposed to various types of training loads, reps, and sets, some of which can exceed their threshold of tolerance. As a result, the ability to adapt to the desired training load decreases and detracts from overall performance.

When athletes drive themselves beyond their physiological limits, they risk going into a state of fatigue—and the greater the level of fatigue, the greater the training aftereffects such as low rate of recovery, decreased coordination, and diminished power output. Personal factors, such as stress from work, school, or social situations, can also increase levels of fatigue during training.

MUSCLE FATIGUE

Fatigue can be defined as an inability to maintain the expected force and power output, resulting in reduced work capacity (Maassen 1997; Powers and Howley 2009). Such fatigue depends on many factors, including a person's state of fitness, fiber-type composition, and sport. For example, fatigue in an endurance-trained athlete is different from fatigue in a power-trained athlete. Cross-sectional studies reveal that the training background of power-trained athletes and endurance-trained athletes has an impact on the functional organization of the neuromuscular system (Garrandes et al. 2007). These data demonstrate that neuromuscular functioning adjusts in response to the contraction type principally used in the sport activity.

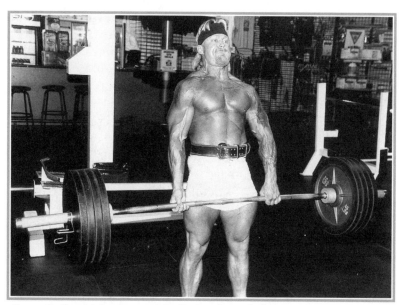

Trevor Butler driving beyond the limits of muscle fatigue.

Central and Peripheral Nervous Systems

Muscle fatigue can be broken into central and peripheral components. Central nervous system (CNS) fatigue is related to events of neural input to the higher brain centers and central command centers, to recruitment of the alpha motor nerve pool, and to the alpha motor nerves themselves. CNS fatigue results from either a reduction in the number of functioning motor units involved in the activity or a reduction in their firing frequency (Hubal, Rubinstein, and Clarkson 2007). Peripheral nervous system (PNS) fatigue involves the neuromuscular junction, the process of excitation–contraction (EC) coupling (which involves the activation of the surface membrane), the propagation of that activation down the T tubules (which brings the activation into the depths of the cell), the release of calcium, and the activation of contractile elements involved in the generation of force and power. Impaired peripheral muscle function could result from damaged contractile proteins, a damaged sarcolemma (the cell membrane surrounding the muscle fiber), disrupted excitation–contraction coupling, and an altered intracellular environment, such as altered pH or ATP levels (Hubal, Rubinstein, and Clarkson 2007).

The central and peripheral nervous systems play an important role in fatigue, since temperature as well as psychological factors (e.g., incentive and stress) can cause fatigue. In a study by Nybo (2008), the physiological mechanisms involved with hyperthermia-induced fatigue primarily relate to changes in the CNS that lead to central fatigue. According to Amann et al. (2008), the importance of psychological factors, which eventually also involve neurobiological changes, and all the various aspects of skeletal muscle metabolism must certainly not be overlooked in relation to muscular fatigue.

The CNS and peripheral nervous systems have two basic processes for modulating muscle function: excitation and inhibition. Throughout training, the two processes constantly alternate. For stimulation, the CNS sends a nerve impulse to the working muscle, causing it to contract and perform work. The speed, power, and frequency of the nerve impulse directly depend on the state of the CNS.

The nerve impulses are most effective (as evidenced by good performance) when controlled excitation prevails. When the opposite occurs, as a result of fatigue, the nerve cell is in a state of inhibition, and the muscle contraction is slower and weaker. The force of contraction relates directly to the electrical activation sent by the CNS and the number of motor units recruited; as fatigue increases, the recruitment of motor units decreases. Nerve cells cannot maintain working capacity for a very long time. Under the strain of training or demands of competition, the working capacity decreases. If high intensity is maintained in spite of fatigue, nerve cells assume a state of inhibition to protect themselves from external stimuli. Fatigue, therefore, should be seen as the body's way of protecting itself against damage to the contractile mechanism of the muscle.

Skeletal muscles produce force by activating their motor units and regulating their firing frequency, and these factors must progressively increase to enhance force output. The body can neutralize fatigue to some degree by signaling motor units to change their firing frequency, thereby permitting muscles to maintain force more effectively under a certain state of fatigue. If the duration of sustained maximum contraction increases, the frequency of motor unit firing decreases, and inhibition becomes more prominent (Nybo and Nielsen 2001).

One study demonstrated that in a 30-second maximum voluntary contraction, firing frequency decreased by 80 percent from beginning to end (Marsden, Meadows, and Merton 1971). Other studies reported a decrease in the firing rates of most motor units during a short-lasting fatiguing task (Deluca and Forrest 1973; Garland et al. 1994). A later study by Adam and Deluca contradicted these findings by demonstrating this initial decrease was followed by an increase as the muscle continued to contract and progress toward exhaustion (2005). A more recent study concluded that substantial changes in motor unit activity were found after eccentric exercise, which included an increase in motor unit firing rate (Dartnall, Nordstrom, and Semmler 2008). Much information is still needed about the mechanisms responsible for the change in correlated motor unit activity with exercise-induced muscle fatigue and damage.

Sites of Muscle Fatigue

Most research findings point to two sites of muscle fatigue. The motor nerve is the first. The nervous system transmits nerve impulses to muscle fibers via the motor nerves. A nerve impulse has certain characteristics of force, speed, and frequency. The higher the force impulse, the stronger the muscle contraction, giving greater ability to lift heavier loads. Since fatigue greatly affects the force of nerve impulses, rising levels of fatigue lead to declining force of contraction. This is why longer rest intervals (RIs) of up to 7 minutes are necessary for CNS recovery during the maximum strength phase.

The second site is the neuromuscular junction. This is the nerve attachment on the muscle fiber that relays the nerve impulses to the working muscle. This type of fatigue is largely due to increased release of chemical transmitters from the nerve endings (Bigland-Ritchie et al. 1982; Tesch, Colliander, and Kaiser 1986; Kirkendall 1990). After a set, a 2- to 3-minute rest interval usually returns the electrical properties of the nerve to normal levels. After work of powerful contractions (such as maximum strength training), however, a rest interval of longer than 5 minutes is needed for sufficient recovery to occur.

Metabolic Sources of Fatigue

The complex cycle of muscle contraction is triggered by the nerve impulse that depolarizes the surface membrane of the muscle cell and is then conducted into the muscle fiber. This is followed by a series of events in which calcium is bound together with protein filaments (actin and myosin), resulting in contractile tension. The functional site of fatigue is suggested to be the link between excitation and contraction, which results in either reducing the intensity of these two processes or in decreasing the sensitivity to activation. The flow of calcium ions affects the mechanism of excitation–contraction coupling (Duhamel et al. 2007).

The sarcoplasmic reticulum, made up of lateral sacs contained in the myofibrils of muscle cells, stores calcium needed for muscular contraction (Powers and Howley 2009). With each muscular contraction, calcium is released from the sarcoplasmic reticulum. An impairment in the release of calcium contributes to various types of muscle fatigue. The evidence is now strong that a decline in the rapidly releasable calcium in the sarcoplasmic reticulum can contribute to the reduced calcium release occurring during fatigue (Duhamel et al. 2007; Head 2010).

During vigorous exercise, inorganic phosphate (Pi) concentration levels within the muscle cell rise. Inorganic phosphate may enter the sarcoplasmic reticulum and bind to calcium to form a precipitate (CaPi), thus reducing the amount of releasable calcium in the sarcoplasmic reticulum (Allen, Lamb, and Westerblad 2008). Other mechanisms also contribute to the decline of sarcoplasmic reticulum calcium release during fatigue. There is increasing evidence that glycogen is an essential requirement for normal excitation–contraction coupling, and that when glycogen levels decline, this also inhibits sarcoplasmic reticulum calcium release. It is evident that these factors contribute to the various aspects of fatigue (Allen, Lamb, and Westerblad 2008).

Lactic Acid Accumulation   Bodybuilders predominantly use the anaerobic energy system, which produces high levels of lactic acid. This is the major end product of anaerobic metabolism (i.e., glycolysis). The biochemical exchanges during muscle contraction result in the release of hydrogen ions, which in turn cause acidosis (lactate fatigue), which seems to determine the point of exhaustion (Powers and Howley 2009).

Increased acidosis also inhibits the binding capacity of calcium through inactivation of troponin, a protein compound. Since troponin is an important contributor to the contraction of the muscle cell, its inactivation may expand the connection between fatigue and exercise. The discomfort produced by acidosis can also be a limiting factor in psychological fatigue.

The long-held view that lactate accumulation has a detrimental effect on exercise performance is challenged by newer findings, indicating that lactate is more likely to have an indirect effect on muscle fatigue. Lactate is an important fuel for contracting skeletal muscle and not, as previously believed, merely a metabolic by-product. This by-product was previously thought to be destined for the Cori cycle, or the process by which lactate formed in the muscle during exercise is transported via blood to the liver and converted to glucose (Powers and Howley 2009).

In a study by Lamb and Stephenson (2006), lactic acid does not cause fatigue but actually helps delay the onset of fatigue in two ways: (1) by offsetting the negative effects of raised extracellular potassium on membrane excitability and (2) by inhibiting the sarcoplasmic reticulum calcium pump that would help increase cytoplasmic calcium and consequent force of the muscle contraction. Lactic acid accumulation appears to be an advantage during contractile activity; however, reduced calcium uptake would increase basal intracellular calcium, which is thought to be important in causing low-frequency fatigue (Westerblad et al. 2000).

Although some of the new research findings suggest that lactate accumulation is not detrimental to exercise performance, fatigue is a reality that must be accepted during training. If you correctly design your training program, you will increase your threshold to tolerate fatigue. Well-trained athletes are always capable of working more, with higher efficiency, and with visible results. Equally important is to avoid fatigue by applying some of the techniques suggested in this book, among which a periodized program is essential.

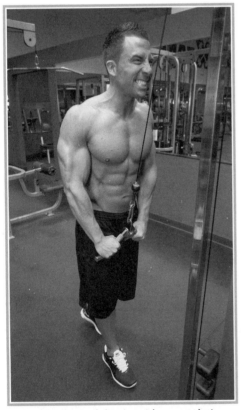

Training through lactic acid accumulation.

Depletion of ATP-PC and Glycogen Stores   Fatigue is experienced in the energy system when phosphocreatine (PC), muscle glycogen, or the carbohydrate stores are depleted from the working muscle (Conley 1994). The result is that the muscle performs less work, possibly because its cells are consuming ATP faster than they are producing it. Endurance capacity during prolonged moderate to heavy bodybuilding activity varies directly with the amount of glycogen in the muscle before exercise, indicating that fatigue occurs as a result of muscle glycogen depletion (Fox, Bowes, and Foss 1989). For high-intensity sets, the immediate source of energy for muscular contraction is ATP-PC. Rapid depletion of these stores in the muscle will certainly limit the ability of the muscle to contract (Sherwood 1993). Muscle ATP loss with exercise is directly correlated to muscle damage and fatigue (Harris et al. 1997).

When an athlete performs high numbers of reps with prolonged submaximal levels of work, the fuels used to produce energy are glucose and fatty acids. The availability of oxygen is critical throughout this type of training because, in limited quantities, carbohydrates are oxidized instead of free fatty acids. Maximum oxidation of free fatty acids is determined by the inflow of the fatty acids to the working muscle and by the aerobic training status of the athlete. The diet to which an athlete has adapted (see chapter 7) is also an important factor in determining substrate oxidation (fat, protein, or carbohydrate). In other words, diet influences whether fat, protein, or carbohydrate is burned for energy. Poor oxygen-carrying capacity in the blood and inadequate blood flow all contribute significantly to muscle fatigue (Grimby 1992).

MUSCLE DAMAGE

Anyone who has trained knows the feeling of stiffness a few days after an intense workout session. Examining the process at the contractile-fiber level will help you understand muscle recovery from a scientific perspective. Recovery is one of the most important elements of successful training. Two basic mechanisms explain how exercise initiates muscle damage. One is associated with the disturbance of metabolic function, while the other stems from mechanical disruption of muscle cells.

Metabolic damage to muscle occurs during prolonged submaximal work to exhaustion. Direct loading of the muscle, especially during the contraction phases, can cause muscle damage, and that metabolic change may aggravate the damage. The concentric portion of a movement occurs when a muscle is activated and force is produced, resulting in muscle shortening (Powers and Howley 2009) (e.g., the upward movement of a biceps curl). The eccentric portion of a movement occurs when a muscle is activated and force is produced, resulting in muscle lengthening (Powers and Howley 2009) (e.g., the resisting downward movement of a biceps curl). Muscle damage can be attributed to both concentric and eccentric movements.

According to research studies by Evans and Cannon (1991) and Ryschon et al. (1997), the force in concentric contractions is dispersed over a greater number of muscle fibers and requires much more metabolic activity in comparison to eccentric contractions. The maximum ATP production rate is highest in concentric action, suggesting an activation of energy metabolism under these conditions. These data demonstrate an increasing metabolic efficiency in human muscle action from concentric to eccentric action. In a more recent study by Muthalib et al. (2010), the biceps brachii muscle utilizes a lower amount of oxygen relative to oxygen supply to produce greater torque outputs during maximal eccentric contractions compared with maximal concentric contractions. This is most likely related to the greater inherent force-producing capacity of the myosin crossbridges that connect to actin filaments and to lower ATP hydrolysis, the reaction that breaks down ATP into ADP and inorganic phosphate, during eccentric contractions than during concentric contractions.

The eccentric movement utilizes fewer muscle fibers than the concentric movement. Since the eccentric phase tends to recruit fewer muscle fibers, each individual fiber is susceptible to greater physical damage. In a research study by Nosaka, Newton, and Sacco (2002), maximal eccentric muscle contractions produced a greater magnitude of muscle damage compared with continuous concentric contractions. In addition, Howatson and Someren (2008) found that eccentric contractions require a lower metabolic cost per unit of torque compared with concentric contractions.

MUSCLE SORENESS

For years, lactic acid buildup was considered the main cause of muscle soreness (Powers and Howley 2009). It is now understood that lactic acid is rapidly removed from muscle and blood after a workout session. Bond et al. (2005) showed that performing continuous light exercise during exercise recovery removed lactic acid from the blood more rapidly. It is now believed that soreness is caused from an influx of calcium ions into muscle cells (Fahey 1991). Calcium is very important in muscle contraction. It stimulates the fiber to contract and is rapidly pumped back into the calcium storage area (sarcoplasmic reticulum) after completion of the contraction.

Calcium leaks out of the sarcoplasmic reticulum when muscle fatigue is evident. The leakage collects in the mitochondria and inhibits ATP production (Proske and Allen 2005). The accumulation of calcium ions within the muscle fiber causes release of proteases—protein-degrading enzymes that break down muscle fibers. The soreness is primarily due to the formation of degraded protein components, or dead tissue. In response to the damaged tissue, the body initiates a cleanup phase by bringing neutrophils and macrophages (types of white blood cells) to the site of injury. Although these white blood cells clean away damaged tissue, they also participate in the production of free radicals. Free radicals can prolong recovery time and cause further muscle damage (Pedersen, Steensberg, and Schjerling 2001; Close et al. 2005). Antioxidants are chemicals that protect cells from oxidative damage caused by free radicals. Antioxidants are important because they can remove free radicals, which may delay exercise-induced muscle fatigue.

Therefore, it is clear that muscle damage occurs at the time of exercise, as judged by the loss of strength. Some of the consequences, such as pain, swelling, and the release of intracellular enzymes, do not occur immediately (Howell, Chleboun, and Conatser 1992). The delay may represent the natural time course of the inflammatory response to injury and thus will be induced 24 to 48 hours after intense exercise. Delayed-onset muscle soreness (DOMS) is defined as a muscle strain injury presenting with tenderness and stiffness of the muscle during movement. The pain stimulus associated with DOMS includes muscle spasm, connective tissue damage, lactic acid, muscle damage, inflammation, and enzyme efflux (Cheung, Hume, and Maxwell 2003). DOMS is associated with muscle injury, which is characterized as rupture of the muscle fibers themselves or of the connective tissue that transmits the pull of the fiber to the tendon.

DOMS occurs more frequently when athletes use muscles that are unaccustomed to being worked (Powers and Howley 2009). Through various research studies, it has been established that eccentric exercise induces the onset of DOMS more than concentric work (Cheung, Hume, and Maxwell 2003). A general recommendation for preventing DOMS is to slowly incorporate a specific exercise into your training sessions. A pattern of slow progression during the first 5 to 10 training sessions allows you to muscularly adapt to the exercise stress and reduces the incidence of DOMS (Powers and Howley 2009).

RECOVERY FROM STRENGTH TRAINING

Whether recovering from fatigue, overtraining, or just an exhausting training session, athletes should be aware of the various techniques that can speed or ease their recovery. Using these techniques is just as important as training effectively. As athletes continually strive to implement new loads into their training programs, they often do not adjust their recovery methods to match the new loads. This imbalance can lead to serious setbacks. Approximately 50 percent of an athlete's final performance depends on the ability to recover effectively and quickly.

It is vital for athletes to be aware of *all* the factors that aid the recovery process because it is the *combination* of all the factors that leads to the most successful recovery. The main factors for consideration are as follows.

- Age affects the rate of recovery. Older athletes generally require longer periods of recuperation than their younger counterparts.
- Better-trained, more experienced athletes generally require less time to recuperate, as they have quicker physiological adaptation to a given training stimulus.
- Female athletes tend to have a slower rate of recovery than males, apparently because of differences in their endocrine systems.
- Environmental factors such as jet lag, short-term changes in altitude, and cold climates tend to slow the recovery process.
- Replenishment of nutrients at the cellular level affects recovery. Muscle cells require constantly adequate levels of proteins, fats, carbohydrates, and ATP-PC for efficient general cellular metabolism as well as for production of energy (Fox, Bowes, and Foss 1989).
- Negative emotions such as fear, indecisiveness, and lack of willpower tend to impair the recovery process.
- The recovery process is slow and depends directly on the magnitude of the load employed in training.

Recovery time depends on the energy system being used. Table 4.1 provides recommended recovery times after exhaustive strength training. These are general guidelines; you will need to determine your ideal recovery times. The timing of recovery techniques strongly influences their effectiveness—whenever possible, they should be performed *during and after* each training session (Bompa 1999).

TABLE 4.1	Suggested Recovery Times After Exhaustive Training
Recovery process	**Recovery time**
Restoration of ATP-PC	2-4 min
Restoration of muscle glycogen: After prolonged exercise After intermittent exercise (such as strength training)	10-48 hours 24 hours
Removal of lactic acid from muscle and blood	1-2 hours
Restoration of vitamins and enzymes	24 hours
Recovery from high-intensity strength training (both metabolic and CNS to reach overcompensation)	2-3 days
Repayment of ATP-PC debt and oxygen debt (faster portion)	2-3 min
Repayment of lactic acid debt and oxygen debt (slower portion)	30-60 min

The recovery process after strength training and bodybuilding prompts the onset of symptoms associated with muscle damage. These include muscle soreness and stiffness, muscle swelling, decreased range of motion, and decrease in muscle force output. With the intention of increasing the dynamics of muscle, athletes utilize numerous recovery techniques. Research has shown that performing a few light sets with the damaged muscle group may decrease muscle soreness and induce the earlier onset of muscle recovery (Saxton and Donnelly 1995; Sayers, Clarkson, and Lee 2000). Recovery techniques, such as massage, heat and cold therapy, and stretching (see figure 4.1), can be used to increase the muscle recovery process.

REST INTERVALS

It is during the rest intervals between sets, not during exercise, that the heart pumps the highest volume of blood to the working muscles. An inadequate RI diminishes the amount of blood reaching the working muscles; without this supply of fuel and oxygen, the athlete will not have the energy to complete the planned training session. Table 4.2 provides guidelines for the length of rest intervals between sets.

A short rest interval between sets causes an increased reliance on the lactic acid (LA) system for energy. The degree to which ATP and PC, a high-energy compound stored in muscles, are replenished between sets depends on the duration of the rest interval. The shorter the RI, the less ATP-PC will be restored and, consequently, the less energy will be available for the next set. If the RI is too short, the energy needed for the following sets is provided by glycolysis, the anaerobic metabolic

TABLE 4.2	A Guideline for RIs Between Sets for Various Loads		
Load percentage	**Speed of performance**	**RI (min)**	**Applicability**
101-105 (eccentric)	Slow	4-7	Improve maximum strength and muscle tone
80-100	Slow to medium	3-7	Improve maximum strength and muscle tone
60-80	Slow to medium	2	Improve muscle hypertrophy
50-79	Fast	4-5	Improve power
30-49	Slow to medium	1-2	Improve muscle definition

Reprinted from Bompa 1996.

Figure 4.1
RECOVERY TECHNIQUES

MASSAGE THERAPY

Massage therapy is the therapeutic manipulation of the soft tissues of the body with the goal of achieving normalization of those tissues. Massage can have mechanical, neurological, psychological, and reflexive effects. It can be used to reduce pain or adhesions, promote sedation, mobilize fluids, increase muscular relaxation, and facilitate vasodilation.

Physiological Effects

- Mechanical pressure on soft tissue displaces fluids.
- Once mobilized fluid leaves the soft tissues, it enters the venous or lymphatic low-pressure systems.
- Massage causes the release of *histamine*, causing superficial vasodilation to assist in washing out metabolic waste products. Venous return increases, which subsequently increases stroke volume.
- Other blood compounds that show increases through massage include myoglobin, creatine kinase, and lactate dehydrogenase.
- Massage may decrease markers of inflammation.
- Massage may decrease muscle spasm and increase the force of contraction of skeletal muscle.
- Decreased spasm, decreased muscle soreness, and increased endurance may result from the wash out of metabolic waste products by fluid mobilization and increased blood flow.

HEAT THERAPY

Heat therapy involves local heating of muscles or joints—usually 15 to 20 minutes with heat on the affected area followed by 15 to 30 minutes of rest (without the heat). Heat therapy can be achieved using a variety of energy sources:

- High-frequency currents, such as shortwave diathermy (deep heat)
- Electromagnetic radiation, such as microwaves (deep heat)
- Conductive heat, such as hot water baths, hot packs, electric heating pads, or warm compresses (superficial heat)

Physiological Effects

- The local effects of heat therapy are due to the elevated temperature response of cellular function.
- Locally, there is an increased blood flow with associated capillary dilatation and increased capillary permeability.
- Initial tissue metabolism increases, and there may be changes in the pain threshold.
- Distant changes from the heated target location include reflex vasodilatation and reduction of muscle spasm, due to skeletal muscle relaxation.

COLD THERAPY (CRYOTHERAPY)

Cryotherapy involves local cooling of muscles or joints—usually 10 to 15 minutes of cold applied to the affected area followed by 15 to 30 minutes of rest (without the cold). The most common forms of cryotherapy include ice packs, ice baths, Cryogel packs, and ice massage.

Physiological Effects

- Cryotherapy decreases soft tissue swelling by
  - decreasing circulation to the injured site by constricting blood vessels in and around the site, causing the blood to become more viscous, or resistant to flow, and
  - decreasing local fluid accumulation and promoting the absorption of excess fluid.
- Cryotherapy can also decrease hemorrhaging and decrease muscle spasms and pain.

STRETCHING

Flexibility refers to the absolute range of movement in a joint, which can be increased by stretching.

Physiological Effects

- Stretching enhances development of proprioception.
- Stretching reduces muscle soreness and muscular tension.

Information on massage, heat therapy, and cryotherapy was partially adapted, with permission, from materials developed by Greg Wells, PhD (www.drgregwells.com).

REST INTERVAL CUES

- A 30-second RI restores approximately 50 percent of the depleted ATP-PC.
- An RI of 3 to 5 minutes or longer allows almost an entire restoration of ATP-PC.
- After working to exhaustion, a 4-minute RI is not sufficient to eliminate lactic acid from the working muscles or to replenish the energy stores of glycogen

pathway that produces lactic acid and hydrogen ions (H^+) as its by-product, which contribute to acidosis (Powers and Howley 2009). Increased acidosis inhibits the binding capacity of calcium through inactivation of troponin (a protein compound). Its inactivation may increase the connection between fatigue and exercise. Also, the discomfort produced by acidosis can be a limiting factor in psychological fatigue. Although recent studies challenge the old theory that lactate accumulation has detrimental effects on exercise performance, it is still evident that lactate may have an indirect effect on low-frequency muscular fatigue.

Several factors influence the appropriate duration of the rest interval between sets:

- Type of strength the athlete is developing
- Magnitude of the load employed
- Speed of contraction
- Number of muscle groups worked during the session
- Level of conditioning
- Amount of rest taken between training days
- Total weight of the athlete (heavy athletes with larger muscles usually regenerate at a slower rate than lighter athletes)

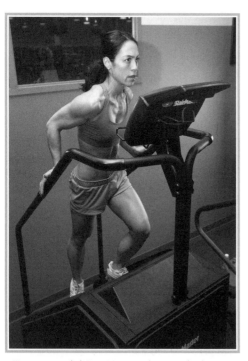

Fitness model Sue Ling understands that aerobic training helps an athlete's recovery process.

Most athletes do nothing during the rest interval to facilitate recovery between sets. There are, however, some things you can do to enhance both the rate and completeness of recovery:

- **Relaxation exercises.** Simple techniques, such as shaking the legs, arms, and shoulders or getting a light massage, are effective for facilitating recovery between sets. Exercises using heavy loads cause an increase in the quantity of muscle protein, which causes muscle rigidity (Baroga 1978). These basic recovery techniques aid in its removal by improving blood circulation within the muscle.

- **Diverting activities.** Diversions involve such activities as performing light contractions with nonfatigued muscles during the RI (Asmussen and Mazin 1978). Such physical activities can facilitate a faster recovery of the prime movers. The message of local muscle fatigue is sent to the CNS via sensory nerves. The brain then sends inhibitory signals to the fatigued muscle that reduce its work output during the RI. As the muscle becomes more relaxed, its energy stores are more easily restored.

Aerobic activity is an important consideration for the rest interval between strength training sessions. An athlete's fitness level and recovery ability influence the rest interval.

Well-conditioned athletes recover more quickly than those with lower fitness levels. We strongly recommend that strength trainers and bodybuilders train their aerobic systems through cardiorespiratory training in addition to training their muscular systems. Another benefit of aerobic training is that it helps bodybuilders and strength trainers stay relatively lean throughout the entire annual plan, not just during contest preparation.

The energy source used during training is probably the most important factor to consider when planning the rest interval between sessions. For example, during the maximum strength phase, when you are taxing primarily the ATP-PC system, daily training is possible because ATP-PC restoration is complete within 24 hours. If, on the other hand, you are training for muscle endurance (for muscle definition), you should schedule workouts every second day—it takes 48 hours for the full restoration of glycogen. Even with a carbohydrate-rich diet, glycogen levels will not return to normal levels in less than 2 days.

NUTRITION SUPPLEMENTS FOR RECOVERY

Energy supplements can prevent or alleviate various aspects of fatigue (see the preworkout stack and workout stack discussions in chapter 8). A large number of nutritional supplements can positively affect the immune system and can help recovery and both prevent and treat injuries due to overtraining. An example of a comprehensive, multifaceted, synergistic supplement that can be useful for all these conditions is Joint Support (see www.MetabolicDiet.com), which contains the following ingredients:

Betaine HCl

BioCell Collagen II (includes chondroitin sulfate and hyaluronic acid)

Boron

Boswellia serrata extract

Bromelain

Calcium

Cayenne

Ginger

Glucosamine sulfate

Glutathione

Harpagosides

Kavalactones

L-arginine

L-methionine

Magnesium

Manganese

Methylsulfonylmethane (MSM)

N-acetylcysteine

Niacin

Omega-3 fish oil (EPA, DHA)

Papain

Quercetin dihydrate

Rutin

Shark cartilage

Silicon

Stinging nettle extract

Turmeric

Vitamin C

Vitamin D

Vitamin E

White willow

Yucca extract

Zinc

Although most soreness results from muscle tissue trauma, stress is also induced on tissues connected to the muscles, including bones, tendons, and ligaments. These tissues are also subject to aging. Connective tissue trauma is a major source of physical discomfort in athletes. This is not surprising, considering that connective tissue is widely distributed in the body—it forms our bones, surrounds our organs, holds our teeth in place, cushions and lubricates our joints, and connects the muscles to our skeleton.

Most connective tissue injuries involve damage to structural components of the tissue. In sports activities, injuries are classified into two types: acute and overuse injuries. Acute trauma occurs from lacerations and from partial or complete rupture of the tissue. Overuse injuries, the most common, result from chronic overloading or repetitive motion.

Inflammation is the most prominent symptom of both types of injuries. Although inflammation is a natural part of the healing process, chronic inflammation may lead to increased tissue degradation and interfere with the repair process. Indeed, chronic inflammation is a major factor in several connective tissue diseases, especially within articular joints. Pharmaceuticals are often used to manage or alleviate symptoms of connective tissue inflammation—yet many of these substances may alter the healing process, and they offer only temporary relief. Many of these medications cause side effects (such as gastrointestinal upset) and may even accelerate joint degradation in the long run.

Over the centuries, herbal remedies have been used to alleviate symptoms of tissue stress. They have also been shown to rebuild tissue and restore function in joints. Many of these natural substances aid in recuperation, help heal sore muscles and joints, increase recovery from injuries such as strains and sprains, and help strengthen musculoskeletal support tissues.

PART TWO

MAXIMIZING NUTRITION
FOR MUSCLE GROWTH

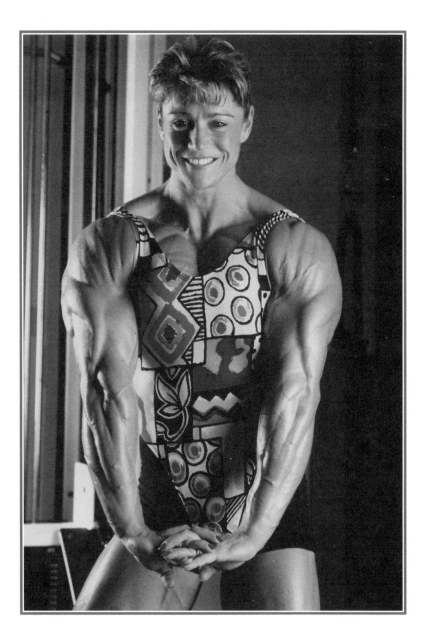

Nutrition and the Metabolic Diet

Over the past six decades, nutrition has been increasingly recognized as an important part of any sport, including bodybuilding and the power sports. In the past, many believed athletes did not need to eat any differently from anyone else—after all, our diets (at least if they were carefully planned) provided everything athletes needed to develop their bodies and compete. Overwhelming scientific and medical information has demonstrated, however, that special approaches to nutrition are vital for athletic success.

This chapter discusses the special nutrition needs of bodybuilders and how you can use diet and nutritional supplements to maximize your muscle mass and strength gains and to minimize your body fat. It is obvious that those who exercise regularly need more calories than those who are sedentary. But it is not so obvious that they need more protein and other macronutrients, micronutrients, and nutritional supplements. Additionally, we must consider just what it takes to maximize gains in muscle and strength and to minimize body fat.

THE METABOLIC DIET

In the past, most bodybuilders and power athletes followed nearly year-round diets that were high in protein and complex carbohydrates and low in fat. The only thing that varied (except when they fell off the diet) was the calories—higher when they were trying to gain muscle mass and lower when they were getting lean. The staple diet, especially among bodybuilders, consisted of a lot of high-protein foods, such as egg whites, broiled or baked skinless chicken, tuna packed with water, and of course lots of oatmeal and rice.

Since Mauro Di Pasquale introduced the metabolic diet, many power athletes, and especially bodybuilders, have gotten off the high-carbohydrate, low-fat diets. The revolutionary metabolic diet manipulates lean body mass and body fat. It does this by effecting metabolic changes and altering the body's anabolic and catabolic hormones and growth factors.

The metabolic diet is easy to follow, and it has three main benefits:

1. It stimulates your metabolism to burn fat instead of carbohydrate as its primary fuel.
2. It maintains the fat burning as you lower your caloric intake so that your body obtains its energy mainly from fat instead of glycogen or muscle protein.
3. It spares and maintains protein, allowing you to build muscle mass.

The first step in the metabolic diet is to switch your metabolism to burn fat as its primary fuel. This is done by limiting dietary carbohydrate and consuming ample amounts of fat. After the initial adaptation phase, you shift from a low-carbohydrate diet on weekdays to a higher-carbohydrate diet on weekends. Doing so manipulates the muscle-building and fat-burning processes and hormones. Cycling between a low-carbohydrate and high-fat regimen to a high-carbohydrate and low-fat regimen manipulates the anabolic and fat-burning processes in the body so that they maintain or increase muscle mass while decreasing body fat. You are training the body to burn mainly body fat in preference to carbohydrates and protein.

After your body is fat adapted, you vary your calories to suit your goal. To increase muscle mass, increase your daily caloric intake by consuming more fat and protein. To lose body fat while maintaining muscle mass, slowly decrease both your caloric and fat intake. It's usually a good idea to do a controlled weight gain first and then to drop that extra body fat while maintaining most of the muscle you packed on while you gained weight. When you begin reducing your caloric and fat intake, your body receives fewer calories and less dietary fat so it will increasingly use its fat stores, not muscle, to make up any energy deficits. In some circumstances, your diet may contain only moderate or even low levels of fat, mainly in the form of the essential and monounsaturated fatty acids.

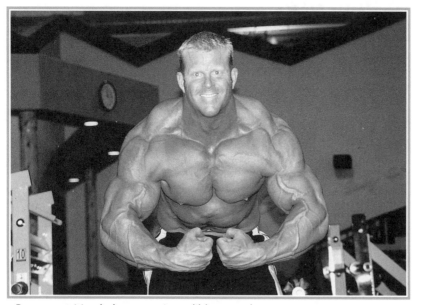

The metabolic diet works because your body learns to burn fat instead of carbohydrate. Your body continues to prefer fats as you drop calories mainly from dietary fat and, depending on your dietary carbohydrate intake, some carbohydrate. You must always keep protein high to spare muscles. As calories drop, body fat becomes the main fuel even if you lower dietary fat dramatically.

Proper nutrition helps create incredible musculature.

PHYSICAL BENEFITS OF THE METABOLIC DIET

One of the advantages of the metabolic diet is an increase in lean body mass without the use of anabolic steroids. The diet does many of the same things hormonally that steroids do, only naturally and without the risks. Another advantage of the metabolic diet is the ability to decrease body fat without sacrificing lean mass.

Decrease Body Fat Without Sacrificing Lean Mass   Unlike the high-carbohydrate diet, when you gain weight on the metabolic diet much less of it is body fat and much more of it is muscle. We have found that eating fat doesn't lead to becoming fat. In fact, high dietary fat is instrumental in increasing lipolysis, or the breakdown of fat, and the resulting loss of body fat. Furthermore, the bodybuilder will maintain more lean body mass during the cutting phase of a diet.

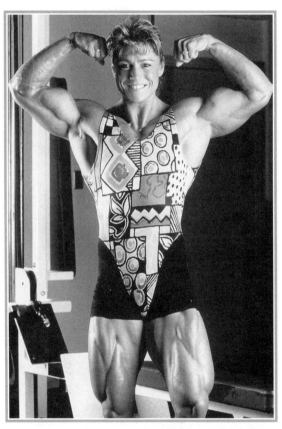

Laura Binetti shows you what decreasing body fat without sacrificing lean mass means.

On a high-carbohydrate diet, if you exercise correctly and do everything else right, you will find that when you lose weight about 60 percent of it is fat and 40 percent is muscle. You may get down to your optimal weight and be ripped, but you are much smaller than you could be. On the metabolic diet, those percentages go way down to 90 percent fat and 10 percent muscle during cutting. With the high-fat diet, you get down to the weight you want but find yourself maintaining a lot more lean body mass. You are bigger and stronger.

Feel Stronger While Losing Body Fat   This stands to reason. Strength is proportional to muscle mass. When you are on a high-carbohydrate diet, sacrificing lean mass to get cut, you are obviously going to feel weaker. Because the metabolic diet cycles in a carbohydrate-loading phase every week to stimulate insulin production and trigger growth, you also do not find yourself getting into the psychological doldrums caused by following one diet all the way through each week. There is a variety in your diet, and this will help you be more energetic and committed than you'd be on the high-carbohydrate diet.

Maximize the Effects of Endogenous Anabolic Hormones   The metabolic diet maximizes the serum levels of testosterone (even in women) (Goldin et al. 1994), growth hormone, and insulin to promote growth and to help firm up and shape your body as you shed fat. It basically conditions your hormonal system to create an endogenous (natural) anabolic (growth producing) environment. You will be surprised at how quickly you will be able to sculpt the body you want as these hormones work together.

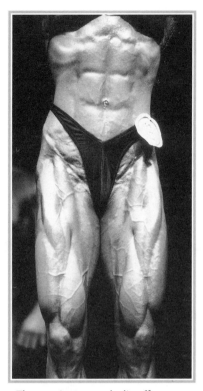

The maximum anabolic effect is achieved when the metabolic diet is carried out to perfection.

The maximization of the three hormones is one of the most remarkable effects of the metabolic diet. Many hormones are reactive to others. For instance, as insulin goes up, growth hormone may decrease. If insulin decreases, growth hormone will increase. The two hormones generally do not work well together, but they can. During and after a workout, it is important to understand that the body decreases in serum testosterone and growth hormone. The metabolic diet attempts to maximize the effect of the three anabolic hormones for 24 hours because contrary to popular belief, you get stronger and form muscle not only after a workout but, if done correctly, during a workout as well. If you can increase both hormones, you will get a better anabolic effect than with an increase in one hormone alone. At the cellular level, the anabolic hormones must be elevated to drive amino acids into the cells for protein formation. The metabolic diet, the weekly cycling it incorporates (carbohydrate-loading phase) to stimulate insulin production, and the utilization of supplements such as Exersol (see www.MetabolicDiet.com) will optimize protein synthesis and maximize growth.

Chapter 8 recommends supplements you can use with the metabolic diet that will help increase insulin sensitivity, testosterone, growth hormone, and insulin-like growth factor 1 (IGF-1) as needed. Your approach to supplements and exercise will be largely determined by how far you want to go in remaking your body. Whatever your goals, you will find the metabolic diet an effective tool in taking the weight off, keeping it off, and making your body look its best.

Increase Strength People on the metabolic diet often find their strength increasing as they are losing weight and body fat. Most bodybuilders find this amazing. They know that when they lose weight, they are also losing muscle and strength. But with the metabolic diet they're losing less muscle, and that, in combination with the fact their bodies are working in an anabolic environment, makes them stronger. They cannot believe it as they watch the fat melt away while their strength increases at the same time.

Decrease Catabolic Activity The metabolic diet results in lower levels of cortisol, a hormone secreted by the adrenal glands that breaks down muscle (catabolism) and uses it for energy. Certain supplements can be added to the diet (see chapter 8) to further decrease muscle breakdown during and after a workout while increasing insulin and growth hormone levels at critical times to promote an anabolic effect. Put simply, you will be breaking down less muscle while adding more.

NATURAL IS BETTER

Using drugs short-circuit your body's normal processes. By providing hormones and other substances from outside the body, you shut down the internal mechanisms that would normally produce those substances. This is easier to understand through the analogy of a factory. If you provide the goods the factory would normally make, then there is no need for the factory to be operational. If the factory is shut down long enough, then sometimes it's hard to get it up and running since you have to round up the workers and raw materials and get everything working at peak efficiency again.

The same things happen to your internal factories when you provide outside hormones and drugs. When the processes involved in making these compounds or in doing the things these compounds do are no longer needed, they are essentially shut down. This can result in a long-term and sometimes permanent imbalance in the body that can be harmful to your health.

An example is the effect of anabolic steroids on males. Their use shuts down the hypothalamic, pituitary, and testicular (evidenced by shrinking testicles) processes involved in the production of testosterone. After the steroids are discontinued, most of the results and advantages of using the drugs are invariably lost while the body is getting back to normal. But in some cases the systems never really return to normal, leaving the athlete in an even worse situation than if he had never taken drugs. On the other hand, by maximizing the stimulation or activation of your internal factories, along the lines that they would naturally be stimulated in the first place, all you are doing is maximizing the input, the operation, and the output of your own body, making it hum along at peak efficiency.

By staying natural, you also prevent the possible short- and long-term consequences of drug use. These include changes in hormonal, metabolic, and homeostatic processes and possible tissue and organ dysfunction. The long-term consequences of using some of the ergogenic and body-composition-changing drugs are yet to be determined but may well result in significant cardiovascular, hormonal, and carcinogenic (cancer producing or promoting) consequences.

MACRONUTRIENTS

Macronutrients are chemical compounds the body needs in order to survive. The three primary macronutrients are carbohydrate, protein, and fat. Carbohydrate and protein are discussed in this section, and fat is discussed in chapter 6.

Carbohydrate

Carbohydrate falls into two categories: simple and complex (see figure 5.1). Simple sugars (simple carbohydrates) include monosaccharides and disaccharides. The two most common monosaccharides are glucose, which is an important energy

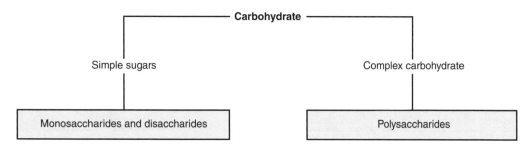

FIGURE 5.1　Simple and complex carbohydrate.

source in living organisms and is a component of many carbohydrates, and fructose, which is a sugar that occurs naturally in fruits and honey. Disaccharides are composed of two monosaccharides. The two most common disaccharides are sucrose, or table sugar, and lactose, or milk sugar. Once sugar is consumed, the liver either converts it into glucose for quick energy or moves it into glycogen or fat storage for later use.

Excessive consumption of this type of carbohydrate might be detrimental to the serious athlete for several reasons. Foods containing simple sugars typically have low nutrition value in terms of delivering vitamins, minerals, and proteins (Wardlaw and Insel 1990).

Polysaccharides make up the complex carbohydrates. As the name suggests, polysaccharides are composed of many (poly) glucose units. They are often referred to as starches and are found in vegetables, fruits, and grains. These carbohydrates are digested slowly and, therefore, do not cause huge fluctuations in insulin or blood glucose levels (Jenkins 1982).

One easy way to choose the right carbohydrate foods while following the metabolic diet is to consult the glycemic index. The foods that do not result in large insulin fluctuations because of slow digestion have low glycemic values. The foods that cause rapid changes in blood sugar and insulin levels have high glycemic values (Jenkins 1987).

Protein

Proteins are composed of chains of amino acids (AAs), which are referred to as "the building blocks of protein." There are 20 different amino acids, of which the body can synthesize 11 (nonessential amino acids) from the food we eat, while the remaining 9 (essential amino acids) must be supplied through the diet (Figure 5.2). All 9 essential amino acids must be present in the body for protein synthesis to occur (Wardlaw and Insel 1990).

It is extremely important for bodybuilders and strength trainers to consume the right foods so all 20 amino acids can work together to form protein. The main concern is obtaining the amino acids the body cannot synthesize—the 9 essential amino acids that must come directly from the diet. The body will take care of the 11 nonessential amino acids. Foods containing all 9 essential amino acids are called *complete proteins*, and these are athletes' friends. Foods that do not contain all 9 essential amino acids are called *incomplete proteins*. Table 5.1 gives a brief listing of some complete and incomplete proteins and their characteristics.

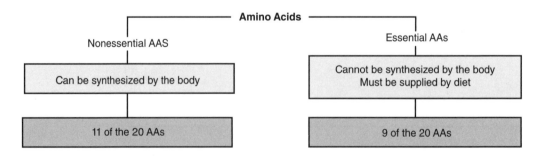

FIGURE 5.2 Nonessential and essential amino acids.

TABLE 5.1	Comparing Complete and Incomplete Proteins	
	TYPE OF PROTEIN	
Characteristics	**Complete protein**	**Incomplete protein**
Contain all 9 essential AAs?	Yes	No
Support body growth and maintenance?	Yes	No, but may support body maintenance
Source	Animal proteins	Plant proteins
Food sources	Beef, chicken, pork, eggs, fish, milk, cheese, yogurt	Soybeans, legumes, tofu, grains, nuts, seeds, vegetables

Although meat eaters can be confident they are getting all the needed amino acids, vegetarian bodybuilders and strength trainers who rely solely on plant proteins must pay particular attention to their protein intake, eating a wide variety of plant proteins to consume all the essential amino acids. Vegetarian athletes must get what they need by combining plant proteins. An example of combining two incomplete protein foods to make a complete package is eating bread and peanut butter. In combination they supply the 9 essential amino acids, while alone they do not.

The biological value (BV) of a protein describes how efficiently body tissue can be created from food protein. According to Wardlaw and Insel (1990), the BV of a food depends on how closely its amino acid pattern reflects the amino acid pattern in body tissue; the better the match, the more completely food protein turns into body protein. If the AA pattern in a food is very different from human tissue amino acid patterns, then the food protein is turned into either glucose (for use as fuel) or fat (for storage) instead of body protein.

Humans and other animals have similar amino acid compositions, while plant amino acid compositions differ greatly from those of humans. Table 5.2 ranks the biological value and net protein utilization (NPU) for many of the main staples of an athlete's diet. Net protein utilization adjusts the BV of a food to account for its digestibility, and because most proteins are almost completely digested and absorbed, the BV and NPU for most protein foods are similar. Again, by eating a wide variety of foods, you can greatly increase the biological value of a meal. This is especially important for vegetarian athletes because, as you can see from table 5.2, for the most part, the foods with the highest BV are animal proteins.

NUTRITION CUES

- Read food labels for macronutrient content.
- Be sure you eat enough protein for your size. Refer to the nutrition sections in chapters 12 through 17.
- Eat a wide variety of protein foods.

TABLE 5.2	Comparative Protein Quality of Selected Foods	
Food	Biological value (BV)	Net protein utilization (NPU)
Egg	100	94
Cow's milk	93	82
Unpolished rice	86	59
Fish	76	—
Beef	74	67
Soy beans	73	61
Corn	72	36
Oats	65	—
Whole wheat bread	65	49
Polished rice	64	57
Peas	64	55
Peanuts	55	55

Adapted, by permission, from G.M. Wardlaw and P.M. Insel, 1990, *Perspectives in nutrition* (St. Louis: Mosby). © The McGraw-Hill Companies, Inc.

THE METABOLIC ADVANTAGE

At this point, a little biochemistry lesson may be in order so you can get a better idea of why the metabolic diet is superior to the competition. Adenosine triphosphate (ATP) is the source of energy for all metabolic activity in the human body. To get the energy the body needs for muscle contraction, breathing, brain cell function, and virtually all other activities, ATP must be generated. People have gotten the idea that glycogen and the glucose that comes from carbohydrate foods are required for the body to produce and replenish ATP and survive.

When carbohydrate foods make up the bulk of your diet, you basically burn the glucose from the carbohydrate (and other sugars that, like glucose, enter the glycolytic pathway) as energy. Glucose enters the bloodstream, and it's either used for immediate energy or stored as glycogen in the liver and muscles. When needed for energy, the stored glycogen is converted back to glucose and used up directly by cells or transported through the bloodstream to other body cells for conversion and use as energy. The glucose not stored as glycogen is made into triglycerides (the storage form of free fatty acids) and stored as body fat.

When fat and protein make up a greater part of your diet, your body no longer relies on those large amounts of glycogen or glucose for energy. A good part of your energy comes from the free fatty acids in your diet or from the breakdown and oxidation of body fat. The body can produce glucose without taking in carbohydrate (by a process called gluconeogenesis), and protein and fat can be used to provide energy and replenish ATP. Instead of burning all the stored glycogen or glucose for energy, the body burns free fatty acids or triglycerides and the glucose that they make. (Chapter 6 discusses good and bad fats as well as concerns such as heart disease and cholesterol levels.)

It is a misconception that you must have dietary carbohydrate to function. This is likely true only in cases where a person may be genetically challenged as far as utilizing fats efficiently. And even in these cases it's unlikely there is a need for extremely high levels of dietary carbohydrate. Also the reasons given for why we need carbohydrate foods are faulty. One of the main reasons cited is that the brain depends on carbohydrates to function properly, but in fact lactate is the preferred substrate for neurons, and these brain cells can also metabolize ketones effectively. As well, other cells in the central nervous system cater to the main brain cells and supply them with energy derived from other nutrients. For example, it has been shown that astrocytes shuttle nutrients to neurons (Magistretti and Pellerin 2000; Deitmer 2001).

Gluconeogenesis

Cellular metabolic flux is dramatically altered by changing the dietary macronutrient content. Some pathways become more active than others, and some processes dominate in the production of energy. In all cases, the body will adapt to the macronutrient content of any diet—no matter how extreme—as long as the diet provides certain essential macronutrients and micronutrients.

There are essential and conditionally essential amino acids and essential fatty acids (see chapter 6 for more on essential fatty acids), but there are no essential sugars or carbohydrates because the body can produce glucose and carbohydrates endogenously. Glucose can be produced as needed by gluconeogenesis. In this process other nutrients, including amino acids and glycerol (which makes up much of our body fat) can be converted to glucose or used directly as energy. Although somewhat complicated, figure 5.3 shows how the body produces glucose internally from other substances including the amino acids, glycerol (source can be from the breakdown of body fat or from the diet), lactate, and pyruvate.

Because there are common pathways for the metabolism of all three macronutrients, variation in the macronutrient content results in adaptations that allow the efficient production of compounds and substrates for energy production and body maintenance. Regardless of the macronutrient mix, the end result and the

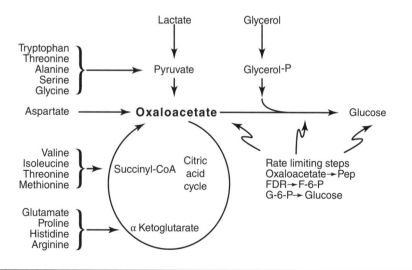

FIGURE 5.3   Entry of precursors into the pathways of gluconeogenesis.

Adapted from Di Pasquale 2002, p. 34.

final pathways are the same. Interconversion of macronutrients, usually at some energy cost (conversion of protein to fats) and with some exceptions (inability to produce glucose from free fatty acids—although you can, to a limited extent, with triglycerides and body fat), is an essential part of energy metabolism. Figures 5.4 and 5.5 show how glucose, free fatty acids, glycerol, and amino acids are broken down to provide energy.

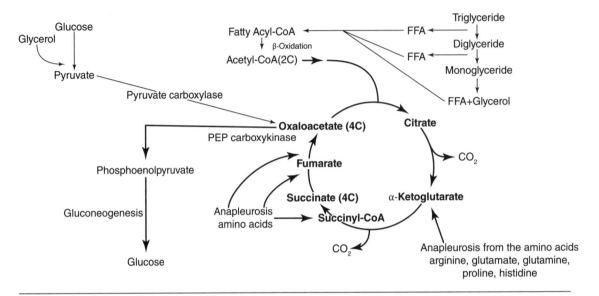

FIGURE 5.4 There is no net glucose synthesis from lipids, except from the glycerol portion—10 percent by weight.

Adapted from Di Pasquale 2002, p. 35.

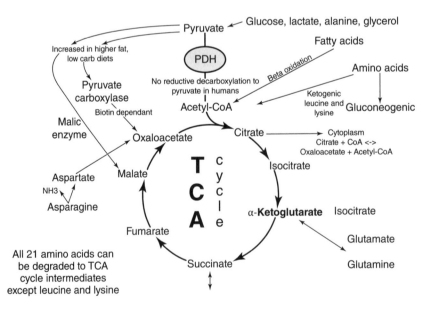

FIGURE 5.5 The metabolic diet controls the major muscle-building and fat-burning hormones in the body to maximize muscle mass and minimize body fat. These hormones include testosterone, growth hormone, IGF-1, insulin, thyroid hormone, and cortisol.

Adapted from Di Pasquale 2002, p. 36.

Lipolysis and Fat Oxidation

The metabolic diet also increases the activity of hormone-sensitive lipase (HSL), the enzyme that breaks down body fat. Adipose tissue lipolysis is stimulated through a cascade of cellular signals, resulting in activation of HSL. Basically, a diet high in fat activates the lipolytic (fat burning) enzymes in your body and decreases the activity of the lipogenic (fat producing) enzymes. Dietary free fatty acids and triglycerides become the body's main energy source. The triglycerides are broken down to free fatty acids, and some of the fatty acids are metabolized to ketones, which in turn can be used for energy by body cells. The use of ketones for energy is especially important to the brain, which can use only glucose and ketones for energy. In short, the free fatty acids and ketones take the place of glucose, and the triglycerides act like glycogen.

When carbohydrates are the main form of energy for the body, the body produces insulin to process it and store it. This is all well and good, but one of the problems with insulin is that it activates the lipogenic (fat producing) enzymes in the body and decreases the activity of the lipolytic (fat burning) enzymes. This leads to an increased storage of body fat and a decrease in the amount of stored fat that will be burned.

The exact opposite occurs on a higher-fat, lower-carbohydrate diet. After undergoing the metabolic shift from being a carbohydrate-burning machine to a fat burner, lipogenesis (the production and laying down of fat on the body) decreases, and lipolysis (the burning of both dietary and body fat for energy) increases. You are burning fat as your primary fuel source instead of using glycogen or breaking down precious protein.

This can have a great effect on overall body fat, and research shows that with a higher-fat, lower-carbohydrate diet, the majority of weight loss is due to the loss of body fat (Schurch, Hillen, et al. 1979; Yancy et al. 2004). In one study of ideal-weight in human subjects, higher-fat diets were accompanied by a very strong lipolytic (fat burning) effect (Kather et al. 1987; Yancy et al. 2004).

In another study focusing on obese subjects, it was found that, when offered high-carbohydrate, relatively low-fat diets or lower-carbohydrate, relatively higher-fat diets, the subjects on the lower-carbohydrate diets lost significantly more fat (Rabast, Kasper, and Schonborn 1987; Brehm et al. 2003). Although prevailing wisdom would predict that the higher-fat diet would simply make people fatter, subjects actually lost more weight on the high-fat diet.

Contrary to what most people believe, fat oxidation is regulated primarily by carbohydrate intake rather than by fat intake (Flatt 1995). Once you have adapted to a higher-fat, lower-carbohydrate diet, a properly designed diet higher in fat and lower in carbohydrate does not result in excessive stored body fat. It actually results in a leaner body composition.

But controlling the formation (lipogenesis) and breakdown (lipolysis) of body fat isn't enough. The fat that is broken down must also be used up by the body for energy (beta-oxidation or fat oxidation) rather than used simply to re-form body fat. Lipolysis is of no use if the fatty acids are not used up. For example, a recent study shows that ephedrine-like compounds increase lipolysis but decrease fat oxidation, so the overall effect may be an increase in body fat. The metabolic diet not only increases fat breakdown but also increases the use of fat as fuel for the body's energy needs. It does this partly by controlling the increase and sensitivity of insulin and partly by increasing growth hormone, IGF-1, and testosterone levels (including an increase in the androgen receptor and binding).

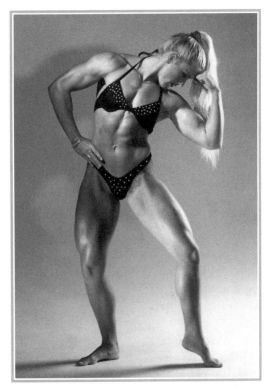

The metabolic diet keeps insulin from yo-yoing, which it does with carbohydrate-based diets.

Insulin Regulation

The metabolic diet, unlike other diets that promote a constant low-carbohydrate intake, does not consider insulin to be the enemy. In fact, insulin is a problem only when it is chronically high or extremely variable, as happens with carbohydrate-based diets. In fact, the metabolic diet makes use of the anabolic effects of insulin while at the same time preventing its bad effects on body fat and insulin sensitivity.

Unchecked, insulin adversely affects body fat by decreasing the breakdown (lipolysis) and increasing the accumulation (lipogenesis) of body fat. What you want to do, and what the metabolic diet focuses on, is to increase insulin at the appropriate time so it works to add muscle mass and maximize the body's anabolic potential by increasing the flow of amino acids into the muscle cells. Insulin also has beneficial effects on protein synthesis, muscle metabolism, and glycogen supercompensation.

What you do not want is fat buildup at the same time. That is why insulin secretion needs to be controlled and limited. Instead of the chronically elevated insulin levels found with the high-carbohydrate diet, the metabolic diet carefully manages insulin during the week so you get its anabolic benefits without packing on all that unwanted fat. The metabolic diet accomplishes this in the following ways:

- It allows only controlled increases in insulin for the desired effects on protein synthesis.
- It reduces the effects of insulin on lipolysis and lipogenesis.
- It provides pulses of insulin and controlled insulin increases at variable times on weekends.

Overall it has been our experience that there is an acute anabolic effect on muscle when a short-term lower-carbohydrate diet is alternated with carbohydrate loading. Cellular hydration is maximized by the water and carbohydrate loading, and insulin sensitivity is increased, leading to an intense anabolic stimulus. The planned fluctuations make for an anabolic effect unparalleled by any other diet. This anabolic effect allows you to gain strength and lean muscle mass.

Insulin, Growth Hormone (GH), Testosterone, and Insulin-Like Growth Factor 1 (IGF-1)

Insulin is produced in the pancreas and is secreted in the blood, where it is bound to carrier proteins and carried to muscles, the liver, and other tissues. The main action of insulin is to regulate the glucose level in the blood. To do this, insulin influences the metabolism of sugars and carbohydrates as well as fats and proteins (Boden et al. 1991). Figure 5.6 shows the sites of insulin action on muscle protein metabolism. Insulin can also influence other anabolic hormones including growth hormone (GH), insulin-like growth factor 1 (IGF-1), and testosterone to further increase the overall anabolic effect.

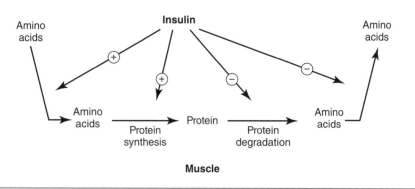

FIGURE 5.6 Sites of insulin action on muscle protein metabolism.

Adapted from Di Pasquale 2002, p. 43.

Growth hormone is very important because it increases protein synthesis and decreases muscle breakdown. During the weekdays when you are on the higher-fat, higher-protein, lower-carbohydrate portion of the diet, insulin levels do not fluctuate wildly as GH secretion increases. Along with stimulating a great environment for body shaping, GH also induces cells to use fat instead of sugar for energy, thus increasing the burning of body fat and limiting its production.

A polypeptide, GH is produced by the anterior portion of the pituitary gland. The metabolic effects of human GH include promotion of protein conservation, stimulation of lipolysis, and fat oxidation (Sjogren et al. 2007). GH acts almost like a "starvation" hormone. When your body's in trouble or you are in a threatened or stressful situation, GH kicks in to mobilize stores of energy in the body to deal with stress and increased energy needs, while at the same time preserving essential muscle mass. GH levels also increase under the stress of exercise. Usually, insulin decreases the secretion of GH, but it appears that the body sees the great increase in carbohydrate and insulin during the weekend portion of the metabolic diet as a stressful situation, much like exercise, and GH can actually increase with insulin. In this way, you potentially get the positive effects of increased GH both during the week and on at least part of the weekends.

Testosterone is the androgenic and anabolic substance produced by the testes. Numerous studies have shown that testosterone increases muscle protein synthesis and enhances strength, size, and athletic performance (Urban et al. 1995; Bhasin et al. 2001). Testosterone, which is critical for increasing muscle mass and strength, also responds well to the metabolic diet. Research in this area has found testosterone is positively linked to dietary fat. For example, premenopausal women placed on low-fat diets experienced decreased levels of both nonprotein-bound estradiol and testosterone (Ingram et al. 1987), and animals fed diets high in cholesterol or fish oil experienced higher testosterone production than those fed with a low-cholesterol diet containing linseed oil (Sebokova et al. 1990). Another study showed that in older men

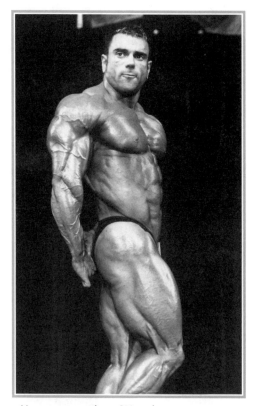

Hormones, such as GH and testosterone, play a key role in a bodybuilder's success.

the consumption of a meat-containing diet (as recommended on the metabolic diet) contributed to greater gains in fat-free mass and skeletal muscle mass with resistance training than did a lacto-ovo vegetarian diet (Campbell et al. 1999).

Recent evidence shows that a low-fat diet results in lower serum basal testosterone concentrations compared with a higher-fat diet in men (Wang et al. 2005) and that increased fat and protein in a diet increases exercise-induced levels of serum testosterone secondary to heavy resistance exercise in younger (Sallinen, Pakarinen, Ahtiainen, et al. 2004) and older men (Sallinen, Pakarinen, Fogelholm, et al. 2007). As well, a low-fat, high-fiber diet decreases serum testosterone levels in men (Dorgan et al. 1996; Wang et al. 2005).

Insulin-like growth factor 1 has been implicated in protein metabolism and in growth and growth processes of many tissues in animals (O'Sullivan et al. 1989; Schoenle et al. 1982). It has a structure similar to insulin (Zapf, Schmid, and Froesch 1984; Blundell et al. 1979) and is thought to mediate most of the anabolic effects of growth hormone (GH) in the body. IGF-1 is produced in the liver, chondrocytes, the kidneys, muscles, the pituitary, and the gastrointestinal tract. The liver is the main source of circulating IGF-1 (Underwood et al. 1986). The IGF peptides are bound tightly to plasma proteins (IGFBPs). Because of this binding, their activity is extended for several hours as opposed to the unbound forms, which can last 20 to 30 minutes.

Levels of IGF-1 and IGFBP-3 (a GH-dependent protein that binds IGF-1) are tied in with GH secretion and increase when GH levels increase. Levels are also age dependent, with low levels in early childhood, a peak during adolescence, and a decline after age 50. As a consequence of protein binding, and thus controlled release, the concentration of IGF-1 remains relatively constant throughout the day, in contrast to fluctuating levels of GH. IGF-1 seems to exert both GH-like and insulin-like actions on skeletal muscles (Fryburg 1994) by increasing protein synthesis and decreasing protein breakdown. Both GH and IGF-1 seem to shift the metabolism toward decreasing fat formation and increasing protein synthesis.

Cortisol

Cortisol is a vital hormone because it diverts glucose utilization from muscles to the brain, facilitates the action of catecholamines (hormones produced by the adrenal gland), and prevents the overreaction of the immune system to injury (Ganong 1988). Cortisol has many actions including stimulating gluconeogenesis (the synthesis of glucose from noncarbohydrate sources); increasing proteolysis (the breakdown of proteins into amino acids) (Simmons et al. 1984) and alanine synthesis; sensitizing adipose tissue to the action of lipolytic hormones (GH and catecholamines); and providing anti-inflammatory action. In addition, cortisol causes insulin resistance by decreasing the rate at which insulin activates the glucose uptake system, likely because of a postinsulin receptor block (Brown, Wallace, and Breachtel 1987; Rizza, Mandarino, and Gerich 1982).

Stress and increased cortisol levels have an adverse effect on serum testosterone levels. A primary anticatabolic effect of exogenous testosterone and anabolic steroids lies in their interference with muscle cortisol metabolism (Hickson et al. 1986). As well, these compounds may prevent the growth-suppressing activity of cortisol (Hickson et al. 1990). Growth hormone also inhibits the muscle catabolic actions of cortisol (Horber and Haymond 1990). In addition, lowering the cortisol level in the blood enhances the response to GH-releasing hormone in healthy adults (Dinan, Thakore, and O'Keane 1994). High levels of cortisol inhibit GH release during exercise by increasing the release of somatostatin, which blocks GH release in the brain.

IGF-1 can diminish the catabolic effects of cortisol without the side effects noted with GH therapy (Mauras and Beaufrere 1995). Cortisol downregulates the IGF-1 mRNA levels, indicating that some of the catabolic effects of glucocorticoids in humans are mediated via a reduced autocrine (signaling in which a cell secretes a hormone) and paracrine (signaling in which the target cells are near the signal-releasing cells) expression of IGF-1 (Swolin et al. 1996). (Messenger RNA, or mRNA, carries genetic coding information to the sites of protein synthesis.) Glutamine directly prevents the cortisol-induced destruction of muscle contractile proteins (Hickson, Czerwinski, and Wegrzyn 1995). Animal studies show that a high-protein, high-fat diet coupled with the use of anabolic steroids will reduce corticosterone-induced muscle breakdown (Ohtsuka et al. 1992).

Normal increases in cortisol stimulate lipolysis, ketogenesis (the process in which ketone bodies are produced as a result of fatty acid breakdown), and proteolysis. Also, the circadian variation in cortisol concentration is of physiological significance in normal humans in that it helps regulate both anabolic and catabolic events (Dinneen et al. 1993). Even mild elevations in serum cortisol within the physiological range can increase plasma glucose concentration and protein catabolism within a few hours in healthy people (Simmons et al. 1984; Shamoon, Soman, and Sherwin 1980). Cortisol (which induces the breakdown of cellular proteins) increases with increased duration of intense exercise. In athletes who are training effectively, basal testosterone levels

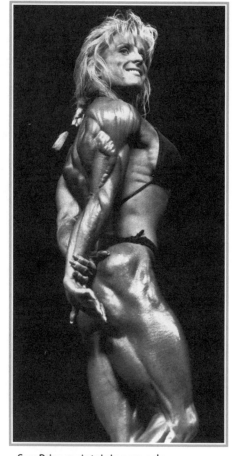

Sue Price maintaining muscle mass while shedding body fat.

rise, as do cortisol levels. Although exercise increases cortisol, well-conditioned athletes show less cortisol secretion during exercise compared with their out-of-shape peers (Deschenes et al. 1991).

PROTECTING MUSCLE PROTEIN

One important by-product of the metabolic shift that takes place when you move from a high-carbohydrate diet to a higher-fat, lower-carbohydrate diet is that fat protects protein in the body. When you are utilizing carbohydrate as your main source of energy, the body tends to save its body fat and will preferentially break down muscle protein to form glucose to burn as energy when the immediate energy stores are exhausted. This is why a significant amount of muscle catabolism can take place in a high-carbohydrate diet.

The fact is that anytime you are exercising and the body needs energy, it will break down what it needs, including muscle, to supply that energy. One of the ways athletes fight this is to sip glucose drinks during a workout. The body will not need to break down muscle as much for energy because it has an outside source of energy constantly coming in. The problem here is that the constant glucose ingestion causes chronically elevated levels of insulin and a decrease in the oxidation of body fat. Instead of losing fat by exercising, you are actually preserving it.

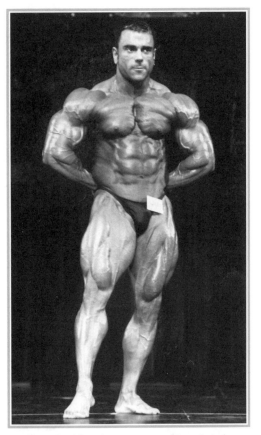

Nelson Da Silva demonstrates his striated physique.

When you are on the metabolic diet, fat works in the same way as glucose. It protects the muscle by serving as an alternative, more available source of energy, and it does this without having to take in more calories since the body has learned to oxidize body fat to provide that needed energy. So now when you exercise you do not need to take in carbohydrate to spare your muscles. Your body will burn up your excess body fat to provide the energy it needs to exercise, at the same time sparing muscle protein.

The concern is catabolism, or the breakdown of muscle tissue. Most people think exercise only creates muscle, but it also breaks it down. Research upholds that the metabolic diet could well also be called "the anticatabolic diet." Along with enabling the body's hormonal system to better burn fat, it decreases the amount of muscle that could be lost during a workout or just during day-to-day activities by protecting muscle protein. This is very important to someone wanting to shape his body for maximum attractiveness and fitness.

Research shows that the ketone bodies (beta-hydroxybuterate and acetoacetate) burned for energy in a higher-fat, low-carbohydrate diet actually decrease protein catabolism (Thompson and Wu 1991). In a study on laboratory rats, a combined treatment with insulin, testosterone, and a high-fat, high-protein diet led to decreased loss of muscle protein caused by the catabolic hormone corticosterone (Ohtsuka et al. 1992). Another study showed higher protein gains and lower fat gains for rats on a high-fat diet (McCarger, Baracos, and Clandinin 1992). The implications for similarly decreased catabolism in humans with the higher-fat, lower-carbohydrate diet are obvious.

Fat distribution also seems more evened out with the metabolic diet. What fat remains on the body seems to be distributed more equally on the frame. You just do not have those pockets of fat that plague some people. Fat is distributed in a more pleasing ratio across the body, making any body-shaping efforts on your part that much easier.

Good and Bad Fats

F atty acids are classified into three groups: saturated, polyunsaturated, and monounsaturated (see figure 6.1). Saturated fatty acids are usually solid at room temperature and are derived from animal sources. Beef and butterfat are high in saturated fatty acids and are good examples of animal sources of saturated fats. Tropical oils, such as coconut oils, kernel oils, and palm oils, also contain saturated fat even though they are not solid at room temperature. They are normally found in processed foods. Milk products such as low-fat or skim milk contain a much lower saturated fat content.

Fats and oils are made up of a number of repeating molecular units. One molecule of fat contains a single molecule of an alcohol called glycerol combined with three molecules of fatty acids. The fatty acids are made up of chains of carbon and hydrogen atoms, with a methyl group (three atoms of hydrogen and one carbon) at one end, chains of carbon and hydrogen atoms in the middle, and a carboxyl group (made up of carbon, oxygen, and hydrogen) at the other end. The hydrogen atoms are connected to each carbon atom, and their number and position determine the degree of saturation of the fatty acid and its shape.

Saturated fatty acids contain carbon atoms that are linked to hydrogen atoms. They are termed saturated fat because they are saturated with hydrogen atoms, and these carbon atoms are all joined by single bonds. Figure 6.2 demonstrates a structure of a fatty acid, butyric acid in butter, and figure 6.3 demonstrates the carbon hydrogen makeup of stearic acid.

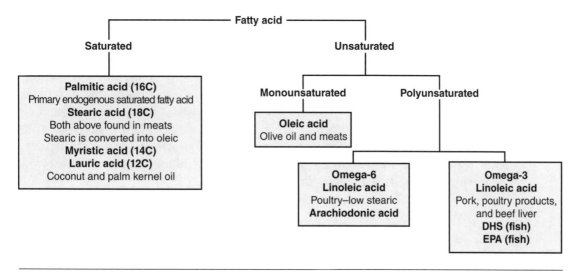

FIGURE 6.1 Common fatty acids.

Reprinted from Di Pasquale 2002, p. 74.

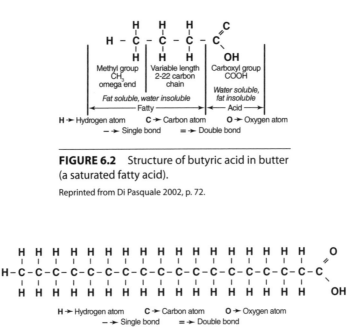

FIGURE 6.2 Structure of butyric acid in butter (a saturated fatty acid).

Reprinted from Di Pasquale 2002, p. 72.

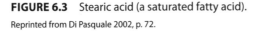

FIGURE 6.3 Stearic acid (a saturated fatty acid).

Reprinted from Di Pasquale 2002, p. 72.

Fats can also be unsaturated. Unsaturated fats are normally found in a liquid state at room temperature. These types of fats come from nuts, vegetables, or seeds. Figure 6.4 shows an unsaturated fat. Note that in the unsaturated fat, one or more double bonds join several of the carbon atoms together. When a double bond is present, each carbon atom will be attached only to a single hydrogen atom. The carbon atoms are no longer connected to the maximum hydrogen atoms and are said to be unsaturated.

A monounsaturated fatty acid contains a single incidence of double bonds along its chain. Monounsaturated fats, such as oleic acid, are found in olive oil and meats. A polyunsaturated fatty acid features two or more connections along its chain where two carbon atoms are double bonded.

The hardness of a fat decreases with the increase in its double bonds. As a result, most of the liquid fats such as vegetable and fish oils are polyunsaturated. Sometimes food producers add hydrogen to the double bonds of a chain to make them less unsaturated in a process called hydrogenation. In this way, vegetable oils can be hardened into shortening for use in cooking. When unsaturated fats are hydrogenated, the resulting fat is composed of substances called trans fatty acids. Many studies show that trans fatty acids raise blood cholesterol levels and are harmful to the heart (Mozaffarian et al. 2006).

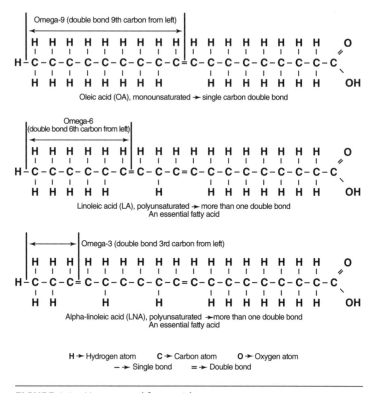

FIGURE 6.4   Unsaturated fatty acids.

Reprinted from Di Pasquale 2002, p. 73.

GOOD FATS

Fat is an important part of a healthy diet. The two essential fatty acids (EFAs) linoleic acid (LA) and alpha-linolenic acid (LNA) (also called omega fats) are critical for health and must be supplied in a person's diet since the human body cannot manufacture them. Linoleic acid (refer to figure 6.4) is classified as an omega-6 fatty acid. Omega-6 fatty acids are polyunsaturated fatty acids that have their endmost double bond six carbon atoms away from the CH3 end of a chain. Alpha-linolenic acid (see figure 6.4) is an omega-3 fatty acid. Omega-3s are polyunsaturated fatty acids with their endmost double bond three carbon atoms from the CH3 end.

Many people do not get sufficient amounts of EFAs in their diets. This can cause health problems because these EFAs are necessary for growth, the integrity of cell membranes, and the synthesis of important hormonelike substances called eicosanoids (see the next section). Additionally, EFA deficiency can lead to high blood pressure, hormonal dysfunction, impaired immune function, coagulation problems, inflammatory changes, dry itchy skin, peripheral edema, and many other conditions.

Most people are deficient in the consumption of omega-3 fatty acids. The omega-3 fatty acids such as LNA, eicosapentaenoic acid (EPA), and docosahexaenoic acid (DHA) are critical to anyone concerned with health and fitness. They increase fatty acid oxidation (fat burning), increase basal metabolic rates, and lower cholesterol. Omega-3 fatty acids also provide an anabolic effect by increasing the binding of IGF-1 to skeletal muscle and improving insulin sensitivity (Liu et al. 1994). As well, fish oils may have important implications for women prone to osteoporosis (loss of calcium from the bones) (Kruger 1995).

EICOSANOIDS

Eicosanoids are physiologically active metabolites (substances produced during metabolism) of EFAs with important effects on the immune, cardiovascular, and central nervous systems. EFAs such as LA and LNA are converted into other fatty acids—EPA, DHA, and dihomo-gamma-linolenic acid (DGLA)—and arachidonic acid, from which the eicosanoids are synthesized. Synthesis of eicosanoids is initiated by signal transduction cascades, which result in the hydrolysis of free arachidonic acid from membrane phospholipids. Since eicosanoids act locally in and around the tissues in which they are produced, they are not hormones but autacoids. Autacoids have hormonelike effects and influence hormonal function. Virtually all cells in the body can form some of the eicosanoids, but tissues differ in enzyme profile and, consequently, in the products they form. Tissues also differ in their ability to be affected by specific eicosanoids. Eicosanoids are not stored to any degree and are synthesized in response to immediate need.

Prostaglandins are eicosanoids that regulate activity in body cells on a moment-to-moment basis and are involved in critical functions such as blood pressure regulation, insulin sensitivity, and immune functions. Many of these findings have yet to be fully identified in research. Although it would be advantageous to be able to direct eicosanoid production so that good eicosanoids are produced preferentially to bad ones, it is difficult to do so because of the complexity of eicosanoid production, actions, and metabolism.

Bad eicosanoids, such as series 2 prostaglandins (PGE-2), which are derived from arachidonic acid, increase platelet aggregation, increase inflammation, and have adverse effects on the cardiovascular system. Thus, it is believed that by inhibiting the enzyme that catalyzes the synthesis of arachidonic acid, less PGE-2 would be formed. More metabolites would be present to produce some of the good eicosanoids, such as series 1 prostaglandins (PGE-1), which have favorable effects on blood clotting and the cardiovascular system. We know that EPA can inhibit the formation of arachidonic acid or the formation of PGE-2 from arachidonic acid. More extensive research needs to be done so we can fully comprehend how these compounds are formed, act, and are metabolized before we can determine how to manipulate eicosanoids.

At present, some strategies using EFAs have been formulated to take advantage of the good eicosanoids. For example, omega-3 fatty acids found in fish oils can decrease production of some arachidonate metabolites and increase levels of certain prostaglandins. The intake of these omega-3 fatty acids has been used to diminish platelet aggregation. It is thought that decreasing your intake of omega-6 fatty acids and increasing omega-3 fatty acids can direct the flow of LA to the good eicosanoids instead of the bad eicosanoids. This may be accomplished by increasing the transformation of LA to gamma-linolenic acid (GLA) or supplementing GLA by using GLA-rich oils. Doing so directs the formation of the good eicosanoids instead of arachidonic acid.

The enzyme responsible for the conversion of LA to GLA is delta-6-desaturase, and many factors can inhibit it. These factors include LNA (the other essential fatty acid), trans fatty acids (see the section Bad Fats), stress, and viral infections. By limiting these factors, more GLA can be naturally formed from dietary LA.

The enzyme responsible for the formation of arachidonic acid from DGLA is delta-5-desaturase, and many factors can inhibit it. These factors include glucagon and EPA. Insulin increases the formation of arachidonic acid from DGLA and thus increases the formation of the bad eicosanoids.

So, in theory, dietary practices can limit the production or transformation of arachidonic acid and encourage the production and transformation of GLA, thus maximizing the production of good eicosanoids over the bad ones. If further substantiated by research, this way of altering eicosanoid synthesis through dietary intake of EFAs would be one of the educated uses of scientific information on eicosanoids.

The metabolic diet discourages excess carbohydrate consumption and encourages good fats in the diet, such as fish, fish oils, and sources of GLA (evening primrose and borage seed oils). At present, this is the most effective way to ensure the correct proportions of EFAs, omega-3s, and omega-6s in the diet.

ESSENTIAL FATTY ACIDS AND THE METABOLIC DIET

EFAs can be beneficial even if a deficiency doesn't exist. If used properly, they can increase overall health, help you avoid heart disease, and help you lose body fat. Overall, the increased processing of foods in our society has significantly lowered the amount of EFAs in the average diet. Foods rich in EFAs are highly perishable and not deemed practical or profitable for most commercial preparations. The extra EFAs you will get from the metabolic diet, as explained here, are just one more reason for giving the diet a try.

As mentioned in the last section, omega-3s play a positive factor in high-fat diets. They are found to a high degree in fish oils (as EPA and DHA) and have been hailed as a major factor in lowering serum cholesterol levels, preventing coronary heart disease (Hodgson et al. 1993; Davidson 1999 ; Harris and Bulchandani 2006), and perhaps even preventing or curing atherosclerosis (Ni, Wu, and Xiao 1994; Simopoulos 2008). Marine oils are a big part of the diets of Eskimo tribes. Although their higher-fat diet would seem to make them prime candidates for heart disease and atherosclerosis, they have been found to be almost immune to cardiovascular problems (at least until Western dietary influences began to intrude on the traditional diet). Studies have centered on omega-3 fatty acids in the fish oils and their cardioprotective capacities as being central to this phenomenon (Henzen 1995).

For people on the metabolic diet, where fat and protein are found in high levels, the omega-3s can provide an excellent hedge against worries about cholesterol. Blood pressure, clotting, immune response, insulin resistance, and triglyceride levels are all positively affected (Simopoulos 1999). Even in cases where dietary cholesterol is increased, omega-3s may aid in actually lowering serum cholesterol (Garg et al. 1989). There is some evidence that in higher-fat diets, aerobic exercise also reduces serum cholesterol (Schurch, Reinke, and Hollmann 1979) and thus may improve the effects of omega-3-rich fish oil on cholesterol.

LNA, EPA, and DHA can also enhance lipolysis (body-fat breakdown) (Awad and Zepp 1979; Parrish et al. 1991) and decrease lipogenesis (body-fat formation) (Belzung, Raclot, and Groscolas 1993; Parrish, Pathy, and Angel 1990). The combined breakdown of stored body fat and decrease in additional body fat can have very positive results for the athlete. You actually end up making less fat and breaking down more of what's already in the body when using these oils. EPA also decreases some of the possible inflammatory effects of using GLA supplements because EPA can reduce arachidonic acid accumulation in some cells and tissues, a side effect of GLA supplementation (Barham et al. 2000).

That is why we wholeheartedly support adding portions of fish and fish oil to your daily diet. And although many foods contain more than one type of fatty acid, plant oils are usually richer in unsaturated fatty acid content than are animal fats. It's not surprising, then, that flaxseed oil, nuts, seeds, and unprocessed vegetable oil are also rich in essential fatty acids.

BAD FATS

There is a very popular misconception that commercial vegetable oils are a good, healthy source of essential and nonessential fatty acids. Nothing could be further from the truth. Most of the vegetable oils you see on the shelf at your local supermarket are very heavily processed. Processing not only removes any useful properties the oil had, such as EFAs or antioxidants, but also can predispose us to certain types of cancers and lower HDLs (high-density lipoproteins, the good cholesterol) (Lichtenstein et al. 1993).

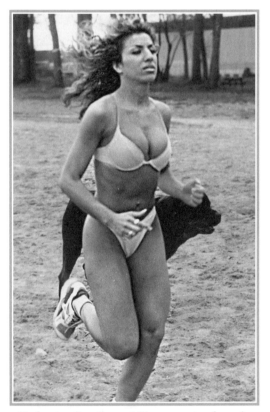

Understanding the nutrition aspects of good and bad fats coupled with cardiorespiratory training makes for a healthy body.

Hydrogenation has been used for decades to change natural oils into fats that are more solid and stable at room temperature, have a longer shelf life, and are easier to use in certain foods and baked goods. Hydrogenation involves heating the oil in a vacuum and then forcing hydrogen through it under pressure. The process is continued until the required level of hydrogen is achieved.

Unfortunately, although hydrogenation and other methods used to refine or change oils, such as chemical solvents, bleaches, and heat, may be healthy for business, they aren't good for our bodies. Trans fatty acids, cross-linked fatty acid chains, and fragments of fatty acid chains produced secondary to hydrogenation can have significant adverse effects on blood cholesterol, increasing the risk of heart disease. By competing with EFAs, these fats lead to EFA deficiencies and subsequently to a host of other health problems including diabetes, cancer, and weight gain. There is also some speculation that trans fatty acids may adversely affect insulin sensitivity, decrease fat oxidation, and increase fat synthesis; all these effects would be counterproductive to anyone on the metabolic diet.

Trans fatty acids are found in refined vegetable oils, shortenings, almost all margarines, and other oil-based foods; almost all fried fast foods; and even baked and prepared snack foods such as cookies, crackers, and chips. Foods containing significant amounts of trans fatty acids usually list hydrogenated or partially hydrogenated products in their list of ingredients. (See appendix A for more information about reading food labels.) Large quantities of unnatural trans fatty acids are also found as food contaminants during excessive heating of cooking oils for deep frying and other mass food preparation procedures that require heat.

Much of the problem resides with the fact that the shape of a fatty acid is essential to its proper functioning. Although trans fatty acids have the same number of carbon and hydrogen atoms as the original fatty acid (known as the cis fatty acid), its shape has been greatly changed. This change in shape, from cis fatty acid to trans, causes competition for existing enzymes. As a result, the cis fatty acids are unable to carry out their proper biological role, which negatively affects cellular metabolism and structure.

The amount of trans fatty acids, and other toxic by-products, found in a food varies according to the extent and nature of the processing. Generally, vegetable oil products that are hard at room temperature (e.g., shortening and margarine) are more riddled with trans fatty acids than products that are liquid at room temperature (e.g., vegetable oil). Several studies have pointed to the adverse health effects of hydrogenated fats and the trans fatty acids in them (especially hard margarines, but even soft margarines are suspect), including an increased incidence of heart problems (Willett et al. 1993), likely secondary to unfavorable changes in serum lipoproteins, a strong risk factor for coronary heart disease (Mensink 1992).

In addition to the well-recognized roles of EPA, the lack of trans fatty acids in the traditional Eskimo staple diet may also be responsible for their cardiovascular health. This diet contains cis forms of the unsaturated fatty acids in physiologically optimal concentrations and is virtually devoid of unnatural and potentially hazardous trans and cis isomers of these fatty acids (Booyens, Louwrens, and Katzeff 1986). These differences in the Eskimo diet would likely ensure that eicosanoids synthesized from dihomo-gamma-linolenic acid, arachidonic acid, and eicosapentaenoic acid are balanced in optimal physiological concentrations.

To sum up, trans fatty acids have been found to raise overall cholesterol levels by increasing LDLs (the bad cholesterol). They also decrease testosterone and insulin response, adversely affect liver enzyme activity, and impair the immune system. They have thus been linked to heart disease, cancer, and other diseases associated with aging. Keep away from these unhealthy fats as much as possible. Instead consume the fats recommended in the next section on good fats.

FATS TO AVOID

- All margarines that are solid due to the high concentration of trans fatty acids. (Liquid margarines that come in a squeeze bottle have a lower concentration of trans fatty acids.)
- Hydrogenated oil products and shortening, which are found in nearly all processed food.
- Baked goods and fried foods, especially fried fast foods.
- Rancid fats and oils of any type. Oils that have been stored too long have likely oxidized and can cause free radical damage in the body.

SOURCES OF GOOD FATS FOR THE METABOLIC DIET

Getting sufficient amounts of good fats helps athletes stay healthy and improve body composition. This section explores several sources of good fats you should include in your diet.

Flaxseed Oil

One of the best-known sources of LNA (and a good source of LA) available is flaxseed oil (also known as flax oil or linseed oil). Hemp oil, another rich source of LNA (and LA and to a lesser extent GLA) is slowly becoming more available. Flaxseed oil consists of 45 to 65 percent LNA, 15 percent LA, and a lesser amount of monounsaturated and saturated fatty acids. Thus, flaxseed oil is an excellent source of LNA and a good addition to any diet, especially the metabolic diet.

Despite its high concentration of LNA, some conflicting pieces of information may limit the usefulness of flaxseed oil. Some studies have shown that increasing dietary LNA (such as with the use of flaxseed oil) elevates tissue EPA concentrations in a predictable manner (Mantzioris et al. 1995). Increased levels of EPA decrease the production of arachidonic acid and its metabolism into bad eicosanoids (Kobayashi, Yokoyama, and Kitamura 1995). However, increased levels of LNA also decrease the production of GLA from LA because LNA inhibits the delta-6-desaturase enzyme that converts LA to GLA and thus decreases the formation of certain good prostaglandins.

It seems that although flaxseed oil is a good supplement to our diets, it shouldn't be overdone. Enough should be used to increase our natural production of EPA but not to decrease the formation of GLA from LA. Thus, as well as some flaxseed oil, we recommend the use of GLA and EPA, as detailed later.

If you use flaxseed oil, then make sure it's fresh. Flaxseed oil, like other perishable foods, will spoil very quickly. That is why it needs to be refrigerated and used soon after opening. Look in any good health food store or nutrition center, and you will find flaxseed oil in the refrigerated section. If you keep it refrigerated, flaxseed oil will generally last up to 6 weeks after it is opened.

A minimum of 1 teaspoon (5 ml) of flaxseed oil per day is recommended to ensure you get the necessary EFAs. Flaxseed oil capsules are also available and generally come in doses of 1 gram per capsule. Thus, you can achieve the daily recommendation through the use of either liquid or capsule format. Fresh unrefined flaxseed oil can also be added to a protein drink or salad (one to three tablespoons) as a tasty way to supplement LNA.

Evening Primrose Oil and Borage Seed Oil

Evening primrose oil and borage seed oil are rich in linoleic acid, vitamin E, and GLA. Evening primrose oil usually contains just less than half the amount of GLA as borage seed oil. DGLA is easily produced from GLA, and the use of GLA supplements may lead to increased production of the good prostaglandins that help fight musculoskeletal inflammation, decrease cholesterol levels and fluid retention, and have beneficial effects on several hormones in the body. Since GLA is a precursor for DGLA, which has been shown to be depleted by steroids, alcohol, and other drugs, it has been suggested that GLA therefore provides protection for the liver.

Thus GLA may be helpful for several reasons. Evening primrose oil, for example, has been used as treatment for a variety of problems including PMS, chronic fatigue syndrome, and arthritis. Since GLA is important for the production of several prostaglandins used to fight inflammation and muscle soreness in the body, it may be of great use to those involved in an advanced exercise program. If you suffer from any of these conditions, you might want to give either oil a try.

In any case, for most of us, it's not a bad idea to supplement our diets with GLA. We recommend at least 500 milligrams of GLA daily. That usually translates to six or more capsules of evening primrose oil or three or more capsules of borage seed oil daily. These products can be purchased in the supplement section of any good health food store. Each of these products will have a label that breaks down the content of the product and will indicate if it should be refrigerated after opening or stored in a dry, cool place.

Fish and Fish Oils

Fish oils belong to the alpha-linolenic omega-3 series of fatty acids and are rich in eicosapentaenoic acid (EPA) as described already. Although the body is able to convert alpha-linolenic acid to the longer-chained EPA and DHA, it does so slowly. It makes good health sense to consume fish oils since they are rich sources of EPA and DHA.

Although they increase fat-burning capabilities and lessen the amount of fat on the body, fish oils also aid in limiting the breakdown of muscle tissue and adding muscle tone for increased body shaping. One of the ways they do this is by increasing insulin sensitivity or decreasing insulin resistance, especially with high-fat diets (Taouis et al. 2002). They may also lower blood cholesterol levels, have vasodilatory effects (widening of the blood vessels), and be protective against (Bartram et al. 1993) and perhaps even therapeutic for (Rose et al. 1995) certain cancers. EPA also seems to decrease the production of arachidonic acid from DGLA, thus decreasing the production of some of the bad prostaglandins.

Fish oil also seems to have significant anti-inflammatory effects and protective effects on joint cartilage, especially for arthritic conditions (Curtis et al. 2000). EPA and DHA seem to have some similar and independent effects on the body. For example, one study found that DHA, rather than EPA, is responsible for the anti-inflammatory effects of fish oil (Tomobe et al. 2000).

The best way to obtain fish oil and thus your complement of its very important omega-3s is to regularly eat fresh fatty fish. For example, 100 grams (3.5 ounces) of Atlantic salmon has about 1,400 milligrams of omega-3 fatty acids (EPA and DHA). Thus half a pound of Atlantic salmon will give you an excellent daily complement of omega-3s.

Any fish—be it shell, freshwater, ocean, or whatever—contains some omega-3 fatty acids. There is evidence, though, that ocean fish is a better source of omega-3s than freshwater fish (except for lake trout). Fish from the colder northern waters such as the North Atlantic are superior to those caught near the equator, and shellfish have lesser amounts of omega-3s than other fish. Of the commonly available fish, the ones that are highest in omega-3s are salmon, herring, sardines, mackerel, and bluefish. One or all of these fish can be eaten three to four times a week.

On the basis of the many studies showing the benefits of fish oil, we recommend that fish or fish oil be consumed every day if possible or, if not, at least every other day. If you have problems with eating fish on a regular basis, use a fish oil supplement, such as salmon oil capsules. Aim for 2,000 milligrams of EPA a day. Fish oil usually contains 20 percent EPA and a lesser amount of DHA, so 10 capsules a day of 1,000 milligrams of fish oil should give you the recommended amount. If desired, or if there is a personal or family history of coronary artery disease, you can consume more fish oil, as there appears to be no adverse metabolic effects of long-term fish oil supplementation (Eritsland et al. 1995).

Be careful to buy fresh fish oil capsules that are in an opaque container. If the capsules are fishy tasting, chances are they are partially rancid and shouldn't be used. Keep the fish oil capsules in the refrigerator and away from light, and use them up as soon as possible, at least within a few months of purchase.

Monounsaturated Fats

Monounsaturated fatty acids are produced by the body and are found in fats of both plant and animal origin. Oleic acid is the main monounsaturated fatty acid. Animal sources of oleic acid include beef, pork, lamb, chicken, turkey, dairy products, eggs, and some fish (e.g., eel and trout). Although it is commonly believed that the fats found in these foods are all saturated, this is not the case. Oleic acid makes up 20 to 50 percent of the fats.

The plant sources of monounsaturated fatty acids include olive, canola (rapeseed), hazelnut, and peanut oils as well as the foods from which these oils are extracted. Nuts, such as almonds, pistachios, and macadamias, and avocados have significantly higher levels of oleic acid than of other monounsaturated fatty acids.

Monounsaturated fatty acids, especially oleic acid, seem to have some advantages over other fatty acids. A significant intake of monounsaturated fatty acids will not increase your risk of heart disease and may even decrease it by their effects on total cholesterol, HDL, and LDL (Wahrburg et al. 1992). The body also seems to have an easier time metabolically handling oleic acid over the other monounsaturated fatty acids.

Canola oil contains erucic acid, which may have some toxic effects. Because of its method of extraction, canola oil contains some deformed fatty acids. Studies also show that, unlike olive oil, which can decrease total cholesterol and LDL, canola oil has no such effect on blood cholesterol (Lichtenstein et al. 1994).

For various reasons, olive oil seems to be one of the better fats to consume on the metabolic diet. But only certain olive oils are candidates. Like any other oil, heat, chemicals, solvents, and other refining processes ruin the health effects of olive oil. The best olive oils are the cold-pressed extra virgin olive oils since these oils are extracted using gentle pressure rather than with heat and solvents.

A body of epidemiological evidence points to the health effects of olive oil (Keys et al. 1986; Katsouyanni 1991). Studies show that olive oil decreases atherogenesis (the formation of fatty deposits on the lining of the artery walls, as in atherosclerosis) (Aviram and Eias 1993). Olive oil seems to be one of the players responsible for the health effects of the Mediterranean diet (Massaro, Carluccio, and De Caterina 1999), perhaps partly because of the antioxidant effects of the absorbable phenols present in olive oil (Vissers et al. 2002; Leenen et al. 2002). Additionally, very few pesticides and chemicals are needed to grow olives; therefore, this source of fat seems to have everything going for it. Olive oil is definitely a useful and necessary part of the metabolic diet.

Saturated Fats

Many of the foods recommended in the metabolic diet, such as red meat, eggs, cheese, and butter, contain saturated fats. These fats do have a tendency to raise total serum cholesterol and LDL levels in some people, especially those with previous blood cholesterol problems. The increase in total cholesterol is mainly from an increase in LDLs, although there is also a small increase in HDLs (McNamara 1992).

However, not all saturated fatty acids have an adverse effect on total cholesterol. For example, stearic acid (the main saturated fatty acid found in beef) and medium-chain saturated fatty acid have little or no effect on total cholesterol. Recent studies show that replacement of carbohydrate with stearic acid (as done to some extent in the high-fat, low-carbohydrate phase of the metabolic diet) has little effect on lipid and lipoprotein concentration in plasma (Denke and Grundy 1991; Katan, Zock, and Mensink 1994). As well, in these studies oleic and linoleic acids had beneficial effects on blood lipids by raising HDL and lowering LDL.

It's important to realize that recent research shows it is the oxidized forms of cholesterol and LDLs that increase the incidence of cardiovascular disease (CVD), including coronary artery disease (Hansen, Pedersen, and Mulvad 1994). Thus, factors that decrease the tendency of LDLs to oxidize (such as consuming monounsaturated and marine oils) can negate the harmful effects a higher-fat diet may have in contributing to cardiovascular disease. Natural fatty acids in the cis configuration do not have the toxic harmful effects seen with the use of trans fatty acids. They are mainly an effective and compact source of energy. Most of us have no real problem with these saturated fats—our bodies know how to deal with them.

Saturated fats are an integral part of the metabolic diet. If used properly, natural saturated fats will help you lose weight and body fat. Any adverse effects they may have on overall blood cholesterol are usually diminished because the body's saturated fat is being utilized as a primary source of energy. Therefore fats do not have the opportunity to do any harm. (See chapter 7 for information about monitoring cholesterol.) Other recommended fats can decrease or eliminate any adverse changes resulting from the metabolic diet to total cholesterol, HDLs, and LDLs.

BUTTER OR MARGARINE?

Most health experts can argue the pros and cons for margarine and butter. Margarine does not contain cholesterol and has high concentrations of monounsaturated and polyunsaturated fatty acids, which reduce LDLs. However, margarine contains trans fatty acids because it has undergone the process of hydrogenation. At one time, trans fatty acids were considered healthier than the saturated fat found in butter. However some studies have found that trans fatty acids are more harmful than saturated fats. Butter is not processed and therefore does not contain trans fatty acids. The negative aspect of butter is that it contains saturated fat. Both saturated fat and trans fatty acids have been found to have adverse health effects on blood cholesterol and heart disease. As is often the case, the key is moderation and portion control.

The key is that when you're fat adapted, your metabolism is different from the standard predominantly carbohydrate-burning system. Dietary fat, such as saturated fat, does not react the same during metabolism. Thus, cardiovascular and metabolic problems that result from high-fat, high-carbohydrate diets will not occur.

Red Meat

Red meat has been maligned now for the past few decades. It seems nothing good can be said about it except it's great barbecued. But the tide is turning, and research is showing that red meat has been undeservedly maligned (Hodgson et al. 2007).

We have always said that red meat is good. And there are several reasons for this. Again, just as with saturated fat, there are too many inconsistencies. After all, red meat has been a staple in our diets since the beginning of our time. So why all of a sudden is it poisonous to us? First, red meat contains as much oleic acid, the same monounsaturated fat as in olive oil, as it does saturated fat. Oleic acid is considered to have significant health effects (Wahle et al. 2004); it is also believed to act as a sensing nutrient and when present decreases appetite (Obici et al. 2002).

Additionally, red meat is one of the best sources of amino acids. It's high in vitamins A, E, and B complex. Vitamin B_{12}, plentiful in meat, is not found in vegetable products. Red meat is loaded with iron that is easily absorbed, unlike the iron in many plant sources. Red meats are also excellent sources of other nutrients including L-carnitine, taurine, conjugated linoleic acid (CLA), coenzyme Q10, potassium, zinc, and magnesium—all vital nutrients, especially for those who want to improve their body compositions.

L-carnitine is primarily found in meat, and red meat is the best source, with about 600 milligrams per 100 grams. Fish contains only 35 milligrams per 100 grams. For athletes, plentiful L-carnitine means not only a larger proportion of lean muscle mass but also increased use of energy-rich fat as fuel during exercise. Conjugated linoleic acid can result in a reduction of overall body fat and an increase in lean muscle metabolism in the body (Gaullier et al. 2004; Eyjolfson, Spriet, and Dyck 2004; Steck et al. 2007.)

Red meat is also one of the best foods for maximizing body composition. A recent study found that women on a low-calorie red meat diet lost more weight and were healthier than those on a low-calorie, low-meat diet (Clifton et al. 2003). Normally with high-protein diets, urinary calcium increases, causing an adverse calcium balance. During this study, no adverse effect on bone metabolism resorption (the process from which calcium is transferred from bone fluid to the blood) occurred. This bone resorption is often a precursor for osteoporosis.

In another study, red meat was shown to have beneficial effects on serum cholesterol and triglycerides, the other important fat (Davidson et al. 1999). At the end of the 9-month study, the red meat group had an average decrease of 1 to 3 percent in "bad" low-density lipoprotein (LDL) cholesterol, an average 2 percent increase in "good" high-density lipoprotein (HDL) cholesterol, and an average drop of 6 percent in their triglyceride levels.

Red meat, with its saturated fat, increases serum testosterone levels. We've seen this in our own clinical studies on patients and athletes we've put on diets, with the emphasis on red meat. And this association has also been shown in some studies (Hamalainen et al. 1983; Hamalainen et al. 1984; Dorgan et al. 1996).

SUGGESTIONS FOR FAT CONSUMPTION

Twenty-five percent of your fat intake should come from olive oil and the EFA-rich foods mentioned in the previous section. These include nuts, seeds, fish, flaxseed oil, salmon oil, and unprocessed vegetable oils. Purchase vegetable oils from an organic supermarket because they will not be processed. If you can afford to buy all your foods in an organic form that is not refined or processed, that would be ideal. The other 75 percent of your fat intake should come from high-quality red meats, chicken, eggs, cheese, pork, shellfish and other fish, and liquid margarine or organic butter. Also, make an effort to buy omega-3 enriched eggs and dairy products. Table 6.1 provides an easy way to judge the various fats in some common foods and oils.

Buy and consume oils that are predominantly monounsaturated (olive oil). Bake, boil, microwave, poach, or steam foods instead of frying them, and consume only fresh foods. Supplement your diet with GLA-containing oils (such as evening primrose or borage see oil), unspoiled fish oil (if your intake of fish is lacking), and to a lesser extent flaxseed oils as discussed previously. Make liberal use of extra virgin olive oil for preparing foods, salads, and protein drinks and in any other way you find palatable.

TABLE 6.1 Fatty Acid Composition of Commonly Consumed Foods

Food	% saturated fat	% mono-unsaturated fat	% poly-unsaturated fat
Butter, cream, milk	65	30	5
Beef	46	48	6
Bacon and pork	38	50	12
Lard	42	45	13
Chicken	33	39	28
Fish	29	31	40
Coconut oil	92	6	2
Palm kernel oil	86	12	2
Cocoa butter	63	34	3
Olive oil	15	76	9
Peanut oil	20	48	32
Cottonseed oil	27	20	53
Soybean oil	16	24	60
Corn oil	13	26	61
Sunflower seed oil	11	22	67
Safflower seed oil	10	13	77

Reprinted from Di Pasquale 2002, p. 95.

chapter 7

Implementing the Metabolic Diet Plan

This chapter explains how to shift your body from a predominantly carbohydrate-burning system to a predominantly fat-burning system through the start-up and assessment phases. You will then be able to manipulate your body's optimal weekday and weekend (carbohydrate-loading period) carbohydrate caloric intake. Once you have achieved this, the metabolic diet can be used to maximize lean body mass and strength through the progression of different training phases.

BEFORE YOU START

Before starting the metabolic diet, you should get a complete physical from your doctor. You should also have a blood workup, including a complete blood count, cholesterol levels (total, LDL, and HDL), TSH (a test for thyroid function), fasting blood sugar, serum uric acid, serum potassium, liver function array, and BUN (blood urea nitrogen). Your doctor may also want to run additional tests.

As for the cholesterol issue, because you are burning fat for energy, much of the cholesterol and saturated fats that could cause a problem are used up in the process. Studies have even shown that along with increasing the utilization of fat as an energy source and providing for weight loss, the metabolic diet can even reduce serum cholesterol (Schurch, Reinke, and Hollmann 1979). In fact, a study published in July 2002 showed that the long-term use of a low-carbohydrate diet resulted in increased weight and fat loss and a dramatic improvement in the lipid profile (decreased cholesterol, triglycerides, and LDL levels and increased HDL levels) (Westman et al. 2002).

It never hurts to keep track of your cholesterol level whenever you change diets and even more so if you have had or have a tendency toward a cholesterol problem. Cholesterol levels are largely determined by individual metabolism and body chemistry, and genetics plays a strong role. If there are cholesterol problems in your family, there is a good chance you may have them too. And if you have a chronic problem with cholesterol, you need to talk to your doctor about how this may be affected by the metabolic diet and what you can do to limit any adverse affects. Frequent monitoring of your lipid status will let you know where you stand and if changes need to be made.

You can make a number of adjustments to the metabolic diet to control your cholesterol intake if needed. Marine oils, flaxseed oil, olive oil, and other nutritional supplements will help. If your serum LDL or HDL levels are adversely affected by the diet at the start (when you are adapting to burning fat as your main fuel) or when you are bulking up and taking in more fat, then the problem may correct itself as you modify the carbohydrate level to suit your metabolism or when you are in the process of decreasing your body fat, such as when you go into a definition or cutting phase. Meat restriction may also be necessary. But again, this is something you need to work on with your physician. If the metabolic diet seems like the answer for you, you will need to put your heads together to devise a plan that lets you benefit from the weight loss and body composition advantages the diet provides while keeping cholesterol in check. Additionally after your body makes the transition from carbohydrates to fats as the main fuel source, fats are not as important as they once were in contributing to dyslipidemia (an abnormal blood lipid profile).

In fact, if you do follow a high-fat diet during the initial fat adaptation or to bulk up, you must then lower the dietary fat levels as you shift gears to burn off that unwanted body fat. To do so, you usually need to gradually decrease your daily caloric intake, drop your dietary fat intake (since you cannot decrease an already low carbohydrate intake), and keep protein levels high to maintain muscle mass. Thus you have to lower your dietary fat intake progressively until you reach your goal. As such, the metabolic diet moves from a high-fat diet to a moderate- and even low-fat diet depending on how low you drop your daily caloric intake. And because you're fat adapted, lowering dietary fats won't affect your ability to use fat as your primary fuel.

So if you are having cholesterol problems, decrease your intake of saturated fats as much as possible and make up any calories that you lack with foods high in polyunsaturated and monounsaturated fats (making liberal use of flax and olive oil), high in protein, and lower in saturated fat. For example, steaks are OK but you have to take off all visible fat. Cutting back on egg yolk consumption while keeping the egg whites is also a good idea.

UNDERSTANDING AND TRACKING YOUR PROGRESS

Along with seeing your physician for a physical and bloodwork, you should weigh yourself and get a body-fat analysis before you begin the diet. Weight loss is important, but so are inches. Use a weight scale once a week to determine your weight, but do not rely on this as the only form of measurement. Losing inches is key and may not be reflected from a weight scale. Rely on the mirror too because a visual perspective always gives clarity as to lean body mass and areas where there is too much body fat. By understanding this, you will be able to keep your enthusiasm high, which is very important for success.

The optimal body-fat percentage for athletes is 10 to 18 percent for women and 5 to 10 percent for men. Please understand that many male and female athletes can be at the lowest percentage levels and be perfectly normal, and it does not affect sports performance. Athletes who are well trained need to worry less about calories because of their ability to burn calories during exercise and ultimately enhance fat burning. Therefore, marked calorie restrictions with intense exercise is not desirable, as excessively depleting body fat stores is unhealthy and counterproductive in regards to maximizing body composition and performance.

Female competitors must be aware of the female athlete triad, which is characterized by disrupted eating habits, menstrual irregularities, and weak bones (onset of osteoporosis) (Kleiner and Greenwood-Robinson 2007). Female bodybuilders are at risk because of the sport's requirement to check weight often and the constant dieting for show appearance. In male athletes, obsessively weighing themselves, overtraining, mirror gazing, and having constant dissatisfaction with one's body is known as body dysmorphia. The obsessive desire to build muscle and avoid gaining fat is understandable in a society geared toward appearance. There is no need to fall into any of these traps on the metabolic diet because your primary fuel source is fat, which allows you to burn it off without sacrificing muscle mass. Eat a healthy, energy-rich diet and become one with your body, understanding exactly what it needs to be successful in your sport.

Overall body-fat percentage can be measured with skinfold calipers. This technique involves measuring fat levels in the body by assessing key fat deposits with the calipers. You can have the skinfold test performed by a professional, or you can do it yourself by purchasing the calipers, along with easy-to-follow instructions. With the calipers you can determine your body-fat percentage by taking skin density measurements of the suprailiac area (see figure 7.1). This area is approximately 1 inch (2.5 cm) above the right hipbone, about 5 inches (13 cm) or so to the right of and just below your bellybutton. As per the diagram, while standing, firmly pinch the suprailiac skinfold between your left thumb and forefinger. Place the jaws of the calipers over the skinfold while continuing to hold the skinfold with the left hand. Then take your measurement as per the instructions and the diagram. Once you have the measurement, refer to the body-fat interpretation chart (included with the calipers) to determine your body-fat percentage.

The best way to measure your progress while you are on the metabolic diet is the metabolic index (MIDx). The MIDx is a ratio derived by considering not only weight and height but also your percentage of body fat. The MIDx takes into account all the variables that other methods cannot. With the MIDx you get a snapshot of your body composition and progress.

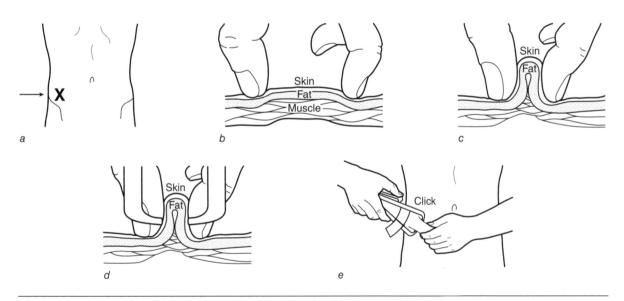

FIGURE 7.1   To complete the skinfold test at the suprailiac site, *(a)* stand up straight, *(b and c)* pinch the skin between your thumb and forefinger, and *(d and e)* place the jaws of the caliper over the skinfold while continuing to hold the skinfold with your hand.

Reprinted from Di Pasquale 2002, p. 99.

LOGGING YOUR DIET

Keep in mind that it's important to document aspects of the diet and their effects on your body. It may be inconvenient and even irritating at times, but if you are interested in getting the most out of your efforts, you need to chart your progress and the ways you respond to changes in the diet. Make notes to yourself on when you begin to smooth out during the weekend, what you were eating, how many calories you were eating, and any other essential information.

Keeping your own diet log will give you a record of what you have done and give you added confidence with the moves you make in training and diet. This is the way you will really dial in the time when you look best and how to get that look. You may back off on the documentation after being on the diet for some time and becoming familiar with it, but you will still want to make at least weekly notes on your findings as you proceed.

The MIDx is very easy to calculate.[*] In fact, just fill in your weight in pounds, your height in inches, and your body-fat level as a percentage into the following formula and do the calculations. Divide your body weight in pounds by your height in inches squared. Then, multiply the results by 7,250, and finally divide the results by your percent body fat (Di Pasquale 2002-2008).

MIDx = {body weight in pounds ÷ (height in inches)^2 × 7,250} ÷ % body fat

If you are using the metric system, use this equation:

MIDx = {body weight in kilograms ÷ (height in meters)^2 × 10.3} ÷ % body fat

As an example, the calculation for an athlete who weighs 185 pounds (84 kg), is 5 feet 6 inches tall (168 cm), and has a total body fat of 10 percent follows:

$$MIDx = \{185\ lb \div (66\ in)^2 \times 7{,}250\} \div 10$$

$$MIDx = \{(185\ lb \div 4{,}356\ in) \times 7{,}250\} \div 10$$

$$MIDx = (.0424701 \times 7250) \div 10$$

$$MIDx = 307.90822 \div 10$$

$$MIDx = 30.8$$

[*]Adapted from Di Pasquale 2002, pp. 100-102.

GETTING STARTED

The low-carbohydrate transition can last anywhere from two to several weeks and allows you to determine if you are an efficient fat user and as such can do quite nicely without too many carbohydrates. If this is the case, then you are all set to carry on with the traditional low-carbohydrate 5-day, 2-day (weekends) shift regimen.

Adaptation Phase

The initial phase of the metabolic diet shows how the body functions under carbohydrate deprivation and is the testing ground to determine an athlete's capability for utilizing fat as the primary fuel source. Those who are efficient fat oxidizers do very well in this phase of the diet. Eventually, the metabolic diet will emphasize low-carbohydrate weekdays and higher-carbohydrate weekend shifts. However, that is not the way it works in the first 12 days. During the adaptation phase, the best approach is few to no carbohydrate foods for the first 12 days. Doing it in this manner will give your body the incentive and direction to make the shift from burning carbohydrates to burning fat as its primary fuel source. It will also provide an immediate indication of whether you are unsuited for low-level carbohydrate consumption.

This phase of the metabolic diet calls for a dedicated higher-fat, high-protein, low-carbohydrate diet from Monday all the way through to the Friday of the next week (a total of 12 days). During that time, you will be limited to 30 grams of carbohydrate maximum per day. If you can handle less—or even zero—carbohydrate, all the better. Fat intake should be set at roughly 50 to 65 percent of calories and protein at 30 to 40 percent of calories (see table 7.1).

During this adaptation stage, you don't really need to change your normal caloric intake—simply substitute protein and fat for your former carbohydrate calories. To do this, replace the carbohydrate you're eating now with protein and fat, and don't change the calorie level at first. (See the section What to Eat later in this chapter for specific food suggestions.)

By beginning the diet with 12 days of high-fat, low-carbohydrate consumption, the metabolic shift will occur quickly, and with certainty, in those who are or can become efficient fat oxidizers. Those who are totally unsuited for bottom-level carbing will be very affected. Symptoms include fatigue and flu-like symptoms where you feel you are coming down with something. Lack of energy, weakness, irritability, and bowel irregularities are common difficulties athletes experience in the initial stages, especially if you are not reacting well to the shift.

TABLE 7.1   **Intake Levels for the Adaptation Phase**

	Carbohydrate intake	MACRONUTRIENT INTAKE AS A PERCENTAGE OF TOTAL CALORIES		
		Fat	Protein	Carbohydrate
First 12 days	30 g	50-65%	30-40%	4-10%
Regular weekday maximum	30 g	50-65%	30-40%	4-10%
Weekend 12- to 48-hour carbohydrate load	No real limit	25-40%	15-30%	35-55%

Assessment Phase

If you are successful with the adaptation phase during the first 12 days, when you come to the second Saturday (the 13th day), you perform a big turnaround. You eat a high-carbohydrate diet anywhere from 12 to 48 hours over the weekend. During this time, as shown in table 7.1, set your fat intake at 25 to 40 percent, your protein intake at 15 to 30 percent, and your carbohydrate intake at 35 to 55 percent. This process is very similar to what athletes call carbohydrate loading. This 14 day period, which includes the 12 day strict carbohydrate adaptation phase followed by the 2 day higher carbohydrate assessment phase is crucial because it allows you to completely understand the diet in its entirety. At this point, you are left with the task of manipulating your optimal weekday and weekend carbohydrate intake levels (metabolic set point).

When the second weekend (days 13 and 14) hits and you are switching to a much higher intake of carbohydrate, insulin levels will rise dramatically. In fact, the higher-fat, low-carbohydrate diet phase makes the insulin response to the high-carbohydrate intake even greater than it normally would be (Sidery, Gallen, and Macdonald 1990; Bhathena et al. 1989). The body's initial instinct is to always be a predominantly carbohydrate-burning system, and thus you get the immediate rise in insulin with the high levels of carbohydrates.

Unfortunately, most people overdo it on the first carbohydrate load and quickly discover the consequences. Symptoms such as bloating and puffiness can occur, which can lead to immediate laying down of excess body fat. This experience, although uncomfortable, can actually be a lesson well learned. In overcompensating for the lack of carbohydrate in the previous 12 days, most people believe they're back-pedaling and have lost any progress they made while low carbing. In fact, this overcompensation provides a learning experience and can teach athletes how to carb up properly on the weekends, especially if you do it consistently and are trying to improve your body composition. Overdoing the carbohydrate weekend, of course, is ideal for the hypertrophy (H) training phase (see chapter 13) and will allow you to add muscle mass and, unless you really overdo it, keep body fat at a manageable level.

The first thing your body does in response to this exaggerated carbohydrate loading is stuff the muscles with glycogen, which makes your muscles fuller looking and promotes protein synthesis by directly stimulating the uptake of amino acids by muscle cells. Your protein intake on weekends is much lower than on weekdays, especially when you become experienced and have been on the diet for some time. It is important to understand that you are getting enough protein during the weekdays to compensate if needed. Protein utilization after relative protein restriction rebounds to higher levels than were present before the restriction (Di Pasquale 1997).

After the initial 2 weeks, including your first carbohydrate-loading weekend, when you begin your regular routine on Monday you will be energized and ready to take on the world. During exercise you will find yourself feeling especially

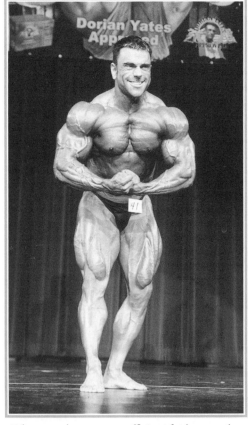

When you become an efficient fat burner, the results are evident.

upbeat, healthy, and motivated. On both Monday and Tuesday your system will be working hard, burning off all the increased glycogen you gained over the weekend and continuing to burn fatty acids. Overall you will experience a rise in fat-burning and body-shaping potential. Then, Wednesday to Friday, with glycogen limited again, you will depend much more on your primary fat-burning metabolism to maximize fat loss and body toning.

The body goes through a large transition during the adaptation phase and during the assessment phase (initial carbohydrate-loading weekend). It is crucial to understand when to stop carbohydrate loading because some people have a tendency to lay down body fat faster than others. As an athlete, you need to be aware of the point at which you begin to feel puffy and bloated. This point will vary greatly from person to person. Some people will hardly feel any response in appetite from the increased insulin. Others, however, will experience wide insulin swings. The huge insulin swings can be a great negative because they cause an increased appetite. For this reason we use 12 to 48 hours as the carbohydrate-loading time on the weekends. This could be cut back to even less than 12 hours for athletes whose appetites become insatiable or for athletes who tend to lay down body fat relatively early in the carbohydrate phase. The important thing is knowing and understanding when you've had enough. The moment you start feeling puffy and bloated, it's time to go back to your weekday high-fat, low-carbohydrate routine.

Granted, it may take you a while to learn when your body is telling you it's time to shift. If you are having trouble with this, make the change earlier in the weekend and see how you look and feel the next week. Experience will eventually teach you to interpret your body signs correctly and know when you are putting on fat. Also, keep in mind that the percentages listed in table 7.1 for fat, protein, and carbohydrate consumption are optimal numbers, at least at first until you find the best numbers for you. If you have never done any real diet planning before, you may have a bit of trouble reaching the targets at first. If so, do not worry. By shooting for the 30-gram carbohydrate limit and 50 percent minimal fat level in the diet during the early weeks, you will make the metabolic shift necessary for initial success.

DETERMINING YOUR METABOLIC SET POINT

The metabolic set point is the level of carbohydrate that suits your metabolism while at the same time maximizes your ability to increase muscle mass and decrease body fat. For athletes and bodybuilders who are efficient fat oxidizers and have little need for dietary carbohydrate, the metabolic diet set point will be low, less than 30 grams and usually approaching zero grams a day. For a small number, the metabolic diet set point may well be high enough that they end up consuming a high-carbohydrate diet. Most people, however, fall somewhere in between, usually between 30 and 100 grams of dietary carbohydrate per day.

By carefully monitoring how your body reacts to the amount of carbohydrate you consume and then making any necessary adjustments in carbohydrate intake, you will eventually arrive at that magic dietary carbohydrate level that is just right for you. To fully understand how the metabolic diet works, you must realize it is a dynamic progression in which you are actively involved. The interactive part of this process allows you to discover enough about your metabolism so that you can achieve your ultimate goals.

If you're feeling tired, you need some help with the carbohydrate part of your diet. When you have to increase the level of carbohydrate, it will take a while before you discover what your carbohydrate set point is. It takes people about 2 months on average to find their ideal dietary carbohydrate level. Once you discover your metabolic set point, you can stabilize your diet to that level for several months while you work on changing your body composition.

It usually takes about 3 or 4 weeks on the phase-shift part of the metabolic diet (the shifting from low carbohydrate during the week to higher carbohydrate loading for some or all of the weekend), to determine if you can survive on this low level of dietary carbohydrate or if you need more carbohydrate at a specific time in the week. To assess the strict part of the metabolic diet (low carbohydrate weekdays and, depending on how long the athlete can carbohydrate load, maybe part of the weekend), focus on the diet 2 weeks at a time. If you feel OK after the first 2 weeks, then you can carry on with the 5-plus weekdays at 30 grams and 1 or 2 days in the carbohydrate-loading weekends.

If you are mildly to moderately tired and otherwise affected, then go through another 2-week adaptation phase to see if things even out. If you are severely affected, then go to a variation diet where you selectively take in more carbohydrate depending on when you are feeling fatigued. If you feel good from Saturday to Wednesday and start to get tired and generally unwell by the time Thursday rolls around, then a Wednesday carbohydrate spike should do the trick. On Wednesday you should increase your carbohydrate to at least 100 grams and usually more. You might try incorporating between .5 and 1 gram of carbohydrate per pound (.5 kg) of body weight and see how you respond.

One word of caution: Do not take in any carbohydrate before working out. Consuming carbohydrate at this time will decrease GH and IGF-1 production and, in effect, increase insulin and decrease the use of body fat as a primary energy source during training.

If you are tired and you do not feel well for most of the low-carbohydrate weekdays, then try increasing the carbohydrate intake by 10 grams per day on the weekdays to see if this helps. If that doesn't help, double the carbohydrate intake to a level of 60 grams per day for as many weeks as it takes for you to function optimally. Most athletes usually level off between 30 and 100 grams per day. Some athletes are metabolically unique and may need to intake more than 100 grams per day. Approximately .5 to 1 gram of dietary carbohydrate per pound (.5 kg) of body weight per day is the norm in those who are relatively poor fat oxidizers. In a small number of cases, it may be necessary to work up to as much as 3 grams of carbohydrate per pound of body weight, depending on the person and the activity he is involved in.

PROBLEM-SOLVING GUIDE

Use the following procedures to dial in your exact carbohydrate needs to make sure you are consuming the optimal (but lowest) level of carbohydrate needed. You are starting on a 2-week adaptation and assessment phase of the strict metabolic diet to see how well you do with 30 grams of carbohydrate on weekdays and carbohydrate loading on weekends. What do you do now?

If you are feeling fine, follow this procedure:

1. Continue with a further 2-week adaptation and assessment phase of the strict metabolic diet to see how well you do.

2. It's now been 4 weeks on the strict metabolic diet assessment phase, and you still feel great. What do you do now? Now your strict metabolic diet begins in earnest: Stay on the schedule of 5 weekdays at 30 grams of carbohydrate and 2 weekend days of carbohydrate loading.

If you're feeling tired, follow this procedure:

1. If you have low to moderate tiredness, you should do another 2-week assessment phase of the regular diet plan (using the weekend and weekday carbohydrate amounts from table 7.1) to see how well you do.

2. If you have moderate to severe tiredness, you need to introduce variations in your diet to overcome this tiredness.

3. Try a carbohydrate spike of an additional 120 grams of carbohydrate just on Wednesday and see how well you do.

4. You did the midweek carbohydrate spike but now you lack energy during training. What should you do? Take 30 to 100 grams of carbohydrate half an hour after training to combat this lack of energy on training days.

5. You still lack energy during training, so what can you do? Increase your daily carbohydrate intake on training days by 30 grams, and do this every week until you feel normal during your workouts.

6. You lack energy all week, so what can you do? Increase your daily intake of carbohydrate by 30 grams.

7. You increased your daily carbohydrate intake by 30 grams for a 1-week period, and you still feel tired all week. So what can you do next? Add another 30 grams of carbohydrate to your daily intake for a 1-week assessment and again every week until you feel normal.

WHAT TO EAT

Tables 7.2 and 7.3 provide a sample 2,500-calorie diet menu for the weekday and a 2,100-calorie diet menu for the carbohydrate-loading weekend. For more weekly and weekend diet plans, please refer to *The Metabolic Diet* by Mauro Di Pasquale (2000). During the weekdays, there are plenty of options for high-fat, high-protein, low-carbohydrate foods, as shown in table 7.4.

Several tips for food preparation will also be helpful. Use a small, inexpensive kitchen scale to measure the weight of the portions you choose to ensure that the daily calorie count is accurate. Also Pam (original, olive oil, or even light oil) can be used for cooking. A spray of .6 seconds is only 4 calories or fewer. The following specific food recommendations can help you make good choices for the metabolic diet:

- **Meats, poultry, and fish.** Virtually any meat is OK, and most of you will focus on steak, hamburger, pork, and other red meats on the diet. In addition, venison, fish (of great importance as you will see later), lamb, shrimp, lobster, chicken, turkey, and other white meats are also OK. So are canned sardines, tuna, shrimp, herring, and anchovies. You can broil, bake, barbecue, roast, or fry these foods. However, don't add any calories while cooking (i.e., use a Teflon pan or Pam when frying instead of adding oil or other fats).

- **Eggs.** If you have a problem with cholesterol you may want to limit your intake of eggs. However, most people can safely eat one to four eggs a day. Whole eggs are great. Deviled eggs can be a good snack food to keep in the refrigerator.

TABLE 7.2 **2,500-Calorie Weekday Diet Menu (30 Grams of Carbohydrate)**

Meal	Food	Calories	Carbohydrate (g)
Breakfast	4 fried eggs with 2 tbsp butter	508	0
	4 slices bacon	140	0
Snack	1/2 cup cottage cheese	90	4
Lunch	9 oz (275 g) ground beef (extra lean)	654	0
	1 tbsp Dijon mustard	15	1
	2 oz (60 g) Parmesan cheese	220	2
Snack	4 cups lettuce greens	200	4
	3 oz (90 g) turkey	133	0
Dinner	8 oz (250 g) chicken	365	0
	1/2 slice whole-grain flax bread (toasted)	60	8
	1/2 cup cabbage, broccoli, and cauliflower mix (steamed)	25	5
	1/2 cup strawberries	20	5
Snack	1 oz (30 g) low-fat cheese	110	1
Total		2,540	30

TABLE 7.3	**2,100-Calorie Weekend Diet Menu (Carbohydrate Loading)**			

Meal	Food	Calories	Carbohydrate (g)	Protein (g)
Breakfast	2 slices whole-grain flax bread (toasted)	200	38	6
	2 tbsp jelly	100	20	0
	1 cup Cheerios cereal	110	20	3
	1 cup skim milk	80	8	8
Snack	8 oz (250 g) apple sauce	220	50	<1
	1 poppy seed bagel (no butter)	195	37.5	4.5
Lunch	2 cups salad lettuce, 1 whole red pepper, 1/2 cup carrots	90	20	2
	2 tbsp low-fat Italian salad dressing	10	0	0
	2 slices whole-grain flax bread (toasted)	200	38	6
	1 tbsp butter	100	0	0
Snack	1 poppy seed bagel	195	37.5	4.5
	2 tbsp jelly	100	20	0
Dinner	1 cup penne vegetable pasta	410	81	10.5
	1/2 cup tomato sauce (organic)	40	7	1
	1/2 cup green beans	25	16	2.5
	2 cups salad lettuce, 1 whole green pepper, 1/2 cup carrots	90	20	2
Snack	1.3 oz (40 g) banana cake	90	20	1
Total		2,155	413	50

TABLE 7.4	**Suggested Weekday Foods**						

Meat		Cheese[1]	Nuts	Vegetables[2]	Condiments	Beverages	Dessert
Steak	Chicken	Monterey Jack	Walnuts	Cucumbers Alfalfa sprouts Lettuce greens	Butter	Water	Jell-O with whipped cream topping[4]
Hamburger	Eggs	Brie	Sunflower seeds		Vinegar	Coffee	
Pot roast	Sardines	Camembert			Oils[3]	Diet soda	
Venison	Tuna	Muenster			Mayonnaise	Tea	
Lamb	Herring	Gruyère			Salt		
Bacon	Lobster						
Pastrami	Salmon						
Sausage	Anchovies						
Turkey	Shrimp						

[1]Full fat, low carbohydrate.

[2]Low carbohydrate only. No beans, corn, carrots, or peas.

[3]Poly- and monounsaturated fats such as ones found in nuts, olive oil, and flax seed oil.

[4]Sugar-free Jell-O with carbohydrate-free whipped cream topping.

- **Cheese.** Almost any kind of cheese is fair game as well. Use the full-fat varieties. Keep in mind that cheese spreads, cottage cheese, and ricotta cheese are higher in carbohydrate. Brie, Camembert, Muenster, Gruyère, and Monterey Jack are very low in carbohydrate and good for the diet.

- **Fruits.** Unlike in some other low-carbohydrate diets, fruits are allowed, even on the low-calorie days. There are a number of low-carbohydrate fruits you can eat, including oranges, apples, cantaloupes, and strawberries.

- **Vegetables.** Vegetables are great to add to the metabolic diet, but be careful of carbohydrate levels during the weekdays. Carrots, corn, onions, and peas have high carbohydrate content.

- **Salads.** Salads are also an excellent source of greens, but you might want to skip the croutons. Five ounces (150 g) of croutons contain 10.4 grams of carbohydrate. During the weekdays, this would be one-third of your daily carbohydrate allowance. Be inventive with your salads. Use combinations of several of the foods in table 16.3 (page 276). Food choices for cutting include asparagus, brussels sprouts, cabbage, celery, cucumber, dill pickles (not sweet pickles), endive, lettuce (Boston, iceberg, Romaine, and so on), mushrooms, radishes, spinach, green beans, and watercress.

- **Nuts and seeds.** Walnuts and sunflower seeds are also good, but keep track of the carbohydrate content.

- **Condiments.** Condiments such as vinegar, oil, and mayonnaise are fine. Butter and liquid margarine are OK, but try to use oil (especially olive oil) and vinegar dressing most of the time. Most other commercial salad dressings are in the vicinity of 7 percent carbohydrate. Mustard, vinegar, lemon juice, soy sauce, chili powder, horseradish, salt, pepper, garlic, basil, cinnamon, nutmeg, curry, and other herbs and spices are OK. Other condiments that are low in carbohydrate are also OK. Ketchup has too much carbohydrate but some steak sauces are OK.

- **Beverages.** As far as what to drink, that is easy too. Permissible beverages include water, diet soda, soda water and mineral water, diet tonic water, and coffee and tea (preferably black or with cream and artificial sweetener only). The general rule is to cut down on beverages with any significant amount of calories, such as juice or sugary soda. Soda water or mineral water on the rocks with a twist of lemon makes a refreshing drink and can be used at outings and parties instead of soft drinks (since few hosts and hostesses provide diet soft drinks but often have club soda, ice, and lemon juice on hand).

  For alcoholic beverages, avoid beer and sweet wines. You can drink dry wines and hard liquors, but be careful—diet pills and alcohol don't mix well. Since both dieting and diet pills may increase the effect of alcohol, it's best to limit your alcohol intake.

Eat fiber, especially during the adaptation and assessment phases. For the first 2 months of the diet, you could have loose or irregular bowel movements as the body transitions during the high-fat diet. For those people who continue to have problems for longer periods, stay on a natural fiber supplement or incorporate a midday salad into the diet.

PROCESSED AND JUNK FOODS

Try to keep away from processed, prepared, and fast foods. Why? Processed food (canned, packaged, bottled, and sometimes even many of the frozen foods) are too high in sugar, flour, starch, fat, and salt. The sugar, fat, white flour, and starch are calories you can do without. Too much salt will bloat you up.

Junk food and fast food don't just come from variety stores and fast food outlets. They're sometimes made right at home. Taking good food and changing it into junk food is easy to do. You just smear it, mix it, dip it, and cover it with salt, ketchup, mayonnaise, grease, artificial color, artificial flavor, and sugar. The best way to kick the junk food habit is not to go to junk food establishments and not to have any junk food in the house.

Another factor to consider is that if you have cravings, you are only putting off satisfying them until the weekend. You can eat basically anything then. We are just partitioning or separating foods here. We are not saying you cannot have lasagna. You just need to wait for the weekend. That is a lot better than other diets where you are basically stranded on a low-fat or, in some cases, low-carb island for the rest of your life.

This can also work for you psychologically. Food you love can give you a goal. Just get to the weekend and you can have that slice of apple pie. You are giving yourself something to look forward to, and it can even be fun. This doesn't present the kind of frustration and boredom you get eating the same thing over and over, week after week, month after month. You do not have to come up with an elaborate set of recipes to keep yourself sane.

When you get to the weekend, eat what you want! Fill up the tank on foods you love, but keep in mind that there must be a balance between healthy and less healthy foods. Satisfy those cravings. Some people will go overboard at the beginning of the diet and eat until they are nearly sick. Most will overdo it to some degree, but this is fine. It gets easier as you go. After being on the diet awhile, most people no longer have the strong desire for ice cream or onion rings. They may eat these foods sometimes, but they do not pig out on them. As athletes start adjusting their diets and dialing them in for maximum progress, they begin to see some real improvement and acquire some real knowledge about the way their bodies work and how adjustments can be made to achieve their goals.

Artificial Sweeteners   Sugar is going to be a problem for people with a sweet tooth. You can end up craving it, especially at the start as you adapt to the diet. While sugar is eliminated during the low carbohydrate part of the diet, you can intake some sugar on the higher carbohydrate loading weekends. However, during the carbohydrate loading weekends, the athlete should not consume too much sugar or simple carbohydrate. Instead, the athlete should ingest more complex carbohydrate, which will fill carbohydrate stores without the higher insulin levels. Appease any cravings along this line with low-carbohydrate drinks and desserts with artificial sweeteners. However, avoid sorbitol and fructose—remember sugar free doesn't necessarily mean carbohydrate free. Make sure to check the labels. You can also put sugar-free Jell-O (no carbohydrate, uses artificial sweetener) to good use. Topping it with carbohydrate-free whipped cream may be just what you are looking for to gain control.

There's still a lot of controversy over the benefits and risks of artificial sweeteners. Sugar, a natural food, is much higher in calories than the artificial sweeteners. Although the sugar industry is trying to downplay the calorie content of sugar, you're best off to use sugar substitutes instead of sugar and to consume foods with artificial sweeteners instead of sugar whenever you can (e.g., drink diet soda instead of regular soda). Let's examine the common types of artificial sweeteners to help you decide which ones to use to curb your cravings when needed.

Stevia is a shrub whose leaves have long been used by the people of South America to sweeten their beverages. It's marketed in the United States as a dietary supplement that provides sweetness without calories. The Food and Drug Administration (FDA) has concluded through some research findings that stevia may be associated with cancer development and may have negative effects on reproduction and energy metabolism. Some research suggests when used sparingly, stevia may cause little harm, but the FDA cannot approve these findings because of the unsubstantiated research in this area. For this reason, the FDA, the European Union, Canada, and the United Nations will not approve the extensive widespread use of this product in the world community.

Saccharin is made from petroleum products and is about 300 times sweeter than sugar. Canadian studies show that saccharin may be a weak cancer agent. Cyclamate is a synthetic chemical; although not as sweet as saccharin (it is 40 times sweeter than table sugar), it does not leave the bitter aftertaste familiar to saccharin users. As with saccharin, some research studies show it may have cancer-causing potential. Cyclamates may also have mutagenic properties (causing genetic damage).

DINING OUT

Eating out at restaurants while following the metabolic diet is no problem, even on weekdays, if you develop the right approach for this lifestyle. Athletes who have been on the diet for years can look a waiter in the eye and say, "I want a T-bone steak and nothing else!" Most often the waiter will look back and say, "But you get a baked potato, vegetables, bread. . . ." The athletes will break in and repeat, "Nothing else." You will need to do the same, break in and repeat. Waiters may have a little difficulty understanding this at first, but usually, with repetition, the point will sink in.

The fact is you don't want extras on your plate. During the week, you should be staying away from those carbohydrate foods, so keep them out of sight and out of mind. Leave them off your plate; otherwise, you might be tempted to "sample" them. (See appendix A for information about hidden carbohydrate.) The meat is fine, it sticks to your diet, and you will feel good. Order what you want regardless of what the waiter says. If he tries to tell you that you're wasting your money, tell him he's wasting his time.

On the weekend, everything is different. All those breads, potatoes, and salads are fair game. Depending on how your diet is structured, you can order them twice. Just keep them off your plate during the week.

Aspartame is now the main sugar substitute used in North America, although saccharin and cyclamates are still widely in use (the United States restricts the use of cyclamates and allows saccharin to be used freely, while in Canada the opposite is true), and sucralose and acesulfame K are making headway. Aspartame (sweeter than cyclamate but not as sweet as saccharin) is a human-made substance made of three products—two naturally occurring amino acids, phenylalanine and aspartic acid, and methyl alcohol. All three of the ingredients of aspartame are broken down by the body into natural components—unlike saccharin and cyclamate, which are broken down into synthetic chemicals.

Sodium   Although the metabolic diet allows salt, we usually caution against its overuse—don't overdo the salt in an attempt to compensate for the foods you're not allowed. People with high blood pressure, and those with a family history of high blood pressure or heart disease, should put the salt shaker to rest and make do with the salt that's naturally in many foods or added sparingly while cooking. Women who are prone to fluid retention and bloating and those who experience premenstrual syndrome should also avoid taking in too much salt.

Cutting back on your salt intake may make food taste bland at first, but your taste buds will soon adjust to the lower salt intake. After a while you'll be surprised how much better food tastes when you don't smother it with a layer of salt and the natural flavor comes through.

Those who need to cut back on their salt intake should keep away from foods high in salt even on their higher-calorie days. This includes certain juices (orange juice has much more salt than grapefruit juice), pickles, sauerkraut, canned vegetables, canned fish, diet soda, frozen dinners, ketchup, commercial soups, some cereals and breads, self-rising flours, cured meats, corned beef, olives, baking powder, bouillon cubes, most cheeses, and many other foods.

Also anything that's been processed or changed in some way usually has much higher levels of salt than foods in their natural state. For example, a cup of fresh mushrooms has about 12 milligrams of salt, while cream of mushroom soup has almost 1,000 milligrams. Consider the difference between about 2 ounces (60 g) of pork and hot dogs: The pork has around 50 milligrams of salt, while the hot dogs have more than 1,000 milligrams.

TIMING OF CARBOHYDRATE CONSUMPTION

A real question that comes into play on the higher-fat, low-carbohydrate portion of the metabolic diet is when to eat your carbohydrate during the day. Some people spread their carbohydrate foods out. Others get most of them in one meal. Again, the answer depends on personal preference and finding what optimally works best for you as an individual.

Many people believe our eating patterns have become counterproductive in modern society. The average American eats a lot of carbohydrate during the day, and the insulin and serotonin (a brain neurotransmitter that has been implicated in fatigue) responses can become very pronounced. When they need to be productive and alert, in the early afternoon for instance, they will be sleepy and lethargic from all that carbohydrate and the resulting hormone and neurotransmitter rush.

Carbohydrate lovers are better off saving the carbohydrate foods for later in the day. That is what many people on the metabolic diet do. They minimize carbohydrate during the day and find their energy levels greatly increased as a result. The

PSYCHOLOGICAL CONTROL

Along with hormonal control, you will also find the metabolic diet provides for psychological control. The wide mood swings and irritability that sometimes accompany a carbohydrate-based diet can also increase cortisone. Psychological stress can also be a primary component in decreased testosterone production.

The metabolic diet, in part by controlling insulin, can put a stop to the mood swings and irritability that plague high-carbohydrate diets. It also minimizes the hunger and frustration other diets can create. Let's face it. Any diet can be difficult. Diets involve changing lifestyles, and any change can be stressful. But the flexibility, convenience, and simplicity of the metabolic diet go a long way toward getting rid of the stress that normally accompanies a diet.

carbohydrate at dinner helps them unwind in the evening hours and sleep like a baby at night. A few carboholics reserve their carbohydrate for the evening. They eat almost no carbohydrate during the day so they can have their 30 or so grams at night in the form of ice cream or a chocolate bar. That is OK as long as you do not go over your daily carbohydrate quota.

The ideal time to consume carbohydrate is two hours after exercising. For a few hours after exercise, there is a window of opportunity when hormonal factors are just right for rebuilding muscle. Taking carbohydrate two hours after exercise spikes insulin levels and increases protein synthesis, thus maximizing the effects exercise has on strengthening and toning your body. Once again it comes down to understanding how to achieve the optimal benefits on the lowest level of carbohydrate that can be managed. For most athletes this means not exceeding the suggested 30-gram weekday limit of carbohydrate.

EXPERIMENTING FOR PERSONALIZATION

Personal experience and individual body chemistry will influence how you structure the diet. People will have different responses to the carbohydrate-loading portion. The length of that carbohydrate-loading period may vary greatly as a result.

The 30-gram carbohydrate limit is also not written in stone. It serves as a good guide and should be adhered to when beginning the diet, but some people find they can later increase carbohydrate intake to as high as 50 grams per day and still do fine. Others find that anything over 20 grams makes them feel sluggish. Some people on the higher-calorie diets, mainly in the hypertrophy training phase, can take more than 30 grams and still be OK. Once you have made the metabolic shift, you can experiment to find what works best for you. However, the goal is to find the lowest level of carbohydrate that your system can work with, which in most cases will be around the suggested 30 grams per weekday.

Fat levels may also be experimented with to some degree. Some people find optimal results by going as low as 30 percent fat on the diet, but you must beware. You cannot go too low, especially at first when your body is going through the shift from utilizing fats instead of carbohydrates as its primary fuel.

While taking in a lot of protein helps your body stay in a positive protein balance, you need to consume enough dietary fat to successfully change your metabolism to a fat burning system. Remember, without enough dietary fat, your body will not learn how to use fat as a primary fuel. Your body basically says, "I am not going to get rid of this stuff because I may need it down the road." Limit fat in your diet and your body wants to lay it on as a way of keeping it around. You end up cutting dietary fat but adding body fat (Kather et al. 1987).

The fact is your body needs the fat to adjust to burning fat while at the same time sparing muscle. Increasing dietary fat intake will increase your body's use of both dietary and body fat as a primary fuel by increasing the levels of enzymes needed for increased fat breakdown and decreasing the enzymes involved in storing body fat. The bottom line is you are basically losing body fat by increasing the fat in your diet.

So do not worry too much about your overall fat percentages because they usually take care of themselves unless you mistakenly, at least at first, try to limit your fat intake. Of course you can make some adjustments depending on how you are responding to the diet, but be careful. Remember, if you do not give the body enough fat, you will not make the shift to a fat-based metabolism, and your body will lose its shape, which is exactly what you do not want.

This may sound like nonsense, but it's not. Give the body fat and it will use that fat and burn off the body fat. When you are fat adapted, the body is metabolizing fat as a primary fuel so that even if you cut back on dietary fat, your body will still burn fat and spare muscle, only this time it will get the fat it needs from your body fat.

One of the good things about this diet is that you do not have to become paranoid and keep elaborate charts to consume the proper amount of fat. In fact, if you are diligent about eating red meat and other animal foods, including popular foods such as steak, burgers, ham, fish, pork chops, and consuming oils, such as olive oil and the essential fatty acids, you shouldn't have to worry about hitting the recommended high intake of fat and protein. It will naturally happen.

Again, it's important to realize that individual experimentation will play a large role in the metabolic diet. The diet should be varied to provide the optimal level of performance and success for each person. We are all different to some degree in our body chemistries and needs.

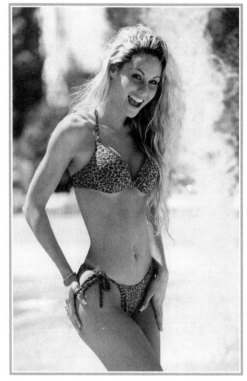

Fitness model Melanie Marden looking lean and sexy.

FINE-TUNING CARBOHYDRATE INTAKE

There are various other ways you can fine-tune the diet so it fits in with your metabolic abilities. Although all of us are able to use fat as our primary fuel, we all have different genetic capabilities. As a result, some of us are efficient fat burners, and some of us are not.

You will know after the first few weeks if you are among the few who have difficulty adjusting and using fats as a primary fuel. These people tend to have a tougher time making the switch, can feel tired, and are easily exhausted by physical activity. It seems they just run out of gas shortly after their weekend carb-up. The reason is their metabolisms prefer carbohydrates to fats and cannot seem to make do on the 5-day, 2-day shift. During the weekend they carbohydrate load and feel OK for the first few days of the week, but when their glycogen reserves are used up, they often feel as if they've been hit by a truck.

Just because your body prefers carbohydrates and cannot operate as well on fats doesn't mean you have to abandon the metabolic diet. It just means you have to change the amount and timing of your carbohydrate intake so that the maximum amount of fat is burned along with the necessary carbohydrates. If you can find the minimum carbohydrate intake you need in order to function normally, then you can benefit from the metabolic diet.

Now let's say you have done the first 2 months but still do not feel right, even though you are using the correct supplements and doing everything right. You may be tired much of the time, especially Wednesday to Friday, and your training may be suffering because you have lost the enthusiasm and stamina you once had. It's time to fine-tune your carbohydrate intake. You can do this in one of several ways.

Increases in Weekday Intake

One way to fine-tune your carbohydrate intake is to gradually increase your daily intake by about 10 grams per day until you reach a level where your symptoms improve. For most people that final level is somewhere between 30 and 100 grams of carbohydrate per day.

Besides finding the baseline carbohydrate level, you also have to determine the best time to consume your carbohydrate foods. It's just as important to time your carbohydrate intake as it is to increase the amount you take in. For people who have to raise their carbohydrate levels, the best time to take the extra carbohydrate is after training. For example, you might want 20 to 30 grams after training along with your posttraining meal or meal-replacement powder.

On the other hand, your low point might be in the evening after you have worked a long day. In this case, a carbohydrate spike right after work might be your best bet. Or you just might want to spread out the extra carbohydrate throughout the day. Do whatever works best for you, keeping in mind that you are looking for the least amount of daily carbohydrate to do the job.

Another important factor is adding the right kinds of carbohydrate. High-glycemic carbohydrate foods are absorbed very quickly and cause a rapid rise in insulin. In most cases, increasing your intake of lower glycemic carbohydrate by increasing your vegetable intake is the best route. For most people, doubling or even tripling the carbohydrate intake in this way helps them over the low-carbohydrate hump and doesn't seem to affect their weight and fat loss while at the same time keeps them from experiencing carbohydrate cravings. If these same people take in carbohydrate from other sources, such as dairy products or high-glycemic foods, it can inhibit their muscle gains and fat loss and make them hungry.

Midweek Spike

Some people find they need a midweek carbohydrate spike to fine-tune their carbohydrate intake. This replenishes their glycogen stores and holds them over until the weekend. You can do the carbohydrate spike in several ways.

One way is to dramatically increase your carbohydrate intake for that day by either taking it in all at once (e.g., a pancake and syrup feed) or spreading it out over the day, using either high-glycemic or low-glycemic foods. One popular way is to do a carbohydrate load lasting an hour on Wednesday morning. During the carbohydrate spike, most people concentrate on loading up with high-glycemic foods and take in between 200 and 1,000 calories in that hour. Once you have had your midweek carbohydrate feed, you should head right back to low-carbohydrate land.

For some people, a midweek jolt of carbohydrate can be very productive for those interested in advanced body shaping or bodybuilding. The increased blood sugar and subsequent insulin spike will increase muscle and liver glycogen dramatically, give you an extra energy "kick," and drive amino acids into muscle cells for increased development. As long as you go right back to the metabolic diet, you will avoid laying down unwanted fat.

In all cases where you increase your carbohydrate intake during the week, it's important to subsequently curb some of your carbohydrate intake over the weekend. That way you will not be overdoing your long-term carbohydrate intake. For example, you might carbohydrate load only one day over the weekend. The idea is to understand what you need to do to create the optimal adjusted working balance.

Short-Term Loading on Weekends

On the weekends you are usually pretty free to take in whatever foods you like. In general, you can increase both your caloric and carbohydrate intake without too much worry over what kinds of foods you eat. However, for some, 2 days of carbohydrate loading may be too much, especially if you go overboard and eat everything in sight. Some people keep their calorie levels at about 2,000 calories per day during the weekdays and jump to 10,000 calories per day on the weekend. Needless to say, this carbohydrate overload on the weekends must be curbed if they are to reach their weight- and fat-loss goals.

Other people can get pretty sensitive to carbohydrate foods and do not feel right after carbohydrate loading. They become bloated, feel tired, and just do not function very well. In these cases, it's best to carb up for just 1 day or even part of a day and then get back on the higher-fat, low-carbohydrate diet. In some cases taking in just one carbohydrate meal may work best. This will make the diet 6 days of high-fat, low-carbohydrate eating and one meal to 1 day of high-carbohydrate eating, but if this works for you then it's the way to go. Again, the length of carbohydrate loading depends on the person. The important thing is to experiment with the length of your weekend carbohydrate load and learn what works best for you.

Eating foods with high glycemic values and less fat will generally lead to a shorter, more intense carbohydrate load. You will almost certainly start to lose tone and retain water, often before the 24-hour mark. By consuming lower-glycemic carbohydrate foods or by combining foods (such as pastas mixed with protein and fat), you will take longer to load. You may want to experiment with both of these approaches to see what works best.

AVOIDING A METABOLIC REVERSAL

Some people cheat on this diet—and they pay for it. They get to Thursday and then suddenly decide they are going to start their carbohydrate load on Friday. They continue the load until Sunday, and guess what? Their bodies shift back to a carbohydrate metabolism. Three days is too much. At that point, you are running a real risk of losing the fat-burning advantage from the diet because of the long-term carbohydrate loading.

One positive of the higher-fat, low-carbohydrate diet is that it is forgiving. If you are at a birthday party in the middle of the week and do not want to be antisocial, you can have that piece of cake. Likewise, business or social events may warrant a high-carbohydrate meal during the week on occasion. Do not worry about it. As long as you get right back on the higher-fat, low-carbohydrate diet, you will not find your body shifting back. After you have been on the diet for a while, it usually takes at least 3 days of continuous carbohydrate loading for your metabolism to start shifting toward becoming a predominantly carbohydrate-burning system.

In fact, the longer you are on the metabolic diet, the more time it seems to take to go back to a carbohydrate metabolism. For those who have been on the diet for years, it may eventually become as difficult to make the switch back to burning glucose for energy as it was to go through the metabolic shift to become a fat burner.

The metabolic diet suppresses the glycolytic pathway used by the body when carbohydrates are the primary energy source. At the same time, the lipolytic (fat burning) pathway is activated. The longer you are on the diet, the more carbohydrate loading it seems to require to fully reactivate the glycolytic pathway. Even if you go out on the road and are forced to change diets for a week, you can generally return to the diet without going through another metabolic shift if you have become a metabolic diet veteran.

VARYING DAILY CALORIC INTAKE

Many bodybuilders have found that if they do the same routine every day, their bodies become used to it and no longer respond. They do not get stronger. They will plateau. You may eventually find this to be true in your own exercise program. It's the same with the metabolic diet.

If you eat the same number of calories every day, you may eventually start to lose the effect of the diet. For this reason you should try to vary calories on a day-to-day basis. Stagger them so that if 2,000 calories a day is your goal, try taking in 3,000 calories one day, 1,000 the next, 2,500 the day after that, and so forth. Table 7.5 provides a 1-week example for a 3,000-calorie diet. Some bodybuilders find they make better progress by keeping the body guessing rather than having it adapt to a fixed daily caloric intake. Being unpredictable keeps your body from making adverse hormonal changes or dropping the basal metabolic rate (BMR) to accommodate a drop in calories.

TABLE 7.5	Staggering a 3,000 Calories per Weekday Diet
Monday	3,500 cal
Tuesday	2,000 cal
Wednesday	3,000 cal
Thursday	4,000 cal
Friday	2,500 cal
Total	15,000 cal (3,000/day)

You can also count your calories on a weekly basis instead of daily. Counting calories on a weekly basis is a good approach if you have difficulty sticking to a daily calorie limit. This approach allows you to take in more calories on some days and fewer on others. If you are strict about your weekly caloric intake, there is no reason not to count calories on a weekly rather than a daily level.

You can also vary those calories on the weekend. A good rule of thumb at the beginning is to increase calories no more than 25 percent over your weekday allotment, but once experienced with the diet, you are on your own. However, you do have to be careful. If you take in a lot of calories, especially the high-glycemic variety, you may find yourself putting on fat very quickly.

INTRODUCING LOW–PROTEIN WEEKENDS

After being on the diet for a while, you may want to treat the weekends as a high-carb, higher-fat exercise while paying less attention to protein. Some people who have been on the diet for an extended period find that a weekend diet of around 40 to 45 percent fat, 50 to 55 percent carbohydrate, and only 7 to 10 percent protein can produce excellent results.

The added fat aids in slowing the release of glucose in the blood, thus preventing sugar rushes and crashes that can leave you feeling spent and irritable. By consuming lower-glycemic foods with increased dietary fat, you will also be able to extend the length of your carbohydrate load and not feel the puffiness and bloating that should signal its end. As for the protein, you are getting enough during the week to get through the weekend with no problems.

Studies show that protein utilization after relative protein restriction rebounds to higher levels than were present before the restriction. Studies also show that in times of protein depletion, the body likely conserves muscle protein and increases the burning of fat stores for energy. This adaptation is usually lost when body-fat stores are near exhaustion (Goodman et al. 1984).

Using Nutritional Supplements

Eating foods as close to their natural forms as possible is the best solution for attaining all your metabolic needs. We have always believed proper dieting refers to the ingestion of vegetables, meats, fish, fats and oils, low-fat dairy products, whole grains, and nuts. These sources are all rich in a combination of important proteins, carbohydrates, fats, vitamins, minerals, fibers, antioxidants, and phytochemicals that athletes require on a daily basis. Unfortunately, in a Westernized society high-pressure jobs, raising families, and social interactions consume a large portion of a person's time. For these reasons, it is recommended that supplements become an integral part of one's daily routine.

Although nutritional supplements can play a vital role in maximizing the effects of exercise, they do not work in a vacuum. They must be coupled with a reasonable lifestyle, proper training routines, and a good diet. Once those three are in order, nutritional supplements can provide an added edge. By using appropriate supplements in the right way and at the right time, you can take athletic performance and body composition to new heights.

Supplements can increase an athlete's anabolic drive and workload capacity and decrease recovery time. Unfortunately, most athletes don't use them properly and thus don't get any significant benefits. Largely because of mistrust and ignorance, people do not use supplements with the same seriousness as they use prescription drugs.

Many supplements gain their anabolic potential in one or more of these ways:

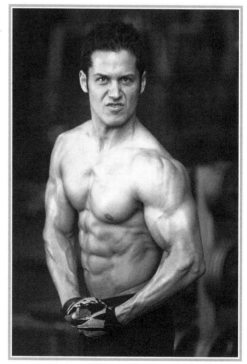

- They increase one's ability to train (e.g., by increasing endurance or by enhancing muscular contraction).
- They increase production of endogenous testosterone, increase growth hormone, or they decrease secretion of cortisol.
- They increase protein synthesis.

Under specific conditions, many nutritional supplements can have positive effects on lean body mass, strength, and endurance. Targeting these supplements is the key to gaining significant amounts of lean body mass and improving athletic performance. The trick to using supplements is to know enough about them in order to use them effectively.

Matt Trudeau believes that nutritional supplements play a vital role in maximizing the effects of training.

BRIEF OVERVIEW OF SOME NUTRITIONAL SUPPLEMENTS

This section provides a brief overview of some of the more popular nutritional supplements to better inform you about their individual properties and about how you can combine them to increase their overall effects on performance and body composition. Many of these nutritional supplements, as either single ingredients or in formulations, can be found in offerings from various supplement companies.

If you already have a balanced diet, then nutritional supplements are not as important for you as for someone whose daily diet is not sufficient. In saying that, you need to comprehend what category you are in. Are you getting a balanced diet with all the necessary food groups, vitamins, and minerals, or are you deficient in these needs?

Vitamins and Minerals

Vitamins and minerals are the metabolic catalysts that regulate biochemical reactions within your body. Many people consume vitamins and minerals, either as part of fortified foods or as supplements. When you mention nutritional supplements, most people think of the daily vitamin pill. The vitamin and mineral "stack" is the most pervasive example of combining a number of supplements together for ease of use and, in some cases, for additive or synergistic effects.

Low intakes of various nutrients can lead to marginal deficiencies. Low intake is a problem in a significant proportion of athletes, especially those watching weight and body composition and who thus do not consume sufficient amounts of many nutrients from foods alone. These deficiencies can be exacerbated by exercise since exercise can increase the need for certain nutrients. For example, lower than normal intake of magnesium along with strenuous exercise, which has been shown to increase the rate of magnesium loss via sweat and urine, can lead to a marginal deficiency. This in turn can impair energy metabolism, muscle function, oxygen uptake, and electrolyte balance (Nielsen and Lukaski 2006; Laires and Monterio 2008).

Stacking vitamin C with quercetin (water-soluble plant pigment) has proven to be an excellent antioxidant and has been shown to increase brain and muscle mitochondrial biogenesis and exercise tolerance, and thus this combination may enhance athletic performance (Davis et al. 2009). Alpha-lipoic acid (a saturated fat derived from octanoic acid) has been shown to enhance insulin sensitivity; decrease postexercise lactic acid concentrations; and have potent antioxidant effects by combining with other vitamins, such as vitamin C, vitamin D, and vitamin E, to have positive effects on the body (Kinnunen et al. 2009). Many nutrients have multiple actions in the body. For example, selenium also has significant anti-inflammatory properties (Duntas 2009).

As noted, problems can arise from exercise-induced mineral loss, which is further enhanced by the fact that many of us don't consume adequate amounts of many essential minerals. For example, one study found an increase in selenium requirements with exercise (Margaritis et al. 2005). Studies show that many athletes, and female athletes, in particular, consume diets that are inadequate for certain key minerals such as zinc, magnesium, copper, and iron. The combination of strenuous exercise and compromised mineral status ultimately leads to low endurance capacity, depressed immune function, and the development of a variety of disease conditions.

Anyone who exercises should consider taking a daily multiple vitamin and mineral supplement. This will ensure they're not suffering from any marginal deficiencies, will provide higher levels of certain nutrients that may offer physiological and metabolic benefits, and will act as a preventative measure against some conditions and diseases (Tuohimaa et al. 2009; Bonjour et al. 2009; Evans 2006; Newman et al. 2007).

Zinc Zinc deficiency in humans is widespread, and athletes may be particularly prone to lower plasma zinc levels (Cordova and Alvarez-Mon 1995; Prasad 1996). Zinc is a constituent of more than a hundred fundamentally important enzymes. A deficiency of zinc can negatively affect nearly every body function (Kieffer 1986).

Especially where a deficiency may be present, supplemental zinc has resulted in increased secretion of growth hormone, IGF-1 (Dorup et al. 1991), and testosterone (Ghavami-Maibodi et al. 1983); and it has been observed to raise plasma testosterone and sperm count (Hartoma, Nahoul, and Netter 1977; Hunt et al. 1992). As well, zinc deficiency can adversely affect the reproductive hormones and as such impair athletic efforts (Oteiza et al. 1995). A recent study looked at the effects of zinc deficiency on physical performance and found that low dietary zinc was associated with impaired cardiorespiratory function and impaired metabolic responses during exercise (Lukaski 2005). Zinc deficiency may also adversely affect protein synthesis. One study on rats investigated the effects of zinc deficiency on the levels of free amino acids in urine, plasma, and skin extract (Hsu 1977). Zinc deficiency adversely affected skin protein synthesis.

A recent study indicates that zinc supplementation in wrestlers prevents production of free radicals by activating the antioxidant system. The authors concluded that physiological doses of zinc supplementation in athletes may beneficially contribute to their health and performance (Kara et al. 2010).

Magnesium Magnesium supplementation has been shown to increase protein synthesis and strength (Brilla and Haley 1992). Another study concluded that insulin sensitivity could be improved by reducing excess body weight, by getting regular physical activity, and possibly by correcting a magnesium deficiency (Lefebvre and Scheen 1995) that has not yet begun to show symptoms.

Calcium Calcium permits the contractile actin and myosin filaments of the muscle cell to associate and produce the force that generates movement. When the neuron innervating a muscle cell signals that cell to contract, calcium is released from the sarcoplasmic reticulum into the region of the contractile filaments, thereby permitting contraction to occur. In one study, supplemental calcium appeared effective in prolonging the time of onset of fatigue in striated muscle (Richardson, Palmerton, and Chenan 1980).

Calcium can prevent muscle cramping during exercise. It is suspected that calcium may also increase growth hormone secretion during exercise. If you feel you need extra calcium, take 500 to 1,000 milligrams of calcium before working out and 500 to 1,000 milligrams during the workout.

Vitamin D Vitamin D is a group of closely related chemicals that regulate absorption of ingested calcium by the intestine. Along with calcium, vitamin D is intimately involved in skeletal homeostasis. But each does much more. Vitamin

D has several vital functions outside this established role. It has been shown to have important implications for general health, immunity, and cognitive function (Adams and Hewison 2008; Ceglia 2008; Buell et al. 2009). Of importance for athletes, vitamin D is intimately involved in body composition, athletic performance, and risk of injury (Bartoszewska, Kamboj, and Patel 2010; Hamilton 2010).

Chromium Chromium is involved in carbohydrate and lipid metabolism. Because the need for chromium increases with exercise (Anderson et al. 1982), and since modern refined foods are low in chromium, athletes may need to incorporate chromium-rich foods or supplements into their diets. If you are engaged in a highly aggressive exercise program, chromium deficiency, even if just marginal, may become a concern (Lefavi et al. 1992). Insufficient dietary chromium has been linked to maturity-onset diabetes and cardiovascular diseases, with supplemental chromium resulting in improvements of risk factors associated with these diseases (Anderson 1986).

Antioxidants

The focus of antioxidant use is on free radicals—highly reactive molecules that possess unpaired electrons. These free radicals play a sizable role in the normal metabolism of food and the use of energy resources during exercise. It is also strongly suspected that they react with the components of body cells in a way that leads to molecular damage and cell death—and, eventually, to aging and death itself. Chemical reactions involving free radicals in the body have been implicated in causing or contributing to cancer, atherosclerosis (hardening of the arteries), hypertension, Alzheimer's disease, immune deficiency, arthritis, diabetes, Parkinson's disease, and various other diseases linked with the aging process. Antioxidants can significantly protect the body from the high free radical concentrations that may lead to these diseases (Packer and Landvik 1989).

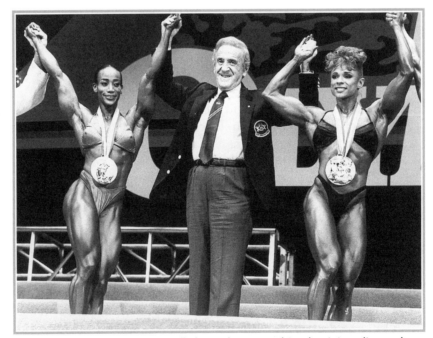

Lenda Murray and Laura Creavalle have always combined training, diet, and nutritional supplements to maintain championship physiques.

A growing amount of data show that heavy exercise can increase the formation of free radicals, which then leads to muscle fatigue, inflammation, and damage to muscle tissue (Reid et al. 1992). Exercise can also decrease the supply of antioxidants. Vitamin E levels, for instance, can decline severely with training, thus depleting the muscle of its most important antioxidant (Gohil et al. 1987).

Emotional stress can raise levels of free radicals just as much as does physical stress (as caused by exercise). During normal conditions, free radicals are generated at a low rate and neutralized by antioxidants in the liver, skeletal muscle, and other systems. But under stress, they greatly increase and can overwhelm the body's ability to neutralize them. Unchecked, they can cause premature aging and breakdown of the body.

Although some recent studies have brought the overall role of antioxidants into some question, the preponderance of evidence still shows that antioxidants can help undo much of the dirty work done by free radicals. If you're following the metabolic diet, and especially if you are exercising as you should, you must make a place for antioxidants in your diet.

Use of Antioxidants by Athletes   Several studies have shown that bolstering antioxidant defenses may ameliorate exercise-induced damage (Packer 1997). For example, one study looked at the effects of resistance exercise on free radical production. Twelve recreationally weight-trained males were divided into two groups. The supplement group received 1,200 IU (international units) of vitamin E once a day for 2 weeks. The control group received placebos. The data indicated that high-intensity resistance exercise increased free radical production and that vitamin E supplementation may decrease muscle membrane disruption (Mcbride et al. 1998).

When used correctly, antioxidants can give an added edge in creating a healthy, fit, and attractive body. They are especially important for those who embark on an advanced, more demanding exercise program. If you are in such an advanced program, you may want to go beyond the minimum amounts provided by multivitamins to maximize the advantages antioxidants can bring.

Although you can consume antioxidants daily, you definitely should consume them, in addition to your daily multivitamin, on days you work out. We also recommend eating a lot of vegetables (especially broccoli, cabbage, lettuce, and leafy greens) and even drinking a glass of red wine with your evening meal. With this combination, most people should cover their antioxidant needs.

Ergogenic Effects of Antioxidants   Skeletal muscle has an amazing capacity to adapt and repair itself. However, significantly increased levels of physical activity, such as intense training, chronic long-duration exercise, and overtraining, limit the body's ability to adapt to tissue damage and will lead to some degree of maladaptation and musculoskeletal tissue changes that are counterproductive to both skeletal muscle function and performance.

Antioxidants form a frontline defense against cell damage caused by free radicals, which are involved in muscle, joint, and tendon damage and inflammation; degenerative arthritis; and even the aging process. The use of antioxidants can reduce free radical damage that occurs when we exercise (Vincent et al. 2006) and can also lessen the ongoing damage to injured tissues caused by free radicals, thus accelerating the healing process. Antioxidants have been shown to enhance aerobic performance (Aguilo et al. 2007).

Antioxidants such as vitamins C and E, selenium, green tea, reduced glutathione, and N-acetylcysteine (NAC) can play an important role in reducing inflammation and fatigue, decreasing tissue damage, and preventing and treating injuries. Various antioxidants, such as vitamin E, have been found useful in the treatment of some forms of arthritis (Sangha and Stucki 1998) and in dealing with the oxidative stress of exercise (Sacheck and Blumberg 2001). Oxidative damage contributes to the pathogenesis of injuries and arthritis, and antioxidants, such as NAC (Zafarullah et al. 2003), have therapeutic value for reducing endothelial dysfunction, inflammation, fibrosis, invasion, and cartilage erosion.

One study found that a combination of two antioxidants, epigallocatechin gallate (EGCG; the main antioxidant in green tea extract) and selenomethionine, had beneficial effects on catabolic and anabolic gene expression of articular chondrocytes (Agarwal, Gupta, and Sharma 2005). The authors of the study concluded that EGCG and selenomethionine regulate chondrocyte metabolism and exert global beneficial effects on articular cartilage.

Various nutrients are necessary for priming the endogenous (originating within the body) antioxidant systems. For example, some minerals (copper, zinc, selenium) contribute to the antioxidant defense system by acting as cofactors for antioxidant Cu-Zn superoxide dismutase and glutathione peroxidase activities.

Supplemental exogenous (originating from sources outside the body) antioxidants interact with endogenous antioxidants to provide protection from the increase in free radicals produced by exercise. Supplemental antioxidants are crucial for those who perform acute and chronic intense or exhaustive exercise and training since this intensity of training produces excessive free radical production and irreparable oxidative damage that overwhelms the endogenous antioxidant system, resulting in irreparable tissue damage, proneness to injury, and ill health.

Compounds With Potent Antioxidant Properties Some antioxidants are particularly potent. Along with an ability to protect muscle tissue, vitamin E also seems to limit arterial damage caused by aging and to minimize the adverse effects of harmful fats on the body (Yoshida and Kajimoto 1989). Vitamin C provides direct protection from free radical damage and also conserves vitamin E (Sies, Stahl, and Sundquist 1992). They work together synergistically in controlling muscle breakdown.

Selenium plays a role in converting fats and protein into energy and provides antioxidant protection when taken with vitamin E. Note that vitamin E not only is an important force in its own right but also is important in enhancing the effects of other antioxidants.

Carotenes come naturally from plants such as carrots, cantaloupes, sweet potatoes, and other orange, green, and yellow vegetables. Many of the carotenes are also called provitamin A because the body converts them into vitamin A. Beyond this, there is evidence that carotenes can also strengthen the immune system and protect against body tissue damage (Bendich 1989).

By far the most well known carotenoid is beta-carotene. What makes it especially compelling is its importance in oxidizing low-density lipoproteins (LDLs) (Lavy, Ben-Amotz, and Aviram 1993). Yet beta-carotene taken by itself can be counterproductive, reinforcing our feelings that antioxidants, or for that matter any vitamin or mineral, should not be used in large doses on their own.

Alpha-lipoic acid (ALA) has potent antioxidant properties intrinsically, secondary to its ability to increase levels of intracellular glutathione and its ability to recycle other antioxidants such as vitamin C, vitamin E, and glutathione (Bast and

Haenen 2003; Packer, Witt, and Tritschler 1995; Jones et al. 2002; Packer, Tritschler, and Wessel 1997; Podda et al. 1994). ALA and glutathione have been shown to have significant effects in decreasing mercury toxicity in the body (Patrick 2002).

ALA has other beneficial effects, such as decreasing proinflammatory cytokines (Packer 1998; Lee and Hughes 2002) and secondary cortisol elevations. ALA also has significant anabolic effects secondary to its beneficial effects on insulin sensitivity and the secretion of growth hormone and IGF-1, all factors involved in maintaining, repairing, and regenerating musculoskeletal tissues (Faust et al. 1994; Burkart et al. 1993; Lateef et al. 2005; Thirunavukkarasu, Nandhini, and Anuradha 2004). ALA is also useful in reversing mitochondrial dysfunction, especially in aging mitochondria (Arivazhagan, Ramanathan, and Panneerselvam 2001; Palaniappan and Dai 2007).

Omega-3 Fatty Acids

Omega-3 fatty acids are long-chain polyunsaturated fatty acids that are converted to a number of active substances in the body such as prostaglandins and leukotrienes; they also are involved in a number of metabolic events. As you learned in chapter 6, linolenic acid is an essential omega-3 fatty acid since the body cannot synthesize it. Other omega-3 fatty acids, however, are synthesized in the body from linolenic acid.

As discussed in chapter 6, the omega-3 fatty acids eicosapentaenoic acid (EPA) and docosahexaenoic acid (DHA) are found in fish oils, which we recommend. Omega-3 fatty acids may increase growth hormone secretion since they are involved in the formation of prostaglandin E1, which in turn is involved in release of growth hormone (GH) (Dray et al. 1980).

Omega-3 fatty acids also provide an anabolic effect by increasing the binding of IGF-1 to skeletal muscle and improving insulin sensitivity, even in diets high in fat, which have a tendency to decrease insulin sensitivity (Liu et al. 1994). As well, they increase fatty acid oxidation (fat burning), increase basal metabolic rates, and lower cholesterol.

Conjugated Linoleic Acid (CLA)

Conjugated linoleic acid (CLA), a mixture of positional and geometric isomers of linoleic acid (LA), is found preferentially in dairy products and meat. CLA is present in cheese, milk, and yogurt that have undergone heat treatment, as well as in beef and venison. Supplementation with 4 ounces (120 g) of cheddar cheese daily was found to increase the ratio of CLA to LA by 130 percent.

CLA appears to have beneficial properties beyond those of linoleic acid. It has shown potential as a powerful anticarcinogen (Ip, Scimeca, and Thompson 1994; Ip et al. 1994) and exhibits potent antioxidant activity (Pariza et al. 1991). CLA may be cytotoxic to human cancer cells in vivo (Shultz et al. 1992). Of importance for those wishing to maximize lean body mass, CLA has possible anticatabolic properties (Cook et al. 1993; Miller et al. 1994).

A team of Scandinavian researchers found that CLA helped overweight and obese people mobilize fat from cells while

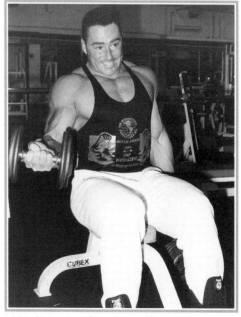

Vito Binetti pushing himself to the limit.

revving up muscle metabolism (Blankson et al. 2000). People taking CLA also saw reductions in total and LDL cholesterol. The authors of the study concluded that consumption of CLA appears to reduce body fat in overweight and moderately obese healthy people.

Caffeine, Ephedrine, and Aspirin

Although a number of studies show that caffeine may favorably affect long-term endurance performance (McNaughton 1986), data on high-intensity, short-term exercise have been mixed (Williams 1991). Still, it seems very likely from an analysis of the biochemical effects of caffeine that it has a beneficial effect on short-term fatigue and muscle fibers in high-intensity, short-term exercise such as weightlifting (Dodd, Herb, and Powers 1993; Jacobson et al. 1992).

Ephedrine is banned by all major sporting federations because it is a powerful stimulant and provides an unfair performance advantage (e.g., delays onset of fatigue, boosts performance). Ephedrine has mild amphetamine-like CNS effects and is used by athletes to enhance training and performance. Aspirin is widely used by athletes for several reasons. It is a common mild pain killer, has anti-inflammatory properties, and has some thermogenic effects. A combination of caffeine, ephedrine, and aspirin is commonly used as a thermogenic cocktail to promote lipolysis (the breakdown of fat) while decreasing muscle breakdown. The result is an increased ratio of lean body mass to fat.

The main hypothesis regarding adding aspirin and caffeine to ephedrine is that the synergism allows for reduced dosages of ephedrine without reducing efficacy. This results in a decrease of side effects, such as cardiac stimulation, from the ephedrine. Whether or not small amounts of aspirin have this effect is open to debate. Nevertheless, aspirin is used widely with the other two compounds.

Although the use of ephedrine and caffeine results in increased lipolysis, there is some doubt as to whether this lipolysis translates into fat loss. Some data indicate that ephedrine, while increasing lipolysis, does not increase the beta-oxidation of fatty acids—the increased lipolysis simply results in increased reesterification of fatty acids and no net change in body fat. This is certainly the case with those adapted to higher-carbohydrate diets, but not with people adapted to higher-fat, low-carbohydrate diets where there is an increased use and oxidation of free fatty acids.

Anticortisol Supplements

Any type of stress—including high levels of exercise, physical or emotional trauma, infections, or surgery—translates into hypothalamic and pituitary changes that result in increased cortisol secretion. Exercise itself, while increasing cortisol, has compensatory anticatabolic effects. Short, intense training sessions tend to result in more moderate cortisol secretion. Well-conditioned athletes show less cortisol secretion during exercise compared with their out-of-shape peers. One measure of overtraining is the ratio of testosterone to cortisol. Elevated cortisol in relation to testosterone is considered indicative of overtraining—that is, if you train properly, your testosterone will rise, while cortisol remains stable.

Vitamin C has some anticatabolic effects that likely involve decreasing exercise-induced cortisol but may also work through its antioxidant action. Conversely, some of the anticatabolic effects of antioxidants may be mediated through a decrease in cortisol. A gram or so of vitamin C, along with some vitamin E (400 IU), beta-carotene (20,000 IU), zinc (50 milligrams), and selenium (50 micrograms) before workouts might be useful.

A supplement has been marketed that may decrease exercise-induced rises in cortisol. According to some studies, phosphatidylserine appears to blunt the pituitary-mediated cortisol response to exercise. Although more research needs to be done to see if the decrease in cortisol translates into increased gains, phosphatidylserine may be of benefit; you may want to include it in your supplement stack, taking 1 or 2 grams before each training session. One caveat: There may be an increase in training soreness, stiffness, and injuries secondary to the cortisol reduction. Consider the benefit-to-risk ratio when using these compounds.

L-Carnitine

L-carnitine appears to increase the body's use of free fatty acids and fatty tissue as an energy source. More fat becomes available for energy, thus saving protein in the muscle cells. Muscle breakdown may also be reduced. Athletes have used doses ranging from 100 to 3,000 milligrams or more per day before training with good effect. However, it seems that at least 2 grams per day (i.e., at least 2,000 milligrams) is needed for the desired effects.

On the other hand it does not appear that carnitine is a limiting factor in the transport and utilization of fatty acids. So while the jury is still out on the effectiveness of carnitine, it makes sense to use it, especially at times when energy output is increased. If you're on an enhanced exercise program, you may at least want to try L-carnitine. Just be sure to look for the name *L-carnitine* on the label. Some manufacturers use a cheaper, less effective form. Some sources, especially the cheaper ones or ones that say they are "professional grade," contain nonpharmaceutical grade L-carnitine, which almost always has significant quantities of toxic D-carnitine.

Creatine Monohydrate

In the early 1980s, as anabolic steroids fell into disrepute, manufacturers began creating products that were supposedly "even better than steroids." In most instances these claims were proven false. Most athletes soon became skeptical that nutritional supplements really did anything at all to improve strength, muscle mass, or athletic performance.

The attitude of most athletes has turned from disbelief to amazement because certain nutritional supplements do work. One of the supplements that helped turn the tide is creatine monohydrate. Although not as effective as high doses of anabolic steroids, creatine works—but it has none of the side effects associated with anabolic drugs. It helps increase muscle mass, provides greater levels of energy, and helps people recover more quickly after an exercise session. The basic mechanism of creatine's action is to help the cells convert ADP to ATP (the cells' basic energy source) at an accelerated pace.

Creatine is used by participants in all kinds of sports, including bodybuilders, Olympic athletes, football players, hockey players, soccer players, softball players, and even tennis players. Potential side effects from overdosing are dehydration, overheating, and kidney damage.

Protein Supplementation

Athletes need higher levels of dietary protein than do sedentary people. Many athletes turn to protein supplements to augment their dietary protein intake. Good sources of dietary protein include eggs, meat, fish, soy, and dairy products. Whole-protein supplements are usually inexpensive and generally contain soybean, milk, and egg protein; hydrolyzed protein with variable amounts of di-, tri-, and polypeptides; and amino acid mixtures.

The consensus is that no valid scientific or medical studies show that supplements of intact protein have an anabolic advantage over high-quality protein foods. Yet there do appear to be certain advantages to the use of whole-protein supplements by some athletes, including the following:

- They are convenient to prepare and store and have a long shelf life.
- They are useful as a protein replacement for those wishing to decrease dietary fat (many protein-rich foods tend to contain fat).
- They enable people to raise their protein intake while minimizing caloric intake.
- They can increase dietary protein in people who cannot eat the volume of food necessary to ensure adequate or increased protein intake.
- In some cases, the cost of protein supplements is lower than corresponding high-protein foods.

Protein supplements have other distinct advantages over whole-food protein in hypocaloric, isocaloric, and hypercaloric diets. Many studies show that protein supplements, including milk and soy proteins, have ergogenic effects (Dragan, Vasiliu, and Georgescu 1985; Dragan, Wagner, and Ploesteanu 1988; Laricheva et al. 1977). These studies found that supplemental proteins significantly improved athletes' physiological condition, led to better sports performance, and resulted in significant increases of lean body mass and strength. Athletes who used dietary protein supplements experienced greater gain in muscle than those who simply took in the equivalent amount of calories. Moreover, protein supplements with other ingredients, such as creatine monohydrate, taurine, and L-glutamine, often enhance gains in lean body mass.

Meal replacement products (MRPs), whether for weight loss or weight gain, give you the standard macro- and micronutrients at different calorie levels. They may be either more or less costly than whole foods you can get at your supermarket. As an all-in-one package, they are usually more convenient and provide better nutrition than many people obtain from junk food meals and high-calorie but nutrient-deficient snacks. For certain effects, the engineered cutting-edge food supplements are better than whole-food protein sources and can be safely and effectively used to increase dietary protein intake and as meal replacements for up to two meals a day. Nevertheless, if you are conscientious about what you buy and eat and are willing to put in the time and effort, you can do as well or better by just buying the whole foods and planning your own diet for weight gain or weight loss.

The best protein supplements are specific combinations of various high-quality proteins. Taking a combination of supplemental protein not only increases dietary protein—which should be even higher when you are trying to lose body fat and weight than at any other time—but also gives your metabolism, thyroid hormone levels, and metabolic rate a boost.

As mentioned previously, it is important to take in at least 1 gram of protein per pound of body weight every day. It's best to spread the intake out in intervals of no more than 3 hours while you are awake. Take some before bed and as soon as you get up to decrease the catabolic effects of the fast that you go through while sleeping. If you wake up during the night, that's a good time to take some more protein to even further decrease muscle catabolism.

Amino Acids

Increased blood levels of amino acids, secondary to a high-protein meal, can cause insulin and growth hormone levels to rise. Increasing these hormones—while increasing amino acid levels but at the same time decreasing muscle catabolism—leads to an enhanced anabolic response.

Studies show that ingestion of branched-chain amino acids modifies the hormonal environment. There is also some information that amino acids (primarily methionine) and the dipeptides methionine-glutamine and tryptophan-isoleucine have a profound anabolic effect: By providing the right reparative elements, these amino acids increase protein synthesis and promote muscle healing. These substances could override or block the increase in glucocorticoid levels in diabetic patients, but further research needs to be performed with diabetic patients to substantiate these findings.

Protein taken after training may increase both insulin and growth hormone and thus have anabolic effects. Increased amino acid availability has been shown to directly influence protein synthesis, especially within a few hours after physical exercise. The rate of protein synthesis, protein catabolism, and amino acid transport is normally increased after exercise and depends on amino acid availability. If there is an increase in the availability of amino acids during this postexercise window, then catabolic processes are more than offset by increased anabolic processes, resulting in an overall increase in cellular contractile protein. Thus it is vital to increase the absorption of amino acids as quickly as possible after exercise.

Food intake can stimulate muscle protein synthesis secondary to increased insulin release, because insulin can

Trevor Butler's training regimen and dedicated dietary habits lead to an enhanced anabolic response.

directly stimulate muscle protein synthesis and, to at least some extent, decrease protein breakdown (Biolo, Fleming, and Wolfe 1995); an improvement in energy balance may affect net muscle protein balance (Butterfield and Calloway 1984). However, the primary way in which one would expect food intake to stimulate muscle protein synthesis is through increased delivery of amino acids to the muscle.

Glutamine

Individual or selectively combined amino acids may also serve as performance supplements. An example is the amino acid glutamine. Glutamine is the most abundant amino acid in the body, making up more than 50 percent of the intracellular and extracellular amino acids. It plays a major role in liver function, serves as cellular fuel to muscle and other tissue in the body, and may regulate protein synthesis (Rennie et al. 1989).

Most important to the serious athlete and fitness enthusiast is glutamine's ability to increase protein production (for muscle building) and decrease protein degradation (resulting in muscle breakdown). Both depend on the size of the glutamine pool in a muscle cell. If it is high, other amino acids won't be forced into glutamine production and will be available for protein synthesis. Skeletal muscle that might have been used to replace glutamine is spared. Glutamine also maintains amino acid balance in the body, thus enabling the body to synthesize more protein and possibly decrease symptoms of overtraining.

Glutamine supplementation may offer a number of advantages to athletes. Exogenous glutamine can spare intramuscular glutamine and result in decreased proteolysis (the breakdown of proteins into amino acids by the action of enzymes) and potentially increased levels of muscle protein. Glutamine can efficiently lead to release of growth hormone and perhaps to higher levels of other anabolic hormones. All these factors strongly suggest that glutamine supplementation may play a major role in enhancing the effects of resistance training.

Branched-Chain Amino Acids

The branched-chain amino acids (BCAAs), including isoleucine, leucine, and valine, have a carbon chain that branches from the main linear carbon backbone. The BCAAs have been investigated for their anticatabolic and anabolic effects. In heart and skeletal muscle in vitro, increasing the concentration of these three BCAAs or of leucine alone reproduces the effects of increasing the supply of all amino acids in stimulating protein synthesis and inhibiting protein degradation (May and Buse 1989).

MAXIMIZING USE OF SUPPLEMENTS

Nutritional supplements can be useful in many ways, provided they are appropriately targeted. Targeting involves using a variety of supplements in tandem (known as *stacking*) to increase the effects of the supplements, using the supplements at the right times, and *cycling* some of the supplements. Cycling ensures that the supplements will do the most good, and it also decreases any tolerance that might develop with long-term uninterrupted use.

Stacking

Nutritional supplements are used for various reasons (e.g., to increase performance and to affect body composition). Since a large number of supplements are available, it is natural that certain ones will be used together to illicit certain effects, which is called stacking. Following are examples of different stacks for different situations.

Preworkout Stack   The purpose of a preworkout or pretraining stack is to maximize energy levels, minimize protein catabolism, increase protein synthesis, increase GH and testosterone levels, and decrease cortisol. An example of a preworkout stack is Resolve, a stack with ephedrine and yohimbine. It includes the following ingredients:

Alpha-lipoic acid	Glutathione
Banaba extract	Inosine
Caffeine USP	L-alanine
Calcium (as calcium phosphate)	N-acetyl cysteine
Cayenne (pepper)	Octacosanol
Chromium	Pyruvic acid
Cinnamon	Taurine
Co-enzyme Q10	Vitamin A
Cordycepic acid	Vitamin C
Dimethylglycine	White willow extract
Ephedrine alkaloids	Yohimbine alkaloids
Ginger	

Workout Stack   An example of a workout stack to be used while training is a training drink. The combination of higher amino acid levels at a time when blood flow is increased appears to maximize muscle protein synthesis. Concentrations of the drink's amino acids and other ingredients should vary depending on whether the training is endurance or for muscle mass and power. In all cases the drink should (1) provide rehydration, electrolyte replacement, energy replacement, and some of the preworkout functions—including increased protein synthesis and decreased muscle catabolism—and (2) decrease overtraining effects and muscle injury.

A good training drink for power athletes should contain at least 30 grams of whey protein isolate (a "fast" protein that results in high systemic amino acid levels—more than 25 percent of them branched). It also would do well to contain the following:

Arginine	Phosphorus
Calcium	Potassium
Creatine	Ribose
Glutamine peptides	Sodium
Leucine	Taurine
Magnesium	

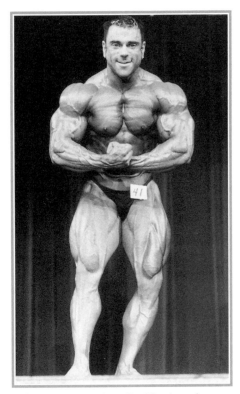

The amazing Nelson Da Silva has always believed that proper stacking, cycling, and timing of nutritional supplements plays a key role in peaking for an important event.

Postworkout Stack Intake of fats, protein, and individual amino acids (and, in particular, certain combinations of amino acids) after exercise can increase ATP-PC storage, protein synthesis, and the anabolic effects of exercise. A proper combination of protein and some fat right after exercise appears to achieve the following benefits, especially if you are following the metabolic diet and are fat adapted:

- Reversing the decreased protein synthesis seen with exercise
- Replenishing muscle glycogen and intramuscular triglycerides
- Increasing protein synthesis and decreasing protein catabolism postexercise
- Raising levels of growth hormone and testosterone
- Increasing the efficiency of recuperation

There are two distinct stages to consider: the time immediately after training and the time 2 to 3 hours later. Immediately after a workout, ingestion of a targeted mixture of amino acids that are absorbed almost immediately induces a strong and rapid increase of aminoacidemia, which in turn acutely stimulates protein synthesis and decreases muscle catabolism. Acute amino acid intake and absorption stimulates the transport of amino acids into muscle, and there is a direct link between amino acid inward transport and muscle protein synthesis (Wolfe 2000). It also appears that a number of amino acids may increase secretion of two powerful anabolic hormones: growth hormone and insulin (Bucci et al. 1990; Iwasaki et al. 1987).

Interestingly, the simultaneous ingestion of carbohydrate and protein decreases the absorption rate of amino acids (Mariotti et al. 2000). You therefore should limit your intake immediately postexercise to amino acids only—no carbohydrate until 2 hours postexercise (Di Pasquale, 2002). Immediately after training, you should ingest amino acids or whey protein powder in order to maximize protein synthesis and stores of intramuscular triglycerides. For more information on postworkout nutrition and the metabolic diet, see chapters 12 through 17.

Ephedra–Caffeine–Aspirin Stack A combination of ephedra, caffeine, and aspirin is used to increase lipolysis and thermogenesis, increase both anaerobic and aerobic performance, and maintain protein synthesis. The net goal is increased lean body mass and less body fat. Many other compounds can be added to this stack to make it more effective for weight and fat loss and for maintaining muscle mass.

Cycling

Athletes cycle nutrient supplements for two reasons. First, they have increased need for certain supplements only at certain phases of training, and it is senseless to waste money on supplements when they will do little good. Second, because the body adapts to certain supplements, they become less useful if they are taken for prolonged periods. Going off the supplements allows the body to return to normal so it will once again get maximum results when the supplements are reintroduced.

The body sometimes adapts only to particular actions of supplements. For example, the ephedra–caffeine–aspirin stack gradually loses its effects on the central nervous system but may not lose its ability to stimulate thermogenesis or to increase oxidation of free fatty acids during exercise. Athletes often cycle creatine, using it only during the most intensive training.

Just as training is most effective when periodized, nutritional supplements can be as well. If you are following a 12-week cycle of training, you might also vary your nutritional supplement intake according to the phase of training. At the beginning, in the first training cycle, you might use only a multivitamin and multimineral tablet—or perhaps some antioxidants, some extra protein, or some meal replacement powders or bars. In the next, more intense phase of training, you may choose to introduce creatine, a pretraining stack, and a posttraining amino acid mix. In the most intense phase of this training cycle, you might want to use some GH- and testosterone-boosting stacks and more comprehensive support in and around training. Chapters 12 through 17 provide additional information on cycling both diet and nutritional supplements.

Timing

The timing of supplement intake can be as important as the supplements taken, often determining whether a certain supplement stack is effective. There is almost always a best time to take supplements for maximum effects; there are ineffective times as well. Timing differs according to the supplement.

Caffeine and certain amino acids, for example, are best taken within a half hour or so of training. A macronutrient mix works best when taken within a few hours of training. GH-boosting formulations work best before training and before sleep.

Timing can also maximize the use of protein supplements. For example, the best times for taking protein supplements are first thing in the morning to put an abrupt end to the catabolic effects of fasting while asleep; after training to take advantage of the increased protein synthesis that occurs after exercise; and immediately before bed to make use of the increased growth hormone secretion during the night and to put off the nighttime catabolic response.

RECOMMENDATIONS FOR SUPPLEMENTING

Use of nutritional supplements is both an art and a science. Even with the scientific information in hand, athletes must experiment to determine how each supplement interacts with their unique metabolisms and with their specific needs and goals. Only you can work out which supplements work best for you and when to use them.

For maximum results from nutritional supplements, use products in which a number of ingredients have been stacked together synergistically and that are designed for specific times and training cycles. For a list of supplements that can be used for specific phases of training, please refer to chapters 12 through 17 or go to www.MauroMD.com.

PART THREE

MAXIMUM STIMULATION
EXERCISES

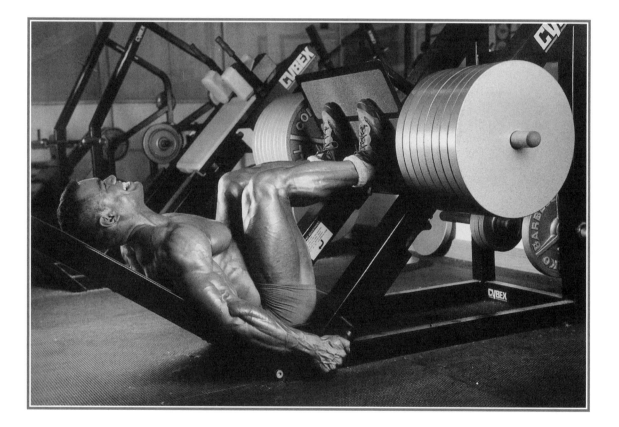

Choosing the Best Exercises

Unlike in strength training, very little research has been done in the area of bodybuilding. Much of the "knowledge" put forth by self-proclaimed experts in the industry is primarily the product of trial and error, scientifically void observations passed on from one generation to the next. Tradition, unsupported by scientific information, has validated and perpetuated a number of myths in the world of bodybuilding and even in that of strength training. In the interest of safety, and for the development of our sport, we took to the laboratory to test some of these myths.

ELECTROMYOGRAPHICAL RESEARCH

Electromyography (EMG) has become an essential research tool, allowing physiologists and medical experts to determine the role of muscles during specific movements (Melo and Cararelli 1994-1995). Electromyography measures the level of excitation (electrical signals) of a muscle group. Muscle contraction is initiated by electrical charges that travel across the membrane of muscle fibers, and this movement of ion flow can be measured at the skin by a surface electromyogram (SEMG) (Kobayashi Matsui 1983; Moritani, Muro, and Nagata 1986). An SEMG is representative of the entire electrical activity of the motor units and the frequency of their firing rates for each muscle being examined (DeLuca et al. 1982; Moritani and deVries 1987).

We conducted a series of studies to find, through EMG recordings, which exercises cause the greatest amount of stimulation within each muscle group and, consequently, to determine which exercises will produce the greatest gains in mass and strength. Figure 9.1 shows the EMG activity during a standing barbell biceps curl, and figure 9.2 shows an example of an EMG test.

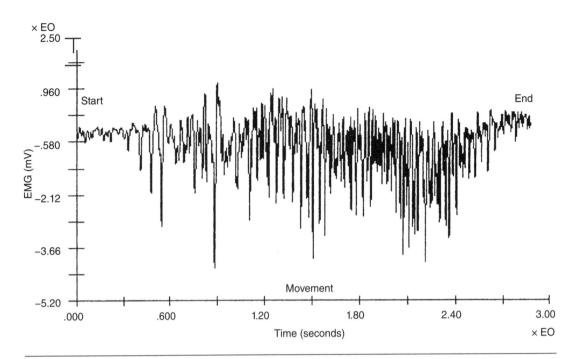

FIGURE 9.1 EMG activity during a standing barbell biceps curl.

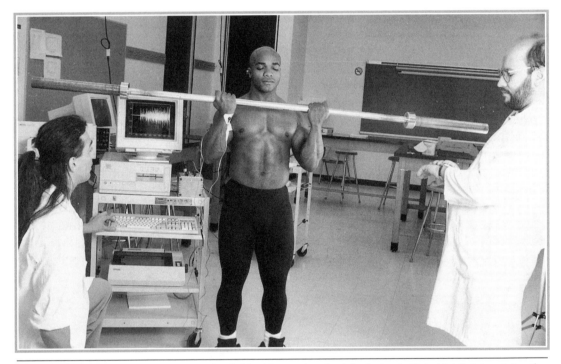

FIGURE 9.2 Coauthor Lorenzo Cornacchia (left) with exercise physiologist Louis Melo (right) determining the EMG activity during a warm-up session of a biceps curl.

Methods

For each study, we used both male and female bodybuilders and strength trainers who were free of neuromuscular disease, had at least 2 years of bodybuilding experience, and had been free of performance-enhancing drugs for at least 2 years. We performed the testing on two separate days. On the first day, 1RM was determined for all exercises. Each subject underwent a warm-up of 10 reps at 50 percent 1RM, 5 reps at 80 percent 1RM, and 2 reps at 90 percent 1RM, with a 5-minute rest interval between sets; 1RM was then performed three times, with a 5-minute rest interval between each repetition. On the second day, the subjects performed 80 percent 1RM five times, with 3-minute rest intervals.

We measured electromyographical activity (EMG) during all exercises, spacing electrodes four centimeters apart over the belly of the muscle group being examined. All EMG data were rectified and integrated (IEMG) for 1 second. For each muscle, the exercise that yielded the highest IEMG determined at 1RM was designated as IEMGmax for the specified muscle. We determined IEMG at 80 percent 1RM by taking the average of the five 80 percent 1RM trials.

We analyzed the data using two one-way repeated-measures analyses of variance to determine which exercise yielded the greatest percent IEMGmax for each muscle. We determined differences between exercises with the Newman-Keuls post hoc test. The purpose was to account for variances in the electrical muscular activation using different exercises to train the same muscle group. The end result would determine which exercise would produce the greatest amount of EMG activation for that muscle group.

Results of EMG Research

The results of our EMG studies show which exercise produces the greatest amount of stimulation within each target muscle group. To comprehend the scientific validity of electromyographical research, it is important to understand the basis for recruitment of muscle fibers and motor units. Entire muscles contain many motor units; each contains a single motoneuron and all of the muscle fibers that it innervates. The number of muscle fibers belonging to a single motor unit can be described as the innervation ratio. The number of muscle fibers and the number of motor units vary widely from muscle to muscle. For example, the lateral gastrocnemius muscle has an innervation of approximately 2,500 to 5,000. The significance of the innervation ratio is largely related to the tension generated in each motor unit (Alway 1997).

Recruitment of muscle fibers within each motor unit begins in the brain, and the signal is sent to the cell bodies in the spinal cord and then finally to the neuromuscular junction. The neuromuscular junction does not provide a true direct connection between the muscle and nerve, but rather an indirect connection. It is similar to a spark plug in a car, where there is a small gap (synaptic cleft) that the electrical signal must "jump" in order to ignite the engine's performance. However, unlike the spark plug analogy, the electrical signal that is passed down the axon does not actually jump the synaptic cleft. Rather, once the electrical signal reaches the end of the axon at the neuromuscular junction, it causes small vesicles to open and flood the synaptic cleft with a neurotransmitter chemical (a substance that transmits the signal from the nerve to the other side of the synaptic cleft) called acetylcholine (Alway 1997).

Acetylcholine crosses the synaptic cleft and binds to receptors in the muscle membrane, and this causes a new electrical impulse to be generated on the membrane surrounding the muscle fiber (sarcolemma). Once the electrical signal (action potential) is generated on the muscle sarcolemma, it travels along this membrane and inside the muscle fiber at each of the open tubes, called transverse tubules, along the sarcolemma. The transverse tubules connect to the sarcoplasmic reticulum (calcium-containing sacs). Once the electrical signal passes from the transverse tubule to the sarcoplasmic reticulum, calcium floods the myofibrils, which then set in motion a series of events leading to the shortening of muscle fibers (sarcomere portions in each fiber). After the action potential has stopped (the electrical signal from the nerve has ceased), calcium returns to the sarcoplasmic reticulum and waits for the next electrical impulse. The more frequently action potentials are sent down the nerve, the more frequently action potentials are formed on the muscle sarcolemmas; and the greater the signal to initiate release of calcium from the sarcoplasmic reticulum, the greater the force that will be generated (Alway 1997).

Tables 9.1 and 9.2 display the results of the EMG studies. Refer to figure 9.3 for anterior and posterior views of the human muscular system and most of the muscles covered by the studies.

TABLE 9.1 IEMGmax Motor Unit Activation

Exercise	% IEMGmax	Exercise	% IEMGmax
STUDY 1: BICEPS BRACHII (LONG HEAD)		**STUDY 4: RECTUS ABDOMINIS**	
Standing dumbbell curl with arm blaster	87	Weighted incline crunch	81
Incline seated dumbbell curl (palms up, lateral rotation)	86	Abdominal crunch (flat bench)	80
Incline seated dumbbell curl (palms up)	84	Weighted crunch	80
STUDY 2: RECTUS FEMORIS (QUADRICEPS)		Ab rocker crunch	72
Safety squat	90	Nautilus crunch	69
Hip belt squat	85	Pulley crunch	68
Leg extension (toes straight)	85	**STUDY 5: ECCENTRIC VS. CONCENTRIC BICEPS FEMORIS**	
Squat (90°)	80	Concentric standing hamstring curl	79
STUDY 3: TRAPEZIUS		Eccentric standing hamstring curl	72
Behind-the-back barbell shrug	59	**STUDY 6: ECCENTRIC VS. CONCENTRIC LATISSIMUS DORSI**	
Front barbell shrug	54	Concentric chin-up	79
Press behind the neck	41	Eccentric chin-up	72

Note: Studies performed in 2001. Data provided by the authors (unpublished).

TABLE 9.2　IEMGmax Motor Unit Activation

Exercise	% IEMGmax	Exercise	% IEMGmax
STUDY 1: PECTORALIS MAJOR		**STUDY 7: TRICEPS BRACHII (OUTER HEAD)**	
Decline dumbbell bench press	93	Decline triceps extension (Olympic bar)	92
Decline bench press (Olympic bar)	90	Triceps press-down (angled bar)	90
Push-up between benches	88	Triceps dip between benches	87
Flat dumbbell bench press	87	One-arm cable triceps extension (reverse grip)	85
Flat bench press (Olympic bar)	85	Overhead rope triceps extension	84
Flat dumbbell fly	84	Seated one-arm dumbbell triceps extension (neutral grip)	82
STUDY 2: PECTORALIS MINOR		Close-grip bench press (Olympic bar)	72
Incline dumbbell bench press	91	**STUDY 8: LATISSIMUS DORSI**	
Incline bench press (Olympic bar)	85	Bent-over barbell row	93
Incline dumbbell fly	83	One-arm dumbbell row (alternate arms)	91
Incline bench press (Smith machine)	81	T-bar row	89
STUDY 3: MEDIAL DELTOIDS		Lat pull-down to the front	86
Incline dumbbell side lateral	66	Seated pulley row	83
Standing dumbbell side lateral	63	**STUDY 9: RECTUS FEMORIS (QUADRICEPS)**	
Seated dumbbell side lateral	62	Safety squat (90° angle, shoulder-width stance)	88
Cable side lateral	47	Seated leg extension (toes straight)	86
STUDY 4: POSTERIOR DELTOIDS		Hack squat (90° angle, shoulder-width stance)	78
Standing dumbbell bent lateral	85	Leg press (110° angle)	76
Seated dumbbell bent lateral	83	Smith machine squat (90° angle, shoulder-width stance)	60
Standing cable bent lateral	77	**STUDY 10: BICEPS FEMORIS (HAMSTRING)**	
STUDY 5: ANTERIOR DELTOIDS		Standing leg curl	82
Seated front dumbbell press	79	Lying leg curl	71
Standing front dumbbell press	73	Seated leg curl	58
Seated front barbell press	61	Modified hamstring deadlift	56
STUDY 6: BICEPS BRACHII (LONG HEAD)		**STUDY 11: SEMITENDINOSUS (HAMSTRING)**	
Biceps preacher curl (Olympic bar)	90	Seated leg curl	88
Incline seated dumbbell curl (alternate arms)	88	Standing leg curl	79
Standing biceps curl (Olympic bar, narrow grip)	86	Lying leg curl	70
Standing dumbbell curl (alternate arms)	84	Modified hamstring deadlift	63
Concentration dumbbell curl	80	**STUDY 12: GASTROCNEMIUS (CALF MUSCLE)**	
Standing biceps curl (Olympic bar, wide grip)	63	Donkey calf raise	80
Standing EZ biceps curl (wide grip)	61	Standing one-leg calf raise	79
		Standing calf raise	68
		Seated calf raise	61

Note: Studies performed and documented in 1998 by T.O. Bompa and L. Cornacchia in *Serious Strength Training* (Champaign, IL: Human Kinetics).

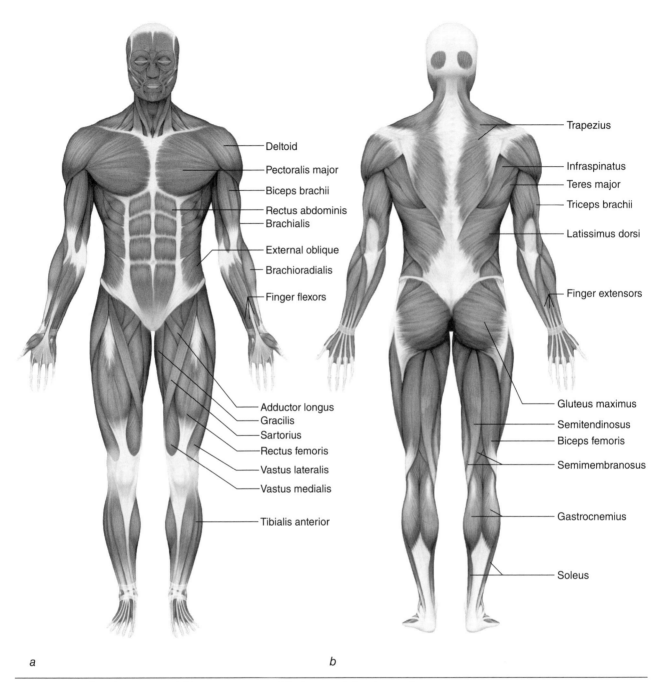

Deltoid
Pectoralis major
Biceps brachii
Rectus abdominis
Brachialis
External oblique
Brachioradialis
Finger flexors

Adductor longus
Gracilis
Sartorius
Rectus femoris
Vastus lateralis
Vastus medialis

Tibialis anterior

Trapezius
Infraspinatus
Teres major
Triceps brachii
Latissimus dorsi

Finger extensors

Gluteus maximus
Semitendinosus
Biceps femoris
Semimembranosus

Gastrocnemius

Soleus

a

b

FIGURE 9.3 The *(a)* anterior and *(b)* posterior views of the human skeletal musculature.

INDIVIDUALIZING A TRAINING REGIMEN

In bodybuilding, muscle hypertrophy correlates directly with tension (force output = high intensity). High-intensity training induces growth when done carefully and correctly. Many bodybuilders shy away from high intensity; or they stop most of their sets before the action becomes quite uncomfortable, choosing to compensate by simply doing more.

Unfortunately, the "more is better" logic is wrong, especially when you are trying to build maximum muscle size as rapidly as possible. When it comes to gaining size and strength, intensity is the bottom line. The harder you work a muscle, the more it is forced to adapt (grow). Lengthening your workouts will have little or no effect on muscle growth; and in most cases adding sets will only cause problems, such as overtraining and muscle atrophy.

The effectiveness of a program is strongly related to its intensity and the exercises performed. Exercises that provide the greatest amount of electrical activity during muscle contraction will produce the highest levels of muscle hypertrophy and strength. The exercises presented in chapters 10 and 11 are recognized for their potential to increase muscular strength and size. Table 9.3 lists all the lower body exercises by body area and the primary and secondary muscles each exercise works. Table 9.4 lists all the upper body exercises by body area and the primary and secondary muscles each exercise works.

It is important to understand, however, that the best program is the one that suits your individual goals. Electromyographic studies have demonstrated that the way in which a muscle responds to an exercise differs among athletes. Many bodybuilders keep plodding along, hoping to make gains using another person's routine or recommendations. They expect to get the same results as the other athlete. This is a mistake.

After you lay the foundation within an all-around routine of basic, gradually progressive exercises (anatomical adaptation), only your personal judgment (or one of a professional trainer) can guide you to outstanding gains. Your body is unique. If our book gives you nothing else but the confidence and independence to listen to your instincts in determining what works best for you, then you will be better off in the end.

The routines you see in muscle magazines are basically worthless. Sure, it is interesting to know how Mr. Olympia prepared for victory; yet his training regimen probably would not work for you. Those articles should be of academic interest only. Many trainees tend to imitate others rather than pay attention to their bodies' responses to various exercises. When bodybuilders discover that a certain exercise or variation works best for them, then they should use it. Follow our training programs; but your ultimate goal should be to maximally build your physique by using your own self-determined training regimen.

TABLE 9.3

Lower Body Exercises

Exercise	Primary muscles worked	Secondary muscles worked	Page #
THIGHS, HIPS, AND GLUTEALS			
Safety squat	Rectus femoris, vastus intermedius, vastus medialis, gluteals, vastus lateralis	Erector spinae, abdominals, hamstrings	146
Seated leg extension (toes straight)	Vastus medialis, vastus lateralis, rectus femoris, vastus intermedius	Abdominals, gastrocnemius	147
Hack squat	Rectus femoris, vastus intermedius, vastus medialis, gluteals, vastus lateralis	Hamstrings, abdominals	148
Leg press	Rectus femoris, vastus intermedius, vastus medialis, vastus lateralis	Gluteals, hamstrings, obliques	149
Smith machine squat	Rectus femoris, vastus intermedius, vastus medialis, gluteals, vastus lateralis	Erector spinae, abdominals, hamstrings	150
Lunge (dumbbells)	Rectus femoris, vastus intermedius, vastus medialis, gluteals, vastus lateralis, hamstrings	Forearm muscles, erector spinae	151
Lunge (Olympic bar)	Rectus femoris, vastus intermedius, vastus medialis, gluteals, vastus lateralis, hamstrings	Forearm muscles, erector spinae, trapezius (upper and lower)	152
HAMSTRINGS			
Standing leg curl	Biceps femoris, semimembranosus, semitendinosus	Gluteals, erector spinae, gastrocnemius	154
Lying leg curl	Biceps femoris, semimembranosus, semitendinosus	Gluteals, erector spinae, gastrocnemius	155
Seated leg curl	Biceps femoris, semimembranosus, semitendinosus	Gluteus maximus (lower part), gastrocnemius	156
Modified hamstring deadlift	Biceps femoris, semimembranosus, semitendinosus, gluteus maximus	Erector spinae, trapezius (lower), teres major and minor, infraspinatus, rhomboids	157
CALVES			
Donkey calf raise	Gastrocnemius	Soleus, hamstrings	159
Standing one-leg calf raise	Gastrocnemius	Soleus, hamstrings	160
Standing calf raise	Gastrocnemius	Soleus, hamstrings	161
Seated calf raise	Soleus	Gastrocnemius	162

TABLE 9.4	**Upper Body Exercises**		
Exercise	**Primary muscles worked**	**Secondary muscles worked**	**Page #**
CHEST			
Decline dumbbell bench press	Pectoralis major (lower chest), anterior deltoids, triceps brachii	Latissimus dorsi, teres major and minor, infraspinatus, rhomboid major, trapezius (upper and lower)	164
Decline bench press (Olympic bar)	Pectoralis major (lower chest), anterior deltoids, triceps brachii	Latissimus dorsi, teres major and minor, infraspinatus, rhomboid major, trapezius (upper and lower)	165
Push-up between benches	Pectoralis major (midchest), triceps brachii	Anterior deltoids, latissimus dorsi, trapezius (upper and lower), rhomboid major, infraspinatus, teres major and minor	166
Flat dumbbell bench press	Pectoralis major (midchest), anterior deltoids, triceps brachii	Teres major and minor, infraspinatus, rhomboid major, trapezius (upper and lower)	167
Flat bench press (Olympic bar)	Pectoralis major (midchest), anterior deltoids, triceps brachii	Latissimus dorsi, teres major and minor, infraspinatus, rhomboid major, trapezius (upper and lower)	168
Flat dumbbell fly	Pectoralis major (midchest)	Latissimus dorsi, triceps brachii, anterior deltoids, medial deltoids, trapezius (upper and lower)	169
Incline dumbbell bench press	Pectoralis minor (upper chest), anterior deltoids, triceps brachii	Medial deltoids, pectoralis major, trapezius (upper and lower), latissimus dorsi	170
Incline bench press (Olympic bar)	Pectoralis minor (upper chest), anterior deltoids, triceps brachii	Latissimus dorsi, medial deltoids, pectoralis major, trapezius (upper and lower)	171
Incline dumbbell fly	Pectoralis minor (upper chest)	Anterior deltoids, trapezius (upper and lower), latissimus dorsi, triceps brachii	172
Incline bench press (Smith machine)	Pectoralis minor (upper chest), anterior deltoids	Pectoralis major, trapezius (upper and lower), latissimus dorsi, triceps brachii	173
Cable crossover	Pectoralis major (midchest and lower chest), anterior deltoids	Latissimus dorsi, trapezius (upper and lower)	174
Parallel bar dip	Pectoralis major and minor, anterior deltoids, triceps brachii	Latissimus dorsi, teres major and minor, infraspinatus, medial deltoids, trapezius (upper and lower)	175
ABDOMINALS			
Abdominal crunch (flat bench)	Rectus abdominis (upper and middle)	Intercostal muscles (sides of your waist)	177
Nautilus crunch	Rectus abdominis (upper and middle)	Intercostal muscles	178
Pulley crunch	Rectus abdominis (upper)	Lower lats, serratus muscles, intercostals	179
Knee-up (flat bench)	Rectus abdominis (lower)	Intercostal muscles	180
Hanging leg raise	Rectus abdominis (mainly lower), serratus anterior	Intercostal muscles	181
Diagonal curl-up	Serratus anterior, rectus abdominis (mainly upper)	Intercostal muscles	182

(continued)

TABLE 9.4   **Upper Body Exercises**   *(continued)*

Exercise	Primary muscles worked	Secondary muscles worked	Page #
BACK			
Bent-over barbell row (Olympic bar)	Latissimus dorsi, trapezius (middle), brachialis, forearm flexors	Brachioradialis, biceps brachii, teres major and minor, rhomboids, infraspinatus	184
One-arm dumbbell row (alternate arms)	Latissimus dorsi, trapezius (middle), brachialis, posterior deltoids, forearm flexors	Biceps brachii, teres major and minor, infraspinatus, rhomboids	185
T-bar row	Latissimus dorsi, trapezius, forearm flexors, brachioradialis	Teres major and minor, erector spinae, infraspinatus, rhomboids	186
Lat pull-down to the front	Latissimus dorsi, brachialis brachioradialis	Biceps brachii, posterior deltoids, teres major and minor, infraspinatus, rhomboids	187
Seated pulley row	Latissimus dorsi, trapezius, rhomboids, erector spinae	Posterior deltoids, biceps brachii, brachioradialis, teres minor, infraspinatus, forearm flexors	188
Front chin-up	Latissimus dorsi, trapezius (upper), biceps brachii, brachioradialis, brachialis	Posterior deltoids, erector spinae, infraspinatus	189
Lat pull-down behind the neck	Latissimus dorsi, trapezius (upper), biceps brachii, brachialis	Forearm extensors, teres minor, infraspinatus, posterior deltoids	190
Back extension	Erector spinae	Gluteals, trapezius (lower)	191
DELTOIDS AND TRAPEZIUS			
Standing dumbbell side lateral	Medial deltoids	Anterior deltoids, trapezius (upper and lower)	194
Standing dumbbell bent lateral	Posterior deltoids	Medial deltoids, trapezius (upper), teres minor, rhomboids, infraspinatus	195
Seated front dumbbell press	Anterior deltoids	Pectoralis major, triceps brachii, trapezius (upper and lower), serratus anterior	196
Seated front barbell press	Anterior deltoids	Pectoralis major, triceps brachii, trapezius, serratus anterior	197
Front barbell shrug (Olympic bar)	Trapezius (upper), rhomboids	Pectoralis major, triceps brachii, trapezius (lower), serratus anterior	198
Standing front dumbbell raise	Anterior deltoids	Forearm extensors, medial and posterior deltoids, rhomboids, pectoralis major	199
Upright row (Olympic bar)	Trapezius, deltoids (anterior and medial)	Biceps brachii, brachialis, forearm flexors	200
Press behind the neck (Olympic bar)	Posterior deltoids, trapezius (upper), triceps brachii	Trapezius (lower), rhomboids, infraspinatus, teres major and minor, latissimus dorsi	201

Exercise	Primary muscles worked	Secondary muscles worked	Page #
BICEPS			
Biceps preacher curl (Olympic bar)	Biceps brachii, brachialis	Forearm flexors	203
Incline seated dumbbell curl (alternate arms)	Biceps brachii	Forearm flexors	204
Standing biceps curl (Olympic bar, narrow grip)	Biceps brachii, brachialis	Forearm flexors, pronator teres, wrist flexors (flexor pollicis longus, flexor digitorum superficialis)	205
Standing dumbbell curl (alternate arms)	Biceps brachii	Forearm flexors, pronator teres, wrist flexors (flexor pollicis longus, flexor digitorum superficialis)	206
Concentration dumbbell curl	Biceps brachii	Forearm flexors, brachialis	207
Standing biceps curl (Olympic bar, wide grip)	Biceps brachii (short head), brachialis	Biceps brachii (long head), forearm flexors, wrist flexors	208
Standing EZ biceps curl (wide grip)	Biceps brachii (short head), brachialis	Biceps brachii (long head), forearm flexors	209
TRICEPS			
Decline triceps extension (Olympic bar)	Triceps (outer and medial heads)	Forearm extensors	211
Triceps press-down (angled bar)	Triceps (outer and medial heads), anconeus	Forearm extensors	212
Triceps dip between benches	Triceps (outer and medial heads)	Anterior deltoids, pectoralis major (lower)	213
One-arm cable triceps extension (reverse grip)	Triceps (outer and medial heads)	Forearm extensors	214
Overhead rope triceps extension	Triceps (all heads)	Forearm extensors	215
Seated one-arm dumbbell triceps extension (neutral grip)	Triceps (inner and medial heads), anconeus	Forearm extensors, posterior deltoids	216
Close-grip bench press (Olympic bar)	Triceps (all heads), pectoralis major (middle and lower)	Latissimus dorsi, anterior deltoids	217
FOREARMS			
Wrist curl (Olympic bar)	Forearm flexors	Wrist flexors	219
Wrist extension (Olympic bar)	Forearm extensors	Wrist extensors	220

chapter 10

Lower Body Exercises

This chapter presents exercises to work the muscles of the lower body. Nearly all of the exercises were chosen based on the results of the EMG studies of the lower body. In each muscle group layout, the exercises are in order from the greatest EMG activation to the least. Refer to the motor unit activation tables in chapter 9.

THIGHS, HIPS, AND GLUTEALS

In bodybuilding, the words *massively carved, ripped, chiseled,* and *separated* describe the perfect pair of thighs. As the foundation of human muscularity, the thighs are clearly the most powerful muscles of the physique.

Squatting can be an excellent exercise for strengthening numerous muscles, bones, ligaments, and tendinous insertion points within the lower body. In fact, for years the squat has been considered the quintessential leg exercise. Unfortunately, because this exercise frequently causes injuries to the lumbar spine and knees, many professional and amateur bodybuilders have reluctantly eliminated conventional squats (with the Olympic bar) from their training routines.

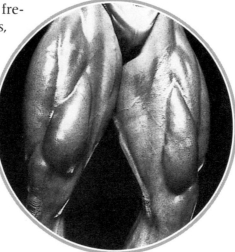

Because squatting leads to substantial gains, however, most strength trainers and coaches were not prepared to witness its extinction; much research was done to develop other, safer squatting methods and equipment. For maximal quad, hip, and glute development, safety squats should be a part of all quad programs. The leg extension is an excellent vastus medialis (quad) exercise.

Safety Squat

Primary Muscles Worked

- Rectus femoris
- Vastus intermedius
- Vastus medialis
- Gluteals
- Vastus lateralis

Secondary Muscles Worked

- Erector spinae
- Abdominals
- Hamstrings

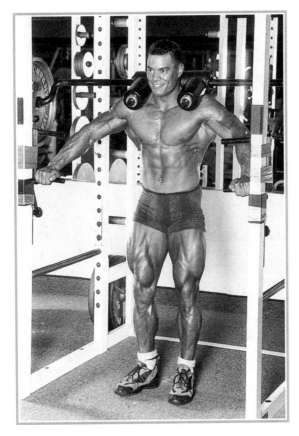

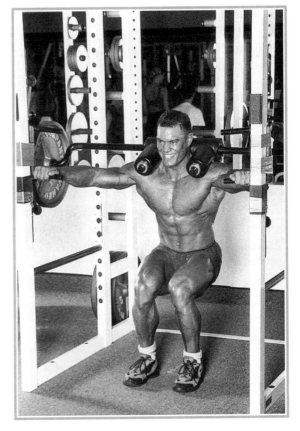

Starting Position

1. Rest the pads of the safety squat bar on your trapezius muscles, and lift the safety squat bar off the squatting holders.
2. Feet should be parallel and shoulder-width apart, with knees slightly bent.
3. Keep the safety squat bar steady on your shoulders, and place your hands on the rack handles.

Exercise Technique

1. Keeping your hands on the rack handles throughout the entire movement, slowly lower your glutes toward the floor by bending the knees.
2. When you reach an approximate angle of 90 degrees, push upward with your quadriceps muscles, allowing them maximal muscle activation.
3. Repeat until the desired number of repetitions is completed.

CUE Using your hands during the safety squat helps you balance and maintain strict squatting form, actually allowing you to spot yourself through your sticking point. This will help you work with heavier loads without fear of sustaining injuries when exerting force through your weakest point.

Seated Leg Extension (Toes Straight)

Primary Muscles Worked

- Vastus medialis
- Vastus lateralis
- Rectus femoris
- Vastus intermedius

Secondary Muscles Worked

- Abdominals
- Gastrocnemius

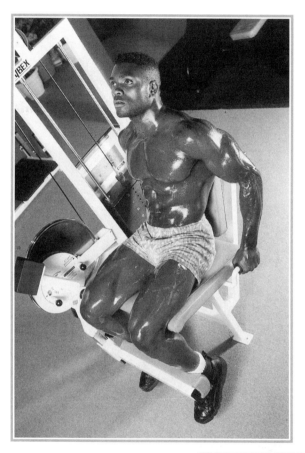

Starting Position

1. Sit on a leg extension machine, and press the back of your knees firmly against the edge of the seat.
2. Place the front of your ankles under the foot pad, and grasp the handles at the sides of the machine.

Exercise Technique

1. Moving only your lower legs, lift the desired weight until your quadriceps muscles are fully extended.
2. Hold this position for 1 second, allowing peak quadriceps contraction to occur.
3. Lower the weight slowly to the starting position, and repeat the movement until you complete the desired number of repetitions.

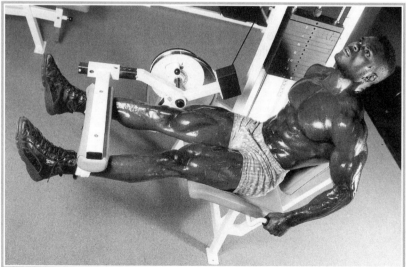

Hack Squat

Primary Muscles Worked

- Rectus femoris
- Vastus intermedius
- Vastus medialis
- Gluteals
- Vastus lateralis

Secondary Muscles Worked

- Hamstrings
- Abdominals

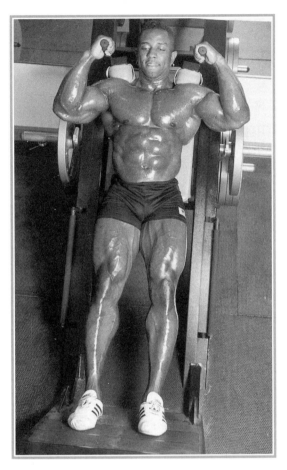

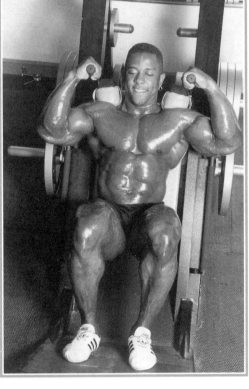

Starting Position

1. Position your body on the hack squat machine with the trapezius muscles under the shoulder pads and your back pressed firmly against the back rest.
2. Place your feet on the angled foot rest, with heels approximately 8 inches (20 cm) apart (varies depending on the person) and toes angled slightly outward.

Exercise Technique

1. Slowly bend at the knees, bringing your torso down toward your heels.
2. When your knees are lowered to an approximate 90-degree angle, push upward to return to the starting position.
3. Repeat the movement until you complete the desired number of repetitions.

Leg Press

Primary Muscles Worked

- Rectus femoris
- Vastus intermedius
- Vastus medialis
- Vastus lateralis

Secondary Muscles Worked

- Gluteals
- Hamstrings
- Obliques

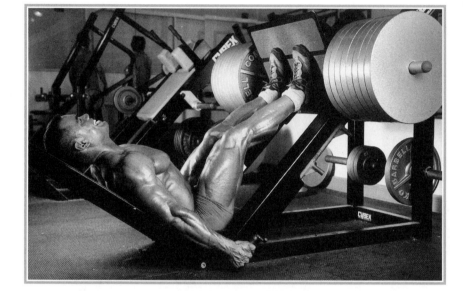

Starting Position

1. Lie on the leg press machine with your buttocks supported on the seat and your back pressed firmly against the back rest.
2. Place your feet flat on the platform with a shoulder-width stance and toes slightly angled outward.
3. Grasp the handles and unlock the weight in preparation to perform the leg press.

Exercise Technique

1. Slowly bend your legs, allowing your knees to travel toward your chest.
2. When your knees have reached an angle slightly greater than 90 degrees (110 to 115 degrees), slowly straighten your legs to return to the starting position (do not lock your knees at the top of the movement).
3. Repeat the movement until you complete the desired number of repetitions.

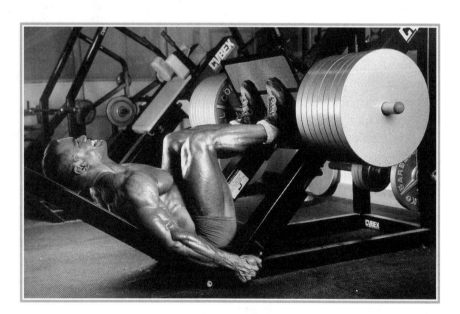

Smith Machine Squat

Primary Muscles Worked	Secondary Muscles Worked
• Rectus femoris	• Erector spinae
• Vastus intermedius	• Abdominals
• Vastus medialis	• Hamstrings
• Gluteals	
• Vastus lateralis	

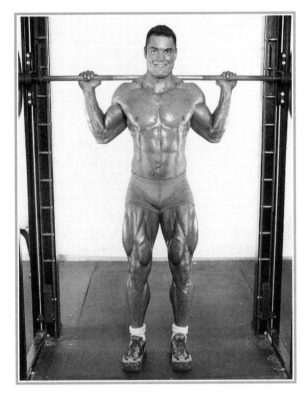

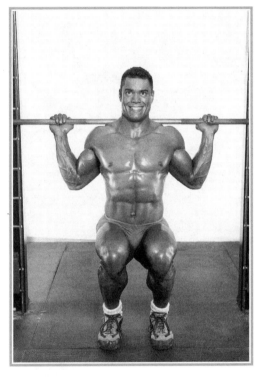

Starting Position

1. Position your body underneath the Olympic bar attached to the Smith machine.
2. Grasp the bar with an overhand grip, with hands slightly wider than shoulder-width apart.
3. At this point, the bar is resting comfortably on your trapezius muscles and your feet are apart in a shoulder-width stance.
4. Unhook the bar from the standards, and step forward slightly with both feet.
5. Remember to keep your back erect and look forward throughout the entire movement.

Exercise Technique

1. Slowly bend your legs until your knees reach a 90-degree angle.
2. Without bouncing at the bottom of the movement, slowly straighten your legs and return to the starting position.
3. Repeat the movement until you complete the desired number of repetitions.

CUE Squatting is an exercise in which technique and balance are of the utmost importance. Squatting inside the Nautilus Smith machine removes the element of balance because the Olympic bar is attached to the apparatus. Despite being considered a revolutionary development in the squatting world, Nautilus Smith machine squats may produce too much strain on the lower back and knees.

Lunge (Dumbbells)

Primary Muscles Worked

- Rectus femoris
- Vastus intermedius
- Vastus medialis
- Gluteals
- Vastus lateralis
- Hamstrings

Secondary Muscles Worked

- Forearm muscles
- Erector spinae

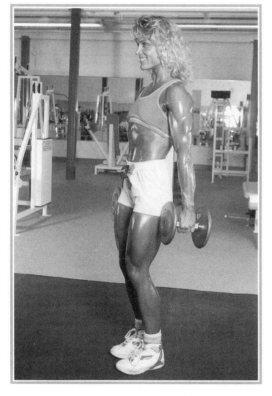

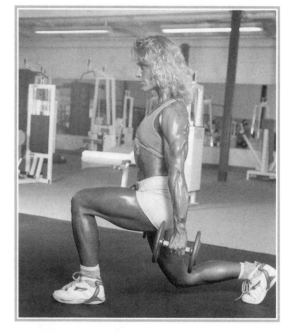

Starting Position

1. Grasp a dumbbell with each hand.
2. Hold the dumbbells at the sides of your body, with arms fully extended (palms facing your torso).

Exercise Technique

1. Step forward with your lead leg (stepping leg), keeping your back erect.
2. Bend the knee of your lead leg until it has reached a 90-degree angle.
3. At this point, the knee of your back leg should be approximately 2 to 3 inches (5 to 8 cm) from the floor.
4. When your back leg is fully lowered, push forcefully with your lead leg and return to the starting position.
5. Repeat the exercise with your other leg, and continue to alternate until you complete the desired number of repetitions.
6. Remember that a shorter lead step places more emphasis on the quadriceps muscles, and a larger step places more emphasis on the gluteal and hamstring muscles.

Lunge (Olympic Bar)

Primary Muscles Worked

- Rectus femoris
- Vastus intermedius
- Vastus medialis
- Gluteals
- Vastus lateralis
- Hamstrings

Secondary Muscles Worked

- Forearm muscles
- Erector spinae
- Trapezius (upper and lower)

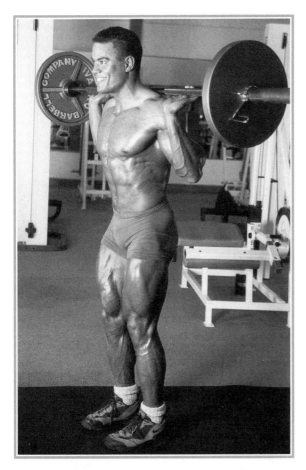

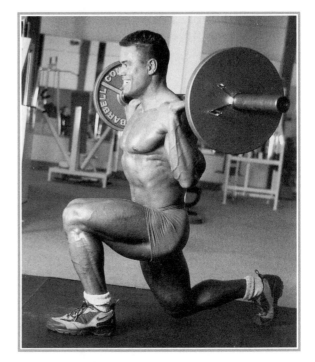

Starting Position

1. Position your body underneath the Olympic bar, and lift the bar from the standards.
2. The bar should be resting on your trapezius muscles, with your hands grasping the bar slightly wider than shoulder-width apart.
3. Take several steps backward, giving you enough clear space to lunge forward.

Exercise Technique

1. Step forward with your lead leg (stepping leg), keeping your back erect.
2. Bend the knee of your lead leg until it reaches a 90-degree angle.
3. At this point, the knee of your back leg should be approximately 2 to 3 inches (5 to 8 cm) from the floor.
4. When your back leg is fully lowered, push forcefully with your lead leg, and return to the starting position.
5. Repeat with the other leg, and continue to alternate until you complete the desired number of repetitions.
6. Remember that a shorter lead step places more emphasis on the quadriceps muscles, and a larger step places more emphasis on the gluteal and hamstring muscles.

HAMSTRINGS

Few people ever talk about the hamstring muscles. Even if you constantly read bodybuilding magazines, very rarely will you encounter professional bodybuilders who discuss hamstrings like they discuss pec training, back blasting, or arm blitzing. However, all bodybuilders will tell you how important the hamstring muscles are to overall leg development. Nothing is more impressive than a bodybuilder who turns to the side to reveal the belly of the hamstring as a massive mound of flesh. Standing, seated, and lying hamstring curls seem to be the best hamstring exercises. The exercises are presented in order for biceps femorus activation (see table 9.1).

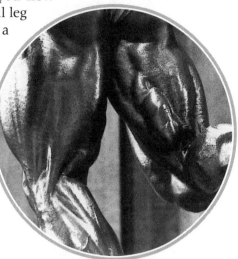

Standing Leg Curl

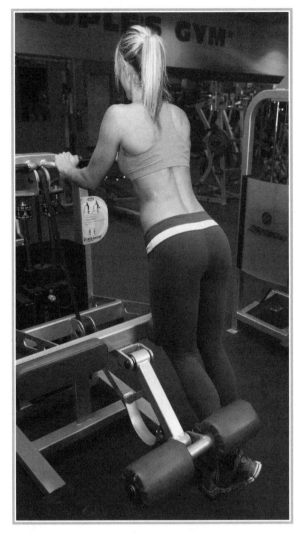

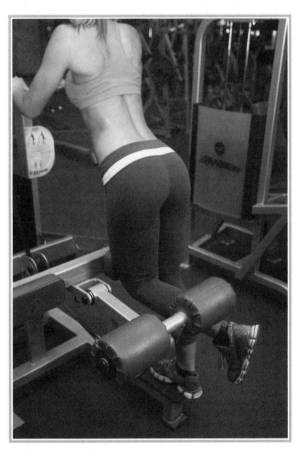

Primary Muscles Worked

- Biceps femoris
- Semimembranosus
- Semitendinosus

Secondary Muscles Worked

- Gluteals
- Erector spinae
- Gastrocnemius

Starting Position

1. Standing on the right side of the machine, place your left quad against the thigh pad and your left heel (calf) under the rectangular ankle pad.
2. With your left hand grasp the bar directly in front of you, and lean your torso slightly forward.

Exercise Technique

1. Slowly raise your foot toward your buttocks.
2. Go as far upward as possible to allow for maximal contraction.
3. Once you reach the top of the movement, slowly lower your leg while resisting against the weight (do not let your foot touch the floor).
4. Repeat until you complete the desired number of repetitions.
5. Reverse your body position, and repeat the exercise for the other leg.

Lying Leg Curl

Primary Muscles Worked	Secondary Muscles Worked
• Biceps femoris	• Gluteals
• Semimembranosus	• Erector spinae
• Semitendinosus	• Gastrocnemius

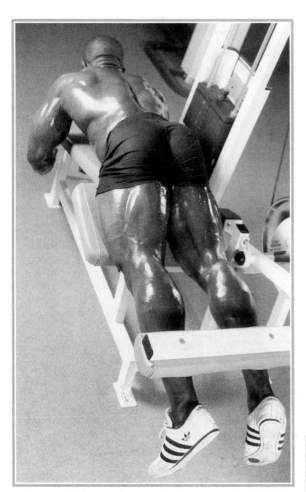

Starting Position

1. Lie facedown on the hamstring curl machine.
2. Slide your ankles underneath the ankle pads, and place your knees at the edge of the bench.
3. Grasp the handles at the top of the machine to keep your body stabilized while performing the set.

Exercise Technique

1. Raise your heels, bringing them toward your buttocks.
2. Go as far upward as possible to allow for maximal contraction.
3. Once you reach the top of the movement, slowly lower your leg while resisting against the weight (do not let the plates touch—keep tension on the working muscles).
4. Repeat until you complete the desired number of repetitions.

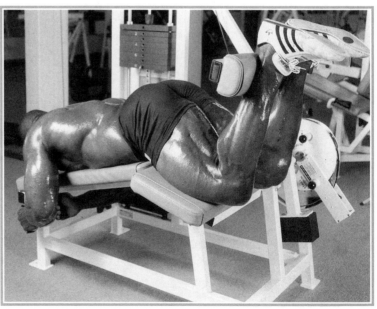

Seated Leg Curl

Primary Muscles Worked

- Biceps femoris
- Semimembranosus
- Semitendinosus

Secondary Muscles Worked

- Gluteus maximus (lower part)
- Gastrocnemius

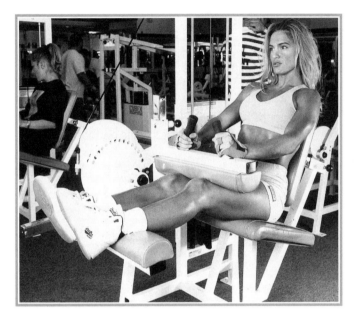

Starting Position

1. Sit on the hamstring curl machine with ankles on top of the ankle pads.
2. Adjust the thigh pad, and lock it down comfortably across your thighs.
3. Keep your back pressed firmly against the back support.

Exercise Technique

1. Bend your knees, bringing the heels under your body and toward your buttocks.
2. Go as far back as possible to allow for maximal contraction.
3. Once your hamstrings are maximally contracted, and while resisting, slowly allow the weight to bring your body back to the starting position.
4. Repeat the movement until you complete the desired number of repetitions.

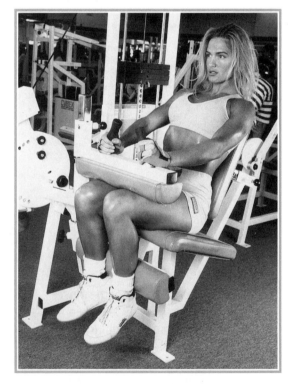

Modified Hamstring Deadlift

Primary Muscles Worked

- Biceps femoris
- Semimembranosus
- Semitendinosus
- Gluteus maximus

Secondary Muscles Worked

- Erector spinae
- Trapezius (lower)
- Teres major and minor
- Infraspinatus
- Rhomboids

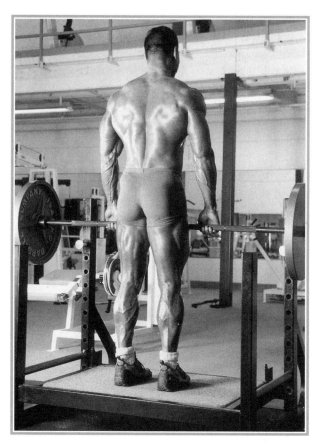

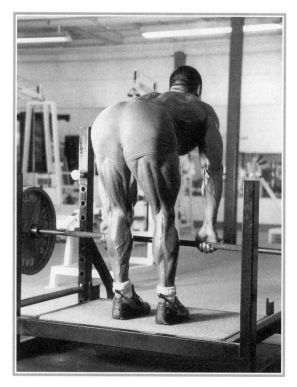

Starting Position

1. Grasp an Olympic bar with hands slightly wider than shoulder-width apart.
2. Hold the bar with arms fully extended at thigh level.

Exercise Technique

1. Keep your back flat, buttocks out, and knees slightly bent.
2. Slowly lower the bar 2 to 3 inches (5 to 8 cm) past your knees.
3. At this point, you should feel a stretch in your glutes and hamstrings.
4. Slowly raise the bar by contracting your glutes and hamstrings and by straightening your torso.
5. Repeat until you complete the desired number of repetitions.

CUE Most lifters perform this exercise incorrectly by bending too far over. Once the hip muscles are fully flexed, the only way to further lower the bar to the shoes is to hyperflex the spine. When this occurs, the lifter places the lumbar spine in a very vulnerable position (career-ending injury or serious complications).

CALVES

All the really great bodybuilders have amazing calves. Some of the greatest body-builders with incredible calf development are Arnold Schwarzenegger, Tom Platz, and Gary Strydom. Many bodybuilders believe the calves are virtually impossible to build because their size is genetically determined. But per-sistence is the hallmark of every champion, especially with stubborn muscles such as the calves. Arnold Schwarzenegger is a prime example of a person with no genetically gifted calf development. He therefore prioritized calf development and used heavy training to develop huge diamond-shaped calves.

If your calves lack width, you should con-centrate your efforts on seated calf raises. Seated calf raises are also excellent for carving deep cuts in the outer sides of your calves. To enlarge your gastrocnemius muscles, you must do plenty of donkey calf, standing calf, and one-leg calf raises.

Donkey Calf Raise

Primary Muscles Worked	Secondary Muscles Worked
• Gastrocnemius	• Soleus
	• Hamstrings

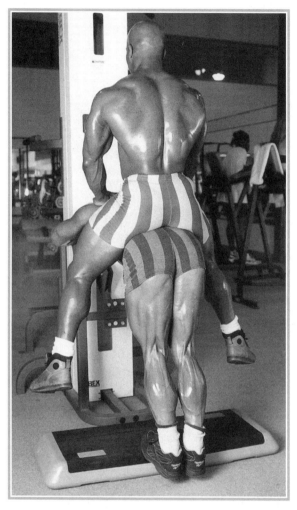

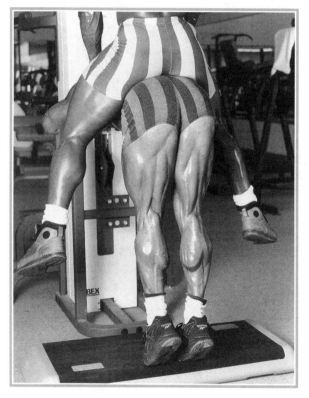

Starting Position

1. Stand with your toes on the edge of a calf board, approximately 3 to 5 inches (8 to 13 cm) in height.
2. Bend forward at the hips until your torso is parallel to the floor, and stabilize your body by holding on to a piece of equipment (e.g., squat rack).
3. At this point, a partner climbs onto your back and straddles your hips.
4. Allow your heels to drop as far as comfortably possible below the level of your toes.

Exercise Technique

1. Raise your torso as high as possible on the balls of your feet.
2. Once you reach the top of the movement, slowly lower your heels as far below the level of your toes as possible, returning to the starting position.
3. Repeat the movement until you complete the desired number of repetitions.

Standing One-Leg Calf Raise

Primary Muscles Worked
- Gastrocnemius

Secondary Muscles Worked
- Soleus
- Hamstrings

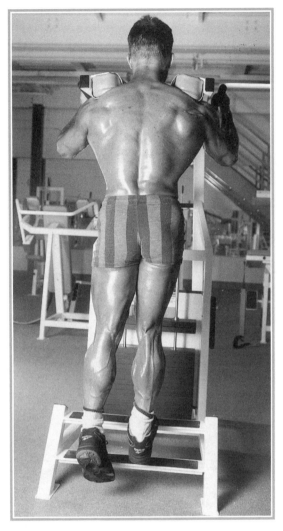

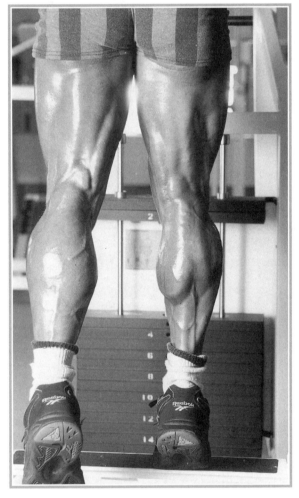

Starting Position

1. Stand on a calf machine with the ball of your right foot at the edge of the platform.
2. Allow your right heel to drop as far below the level of your toes as possible.
3. Place your hands on top of the shoulder pads to stabilize your body.

Exercise Technique

1. Raise your torso as high as possible on the ball of your right foot and toes.
2. Once you reach the top of the movement, slowly lower your heel as far below the level of your toes as possible, returning to the starting position.
3. Repeat the movement until you complete the desired number of repetitions.
4. Repeat for the left foot.

Standing Calf Raise

Primary Muscles Worked
- Gastrocnemius

Secondary Muscles Worked
- Soleus
- Hamstrings

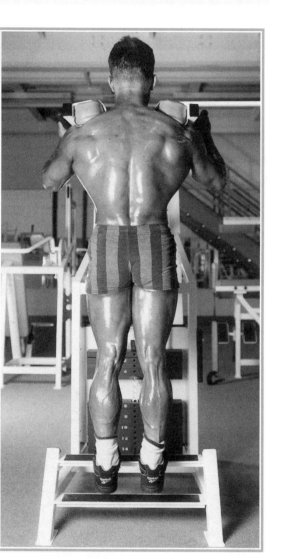

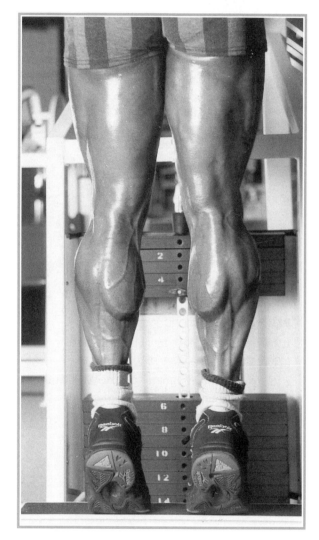

Starting Position

1. Stand on a calf machine with the balls of your feet at the edge of the platform.
2. Allow your heels to drop as far below the level of your toes as possible.
3. Place your hands on top of the shoulder pads to stabilize your body.

Exercise Technique

1. Raise your torso as high as possible on the balls of your feet and toes.
2. Once you reach the top of the movement, slowly lower your heels as far below the level of the toes as possible, returning to the starting position.
3. Repeat the movement until you complete the desired number of repetitions.

Seated Calf Raise

Primary Muscles Worked	Secondary Muscles Worked
• Soleus	• Gastrocnemius

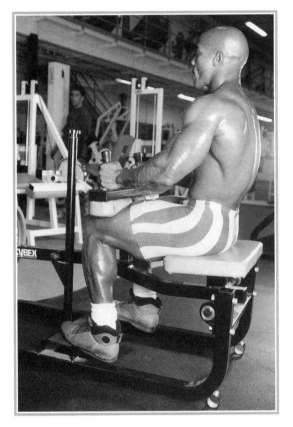

Starting Position

1. Sit on the calf machine with the balls of your feet on the edge of the platform.
2. Hook your knees underneath the pads, and grasp the handles to stabilize your body.
3. Unhook the safeguard for the weight.
4. Allow your heels to drop as far below the level of your toes as possible.

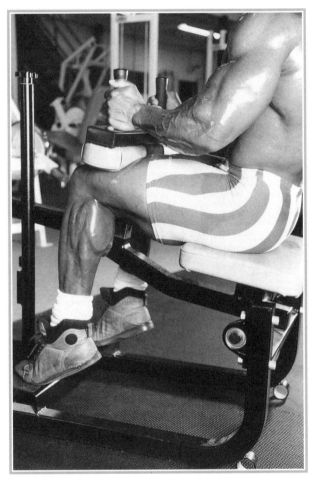

Exercise Technique

1. Raise your heels until your calves are fully contracted.
2. Once you reach the top of the movement, slowly lower your heels as far below your toes as possible, returning to the starting position.
3. Repeat the movement until you complete the desired number of repetitions.

chapter 11

Upper Body Exercises

This chapter presents exercises to work the muscles of the upper body. Nearly all of the exercises were chosen based on the results of the EMG studies of the upper body. In each muscle group layout, the exercises are in order from the greatest EMG activation to the least. Refer to the motor unit activation tables in chapter 9.

CHEST

There is nothing more impressive in the sport of bodybuilding than a pair of striated, slablike pectoral muscles. When you look at competition photos of Arnold Schwarzenegger and Lee Haney, you undoubtedly will conclude that you must beef up your chest if you are ever to win a big bodybuilding title. When these bodybuilders stand relaxed, their chests look twice as thick as their waists from the side.

Many professional bodybuilders look great from the front because they have good pecs; yet from the side view they clearly lack deep rib cages—their chests and waists appear to have about the same thickness. Fully expanding the rib cage is one of the essential factors in developing an impressive chest. The bigger the foundation on which the pectoral muscles are set, the greater the level of development and impressiveness they will achieve.

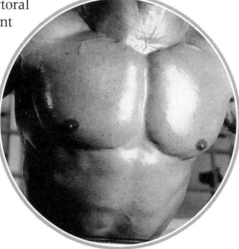

The pecs should be worked from all angles. Certain basic exercises—such as incline flat dumbbell and barbell bench presses and decline barbell bench presses—build muscles on your chest. Flys and pulley crossovers are more effective for shaping and striating the pectoral region. Complete pectoral development results from working all four regions of the muscles: upper, lower, outside, and inside.

Decline Dumbbell Bench Press

Primary Muscles Worked

- Pectoralis major (lower chest)
- Anterior deltoids
- Triceps brachii

Secondary Muscles Worked

- Latissimus dorsi
- Teres major and minor
- Infraspinatus
- Rhomboid major
- Trapezius (upper and lower)

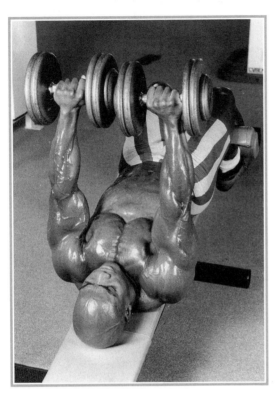

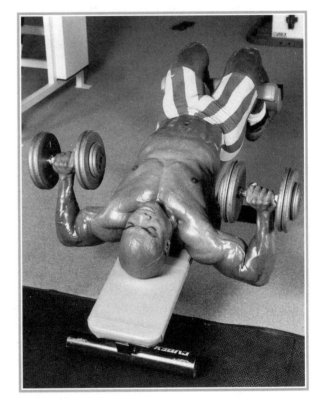

Starting Position

1. Grasp two dumbbells using an overhand grip while sitting at the high end of a decline bench.
2. Secure your ankles and feet underneath the pads.
3. Rest the dumbbells in an upright position on your knees.
4. Lie on the decline bench, simultaneously bringing the dumbbells to the sides of your torso at chest level.
5. Raise the dumbbells to a position of straight arms' length (elbows not locked), with palms facing forward.
6. At this point the dumbbells are directly over your chest, in contact with each other.

Exercise Technique

1. Slowly bend your arms and lower the dumbbells until they are at either side of your chest.
2. Lower the dumbbells to a position where a comfortable but maximum stretch is achieved.
3. Raise the dumbbells from the sides of your chest to the starting position.
4. Perform the desired number of repetitions while keeping the movement fluent, slow, and controlled.

Decline Bench Press (Olympic Bar)

Primary Muscles Worked

- Pectoralis major (lower chest)
- Anterior deltoids
- Triceps brachii

Secondary Muscles Worked

- Latissimus dorsi
- Teres major and minor
- Infraspinatus
- Rhomboid major
- Trapezius (upper and lower)

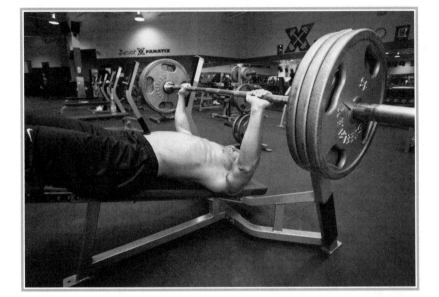

Starting Position

1. Lie down on a decline bench with your back pressed firmly against the padding and feet and ankles secured underneath the pads.
2. Grasp the Olympic bar using an overhand grip, hands 3 to 5 inches (8 to 13 cm) wider than shoulder-width apart, and lift the bar from the standards.
3. Arms should be fully extended (not locked) as you hold the bar over your chest area.

Exercise Technique

1. Slowly lower the bar to touch the nipple line of your chest.
2. Once the bar lightly touches your chest, push it upward to the starting position.
3. Remember never to lock your elbows during this movement. This will allow continuous tension to remain on the working muscles.
4. Perform the desired number of repetitions while keeping the movement fluent, slow, and controlled.

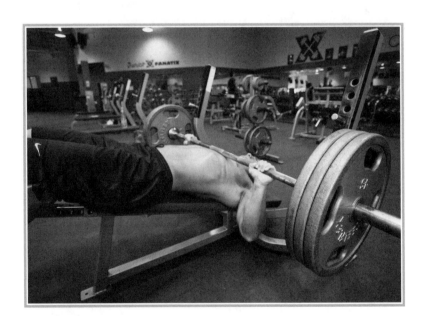

Push-Up Between Benches

Primary Muscles Worked

- Pectoralis major (midchest)
- Triceps brachii

Secondary Muscles Worked

- Anterior deltoids
- Latissimus dorsi
- Trapezius (upper and lower)
- Rhomboid major
- Infraspinatus
- Teres major and minor

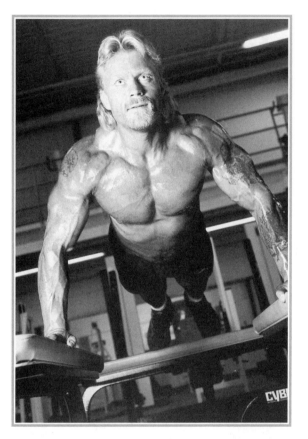

Starting Position

1. Arrange three benches—two parallel to each other and slightly wider than chest-width apart, and one perpendicular to and behind the other two benches.
2. Place both feet on the rear bench and one hand on each of the parallel benches.
3. At this point you are in a supported position, ready to perform push-ups.

Exercise Technique

1. Lower your body as far down between the benches as possible until a comfortable stretch (midchest area) is achieved.
2. Push your body upward to the starting position.
3. Perform the desired number of repetitions while keeping the movement fluent, slow, and controlled.

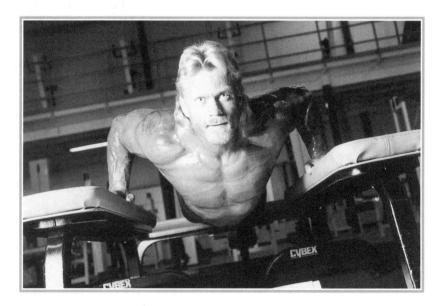

Flat Dumbbell Bench Press

Primary Muscles Worked	Secondary Muscles Worked
• Pectoralis major (midchest) • Anterior deltoids • Triceps brachii	• Teres major and minor • Infraspinatus • Rhomboid major • Trapezius (upper and lower)

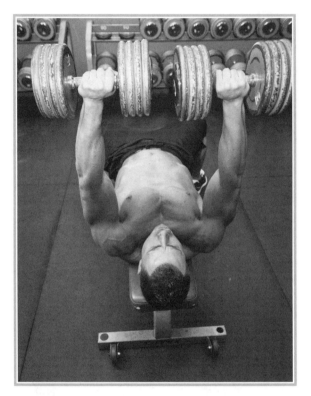

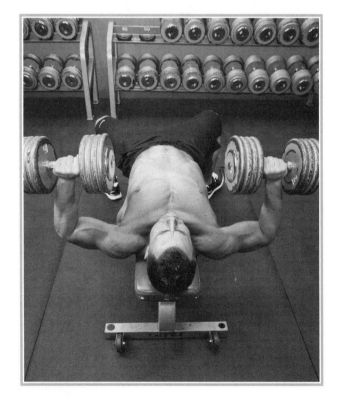

Starting Position

1. Grasp two dumbbells using an overhand grip while sitting at the edge of the flat bench.
2. Rest the dumbbells in an upright position on your knees.
3. Lie on the flat bench, simultaneously bringing the dumbbells to the sides of your torso at chest level.
4. Raise the dumbbells to a position of straight arms' length (elbows not locked).
5. At this point the dumbbells are directly over your chest area, almost in contact with each other, while your palms are facing forward.

Exercise Technique

1. Slowly bend your arms and lower the dumbbells until they are at either side of your chest.
2. Lower the dumbbells to a position where a comfortable but maximum stretch is achieved.
3. Raise the dumbbells from the sides of your chest to the starting position.
4. Perform the desired number of repetitions while keeping the movement fluent, slow, and controlled.

Flat Bench Press (Olympic Bar)

Primary Muscles Worked

- Pectoralis major (midchest)
- Anterior deltoids
- Triceps brachii

Secondary Muscles Worked

- Latissimus dorsi
- Teres major and minor
- Infraspinatus
- Rhomboid major
- Trapezius (upper and lower)

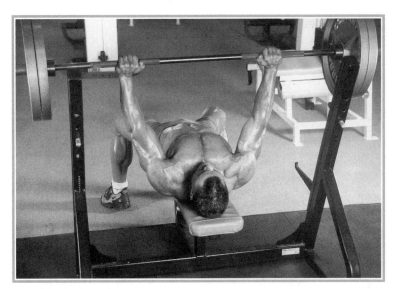

Starting Position

1. Lie on the flat bench, with your back pressed firmly against the padding and feet flat on the floor.
2. Grasp the bar using an overhand grip, with hands 3 to 5 inches (8 to 13 cm) wider than shoulder-width apart, and lift the bar from the standards.
3. Arms should be fully extended (not locked) as you hold the bar over the chest area.

Exercise Technique

1. Slowly lower the barbell to touch the nipple line of your chest.
2. Once the bar lightly touches your chest, push it upward to the starting position.
3. Perform the desired number of repetitions while keeping the movement fluent, slow, and controlled.

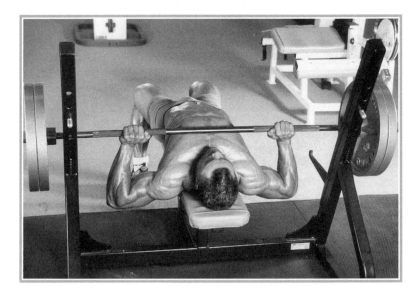

Flat Dumbbell Fly

Primary Muscles Worked

- Pectoralis major (midchest)

Secondary Muscles Worked

- Latissimus dorsi
- Triceps brachii
- Anterior deltoids
- Medial deltoids
- Trapezius (upper and lower)

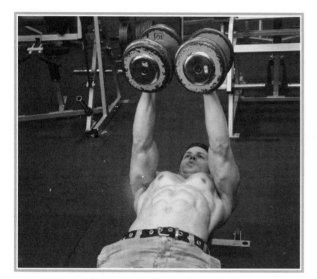

Starting Position

1. Grasp the dumbbells using an overhand grip while sitting at the end of the flat bench.
2. Rest the dumbbells in an upright position on your knees.
3. Lie on the flat bench, simultaneously bringing the dumbbells to the sides of your torso at chest level.
4. Raise the dumbbells to a position of straight arms' length.
5. At this point the dumbbells are directly over your chest, in contact with each other, while your palms are facing inward.
6. Elbows must remain flexed throughout the entire movement.

Exercise Technique

1. Slowly lower the dumbbells in an arc-like motion toward the floor until your chest is comfortably stretched (visualize opening a book).
2. Once you reach this stretch (dumbbells at either side of your chest), return the dumbbells to the starting position, using the same arc-like motion.
3. Perform the desired number of repetitions while keeping the movement fluent, slow, and controlled.

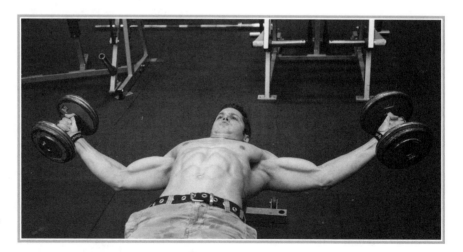

Incline Dumbbell Bench Press

Primary Muscles Worked

- Pectoralis minor (upper chest)
- Anterior deltoids
- Triceps brachii

Secondary Muscles Worked

- Medial deltoids
- Pectoralis major
- Trapezius (upper and lower)
- Latissimus dorsi

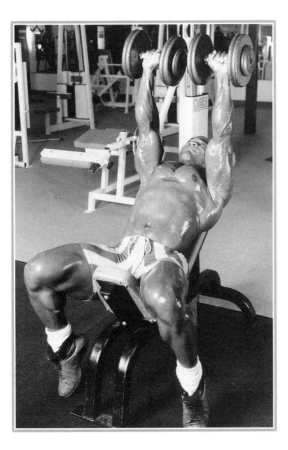

Starting Position

1. Grasp the dumbbells using an overhand grip while sitting at the edge of the incline bench.
2. Rest the dumbbells in an upright position on your knees.
3. Lie on the incline bench, simultaneously bringing the dumbbells to the sides of your torso at chest level.
4. Raise the dumbbells to a position of straight arms' length (elbows not locked).
5. At this point the dumbbells are directly over your upper chest, almost in contact with each other, while your palms are facing forward.

Exercise Technique

1. Slowly bend your arms and lower the dumbbells until they are at either side of your chest.
2. Lower the dumbbells to a position where a comfortable stretch is achieved.
3. Raise the dumbbells from the sides of your chest to the starting position.
4. Perform the desired number of repetitions while keeping the movement fluent, slow, and controlled.

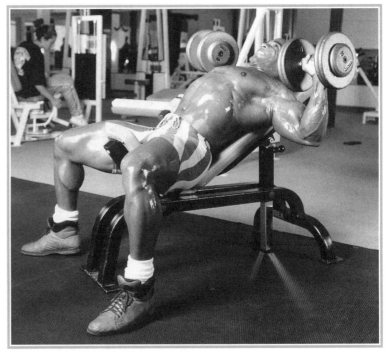

Incline Bench Press (Olympic Bar)

Primary Muscles Worked

- Pectoralis minor (upper chest)
- Anterior deltoids
- Triceps brachii

Secondary Muscles Worked

- Latissimus dorsi
- Medial deltoids
- Pectoralis major
- Trapezius (upper and lower)

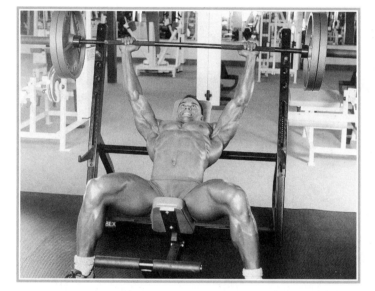

Starting Position

1. Lie down on an incline bench with your back pressed firmly against the padding and feet placed flat on the floor.
2. Grasp the Olympic bar using an overhand grip with hands slightly wider than shoulder-width apart, and lift the bar from the standards.
3. Arms should be fully extended (not locked) as you hold the bar over your chest area.

Exercise Technique

1. Slowly lower the Olympic bar to touch your upper pectoral area.
2. Once the bar lightly touches your upper chest, push it upward to the starting position.
3. Remember: Never lock your elbows. This will allow the tension to remain on the upper chest area.
4. Perform the desired number of repetitions while keeping the movement fluent, slow, and controlled.

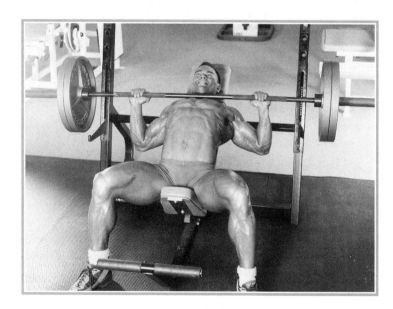

Incline Dumbbell Fly

Primary Muscles Worked	Secondary Muscles Worked
• Pectoralis minor (upper chest)	• Anterior deltoids • Trapezius (upper and lower) • Latissimus dorsi • Triceps brachii

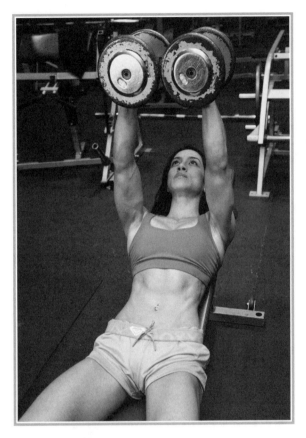

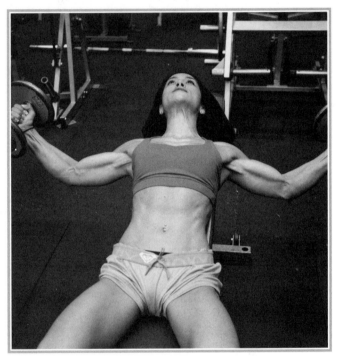

Starting Position

1. Grasp the dumbbells using an overhand grip while sitting on an incline bench.
2. Rest the dumbbells in an upright position on your knees.
3. Lie on the incline bench, simultaneously bringing the dumbbells to the sides of your torso at chest level.
4. Raise the dumbbells to a position of straight arms' length (elbows not locked).
5. At this point the dumbbells are directly over your upper chest, in contact with each other, while your palms are facing inward.
6. Elbows must remain flexed throughout the entire movement.

Exercise Technique

1. Slowly lower the dumbbells in an arc-like motion toward the floor until your chest is comfortably stretched (visualize opening a book).
2. Once you reach this stretch (dumbbells at either side of your chest), return the dumbbells to the starting position, using the same arc-like motion.
3. Perform the desired number of repetitions while keeping the movement fluent, slow, and controlled.

Incline Bench Press (Smith Machine)

Primary Muscles Worked

- Pectoralis minor (upper chest)
- Anterior deltoids

Secondary Muscles Worked

- Pectoralis major
- Trapezius (upper and lower)
- Latissimus dorsi
- Triceps brachii

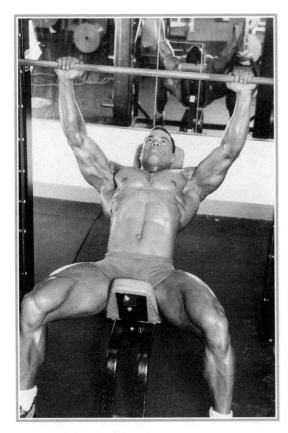

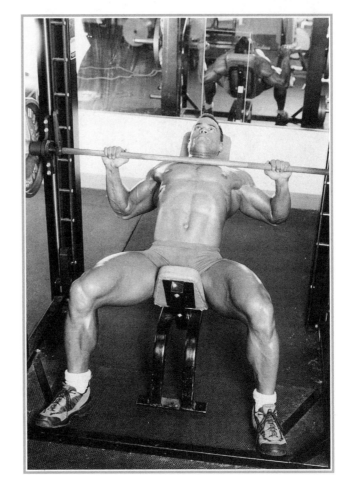

Starting Position

1. Lie down on an incline bench (inside Smith machine workstation) with your back pressed firmly against the padding and feet placed flat on the floor.
2. Grasp the Olympic bar using an overhand grip, with hands 3 to 5 inches (8 to 13 cm) wider than shoulder-width apart, and unlock the bar from the safety standards.
3. Arms should be fully extended (not locked) as you hold the bar over your upper chest area.

Exercise Technique

1. Slowly lower the Olympic bar (Smith machine) to lightly touch your upper pectoral area.
2. Once the bar lightly touches your upper chest, push it upward to the starting position.
3. Remember: Never lock your elbows. This will allow the tension to remain on the upper chest area.
4. Perform the desired number of repetitions while keeping the movement fluent, slow, and controlled.

Cable Crossover

Primary Muscles Worked

- Pectoralis major (midchest and lower chest)
- Anterior deltoids

Secondary Muscles Worked

- Latissimus dorsi
- Trapezius (upper and lower)

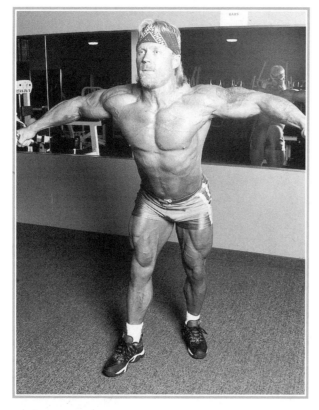

Starting Position

1. Grasp each cable using an overhand grip with palms facing inward.
2. Stand in the middle of the cable machine with feet slightly wider than shoulder-width apart or with one foot slightly in front of the other (use whatever stance you are comfortable with).
3. Keep your back erect and elbows slightly bent throughout the entire motion.
4. To begin the exercise, extend the cables to the point where your chest is completely stretched (arms wide open).

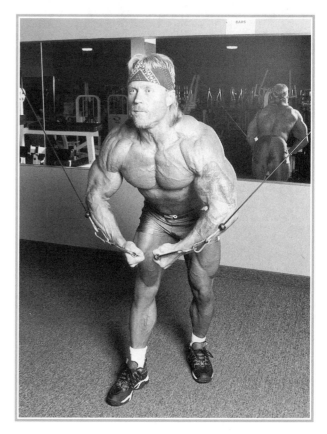

Exercise Technique

1. Move the cables in a downward arcing motion until your hands make contact or nearly make contact (6 to 8 inches or 15 to 20 cm from the front aspect of the pelvis).
2. Hold this position for 1 or 2 seconds to fully contract your pectoral muscles.
3. Slowly resist as you return the cables to their starting position.
4. Perform the desired number of repetitions while keeping the movement fluent, slow, and controlled.

Parallel Bar Dip

Primary Muscles Worked

- Pectoralis major and minor
- Anterior deltoids
- Triceps brachii

Secondary Muscles Worked

- Latissimus dorsi
- Teres major and minor
- Infraspinatus
- Medial deltoids
- Trapezius (upper and lower)

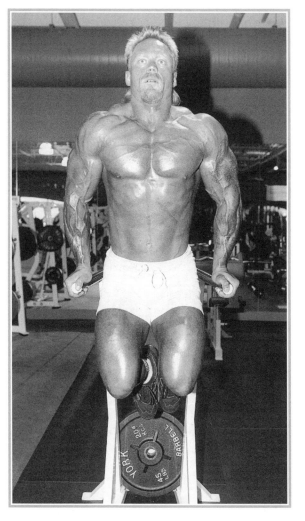

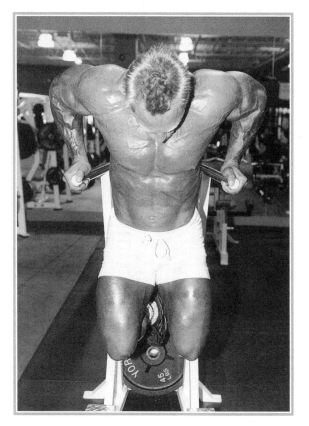

Starting Position

1. Support your body at straight arms' length (elbows not locked).
2. Keep your knees flexed, feet behind you, and torso erect at the starting position.

Exercise Technique

1. Bend your arms, allowing your elbows to travel slightly out to your sides while your torso inclines forward.
2. Lower your body to a point where you achieve a comfortable stretch.
3. When this occurs, slowly push your torso upward to the starting position.
4. Remember: Never lock your elbows.
5. Perform the desired number of repetitions while keeping the movement fluent, slow, and controlled.

ABDOMINALS

The muscle groups that give complete development to the midsection are among the most important, in part because they contribute to the health and integrity of a person's lower back and abdomen. Many lower back injuries result from weak abdominal muscles rather than underdeveloped spinal erectors.

The abdominal muscles are an important part of a competitive bodybuilder's physique. A tightly packed midsection is a characteristic that all panel judges look for. A bodybuilder who enters a competitive stage with great abdominals creates a psychological impact that the evaluating judges and audience cannot overlook. Abdominals that are thickly muscled and tightly defined create a good first impression, resulting in a favorable response throughout the rest of the prejudging and show.

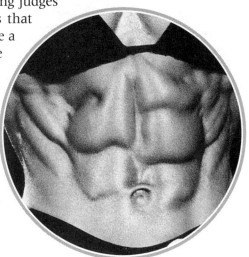

Today men who are competing at 260 to 270 pounds (118 to 122 kg) and women who are competing at 160 to 180 pounds (73 to 82 kg) must have total abdominal development. They should have thick ridges of muscle in the front abdominals, obliques, and intercostals, with deep grooves between the major abdominal groups.

Abdominal Crunch (Flat Bench)

Primary Muscles Worked	Secondary Muscles Worked
• Rectus abdominis (upper and middle)	• Intercostal muscles

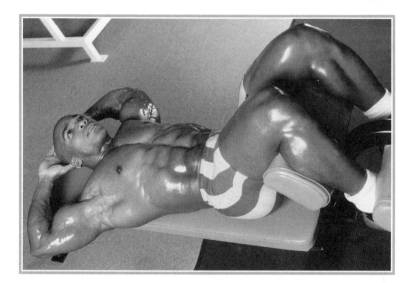

Starting Position

1. Lie flat on an abdominal bench with your knees bent and feet locked under the ankle pads.
2. Place your hands and arms behind your head.

Exercise Technique

1. Use upper abdominal strength to raise your head and shoulders from the abdominal bench.
2. When the rectus abdominis muscles are maximally contracted, hold for 1-2 seconds and return to the starting position.
3. To keep tension on your working muscles, do not allow your torso (upper trapezius and shoulders) to make contact with the bench.
4. Repeat the movement until you complete the desired number of repetitions.

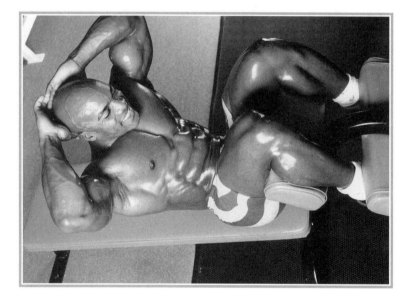

Nautilus Crunch

Primary Muscles Worked

- Rectus abdominis (upper and middle)

Secondary Muscles Worked

- Intercostal muscles

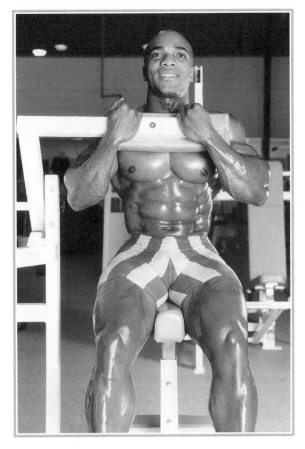

Starting Position

1. Sit on the seat of the crunch machine.
2. At this point, a chest pad should be resting firmly against the chest.
3. Place your hands across the back of the chest padding for support.

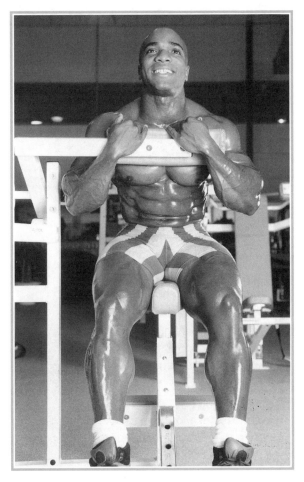

Exercise Technique

1. Bend your torso forward until your abdominals are maximally contracted.
2. Blow all the air out of your lungs as you perform the movement.
3. Slowly return to the starting position, never letting the weighted plates make contact (maintaining tension in the working muscles).
4. Repeat until you complete the desired number of repetitions.

Pulley Crunch

Primary Muscles Worked	Secondary Muscles Worked
• Rectus abdominis (upper)	• Lower lats • Serratus muscles • Intercostals

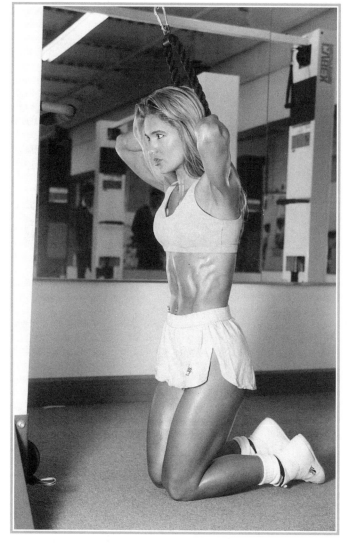

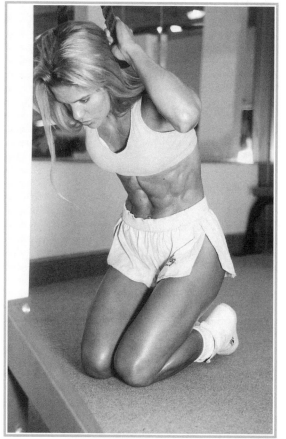

Starting Position

1. Attach a rope handle to an overhead pulley, and grasp the rope handles with an overhand grip.
2. Hold the rope behind your neck, and kneel down approximately 1 foot (30 cm) from the pulley machine.

Exercise Technique

1. Bend over at the waist until your abdominals are maximally contracted.
2. Blow all the air out of your lungs as you perform the movement.
3. Repeat the movement until you complete the desired number of repetitions.
4. The objective is to perform the exercise in a controlled manner and to maintain the tension on the working muscles throughout the entire movement.

Knee-Up
(Flat Bench)

Primary Muscles Worked
- Rectus abdominis (lower)

Secondary Muscles Worked
- Intercostal muscles

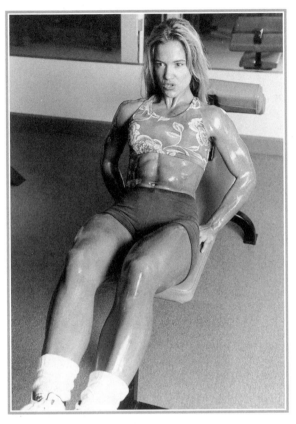

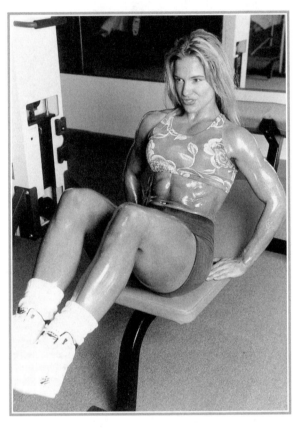

Starting Position

1. Sit on the end of a flat bench, and place your hands behind your buttocks to support your body.
2. Lean back until your torso is approximately at a 45-degree angle to the bench.
3. Extend your legs until they are almost straightened.

Exercise Technique

1. Pull your knees toward your chest.
2. As your knees approach your chest, flex your neck, allowing your head to curl toward your knees (this will ensure maximal abdominal contraction).
3. Return to the starting position.
4. Repeat the movement until you complete the desired number of repetitions.

Hanging Leg Raise

Primary Muscles Worked	Secondary Muscles Worked
• Rectus abdominis (mainly lower)	• Intercostal muscles
• Serratus anterior	

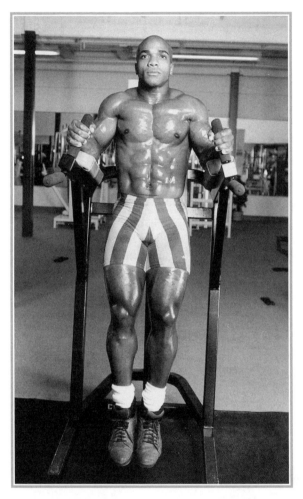

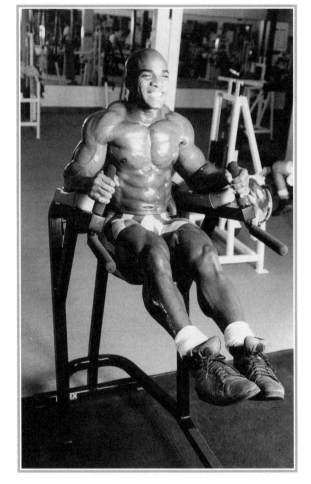

Starting Position

1. Grasp the handles of the hanging leg raise machine and support your body weight with your arms.
2. Allow your torso to hang down in a straight vertical line.
3. Keep your knees slightly bent throughout the entire movement to prevent any unnecessary stress on your lower back.

Exercise Technique

1. Using abdominal strength, slowly raise your legs to the level of your hips.
2. Hold the contraction for a moment, then slowly lower your legs to the starting position.
3. Repeat the movement until you complete the desired number of repetitions.

Diagonal Curl-Up

Primary Muscles Worked

- Serratus anterior
- Rectus abdominis (mainly upper)

Secondary Muscles Worked

- Intercostal muscles

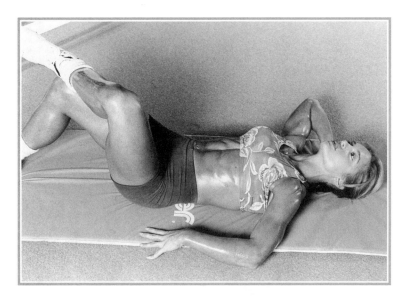

Starting Position

1. Lie down on an abdominal board or floor mat, with your knees bent and feet on the floor.
2. Place your left ankle across your right knee. A triangle should form from their contact.
3. Place your right hand behind your head, and place your left hand on the mat for support.

Exercise Technique

1. Curl your torso diagonally, bringing your right shoulder up toward your left knee.
2. Once you have reached maximal contraction, hold for 1-2 seconds.
3. Return to the starting position (never allowing your shoulders to touch the mat), and repeat until you complete the desired number of repetitions.
4. Reverse body position, and repeat for the other side.

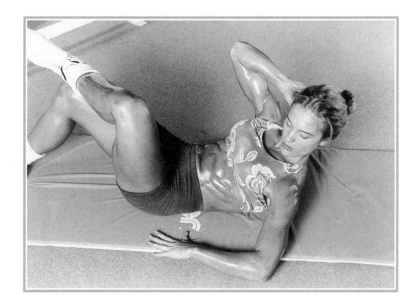

BACK

A front or back lat spread is another impressive feature in bodybuilding. Those wide, thick wings look as if they are ready for flight. All top professional bodybuilders have thick, well-developed latissimus dorsi muscles, and their erector spinae muscles look like huge mounds of flesh. You can work on your wings with these exercises. Back routines are structured around exercises for width, such as lat machine pull-downs and wide-grip chin-ups, and mass exercises, such as bent-over barbell rows, T-bar rows, and one-arm dumbbell rows.

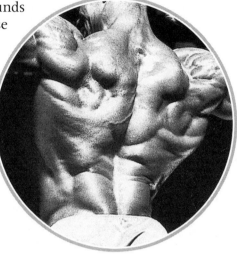

Bent-Over Barbell Row (Olympic Bar)

Primary Muscles Worked

- Latissimus dorsi
- Trapezius (middle)
- Brachialis
- Forearm flexors

Secondary Muscles Worked

- Brachioradialis
- Biceps brachii
- Teres major and minor
- Rhomboids
- Infraspinatus

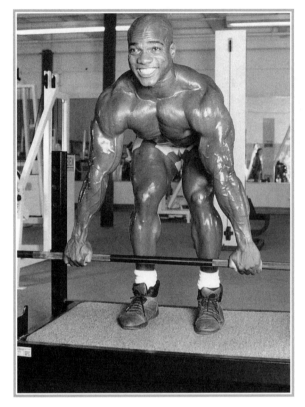

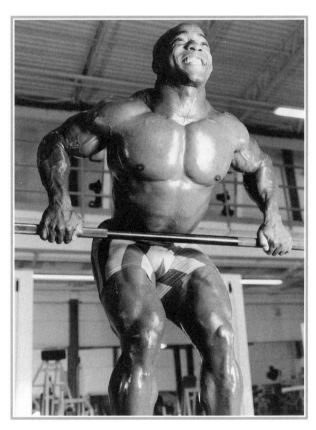

Starting Position

1. Grasp the bar using an overhand grip with your hands approximately 4 to 6 inches (10 to 15 cm) wider than shoulder-width apart, and remove the bar from the standards.
2. Take a shoulder-width stance, and keep your feet flat on the ground.
3. Slowly bend forward at the hips, keeping your back flat and allowing for a slight bend in the knees.
4. At this point, your torso should be parallel to the ground, with arms fully extended, holding the bar.

Exercise Technique

1. Moving only your arms, slowly pull the bar upward, allowing it to touch the lower part of your rib cage. Your torso should not move upward more than 4 inches (10 cm).
2. Lower the weight slowly to the starting position. Repeat the movement until you complete the desired number of repetitions.

One-Arm Dumbbell Row (Alternate Arms)

Primary Muscles Worked

- Latissimus dorsi
- Trapezius (middle)
- Brachialis
- Posterior deltoids
- Forearm flexors

Secondary Muscles Worked

- Biceps brachii
- Teres major and minor
- Infraspinatus
- Rhomboids

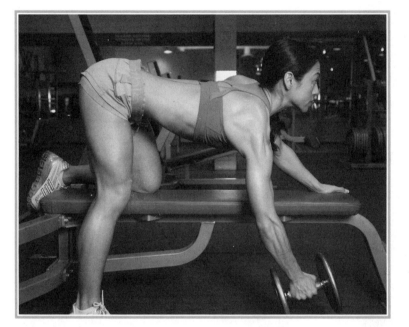

Starting Position

1. Grasp a dumbbell with your right hand using an overhand grip (palms facing your body).
2. Rest your left knee on a flat bench. Your right leg should be flexed with your foot flat on the floor.
3. Bend forward at the hips, and stabilize your body with a straightened left arm.
4. At this point, your torso should be nearly parallel to the floor.
5. The dumbbell in your right hand is at full arms' length.

Exercise Technique

1. Keeping your elbow close to your torso, pull the dumbbell upward in a straight vertical line, allowing it to lightly touch your rib cage.
2. Slowly lower the dumbbell to the starting position. Repeat the movement until you complete the desired number of repetitions.
3. Repeat for the left hand.

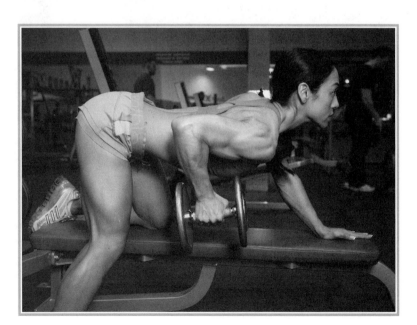

T-Bar Row

Primary Muscles Worked

- Latissimus dorsi
- Trapezius
- Forearm flexors
- Brachioradialis

Secondary Muscles Worked

- Teres major and minor
- Erector spinae
- Infraspinatus
- Rhomboids

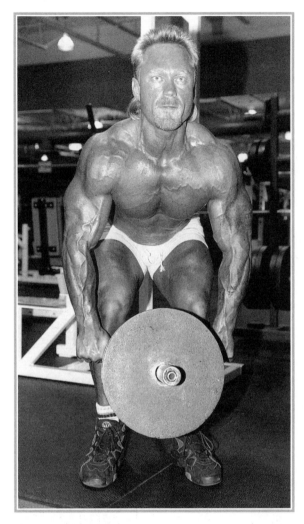

Starting Position

1. Bend forward at the hips, keeping your back flat and knees bent.
2. Grasp the T-bar handles using an overhand grip (palms facing backward).
3. Raise your torso to a position where it is parallel to the floor.
4. Arms should be fully extended.

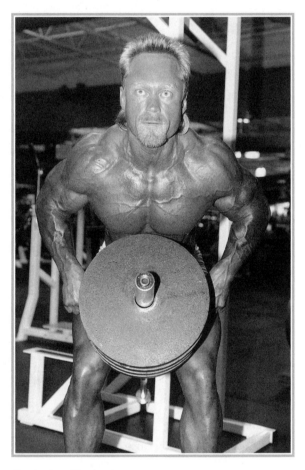

Exercise Technique

1. Pull your hands upward until the weight touches your chest.
2. Your torso should not move upward more than 4 inches (10 cm).
3. Slowly return to the starting position. Repeat the movement until you complete the desired number of repetitions.

Lat Pull-Down to the Front

Primary Muscles Worked

- Latissimus dorsi
- Brachialis
- Brachioradialis

Secondary Muscles Worked

- Biceps brachii
- Posterior deltoids
- Teres major and minor
- Infraspinatus
- Rhomboids

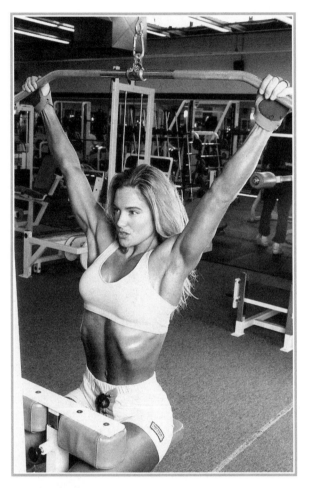

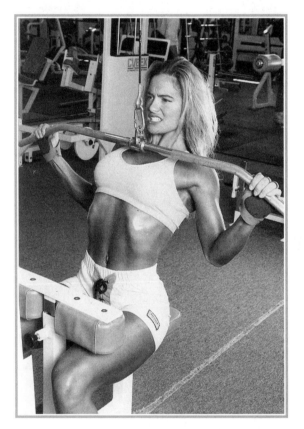

Starting Position

1. Stand in front of the lat pull-down machine and grasp the bar using an overhand grip (wide).
2. Sit down with your feet flat on the floor, back straight, and thighs secured underneath the thigh pads.
3. Arch your torso and lean backward.
4. Your torso remains rigid throughout the entire movement.
5. At this point, your arms are fully extended, holding the lat bar overhead.

Exercise Technique

1. Initiate the movement by pulling your elbows downward and backward.
2. Bring the bar in front of your head until it touches the upper part of your chest; hold for 1-2 seconds.
3. Slowly bring the bar back to the starting position, and repeat the movement until you complete the desired number of repetitions.

Seated Pulley Row

Primary Muscles Worked

- Latissimus dorsi
- Trapezius
- Rhomboids
- Erector spinae

Secondary Muscles Worked

- Posterior deltoids
- Biceps brachii
- Brachioradialis
- Teres minor
- Infraspinatus
- Forearm flexors

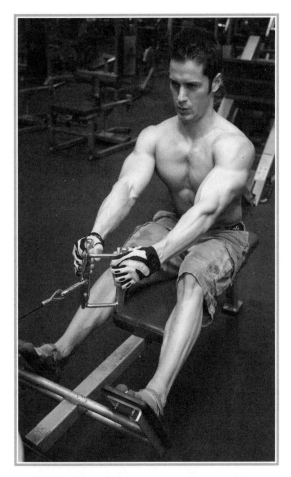

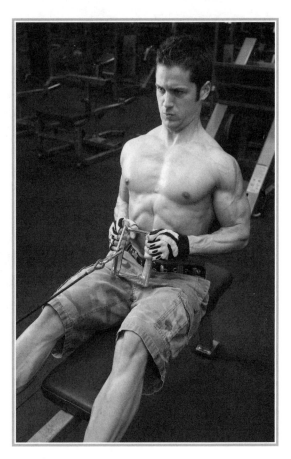

Starting Position

1. Grasp the seated pulley handle with palms facing inward.
2. Straighten your arms, sit on the padding, and place your feet on the floor rests at the front of the machine.
3. Keep a slight bend in your knees throughout the movement.
4. Lean forward, allowing your head to lower between your arms (excellent prestretch for the lats) and keeping your back flat.

Exercise Technique

1. Bring your torso to an erect position, pulling the handle toward your abdominals.
2. To maximally contract your lats, remember to slightly arch your back and keep your elbows close to your torso while pulling the handle toward the abdominals.
3. Return to the starting position. Repeat the movement until you complete the desired number of repetitions.

Front Chin-Up

Primary Muscles Worked

- Latissimus dorsi
- Trapezius (upper)
- Biceps brachii
- Brachioradialis
- Brachialis

Secondary Muscles Worked

- Posterior deltoids
- Erector spinae
- Infraspinatus

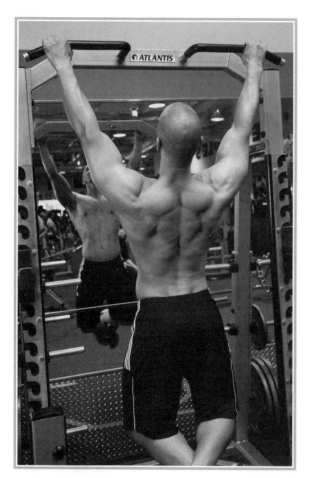

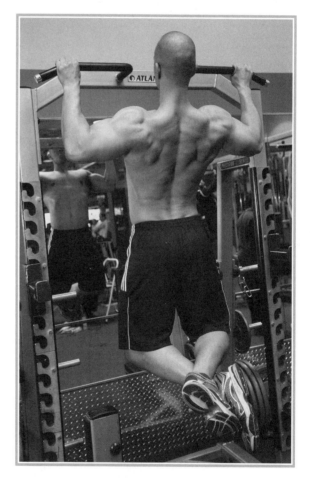

Starting Position

1. Grasp a chin-up bar with an overhand grip approximately 3 to 5 inches (8 to 13 cm) wider than shoulder-width apart.
2. Knees are flexed at a 90-degree angle so your ankles can cross over each other.

Exercise Technique

1. Pull your body up in a vertical line until your chin is parallel to the chin-up bar.
2. Slowly lower your body to the starting position. Repeat the movement until you complete the desired number of repetitions.

Lat Pull-Down Behind the Neck

Primary Muscles Worked	Secondary Muscles Worked
• Latissimus dorsi	• Forearm extensors
• Trapezius (upper)	• Teres minor
• Biceps brachii	• Infraspinatus
• Brachialis	• Posterior deltoids

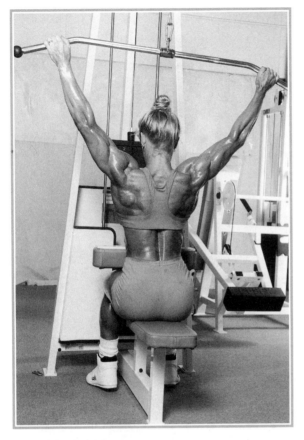

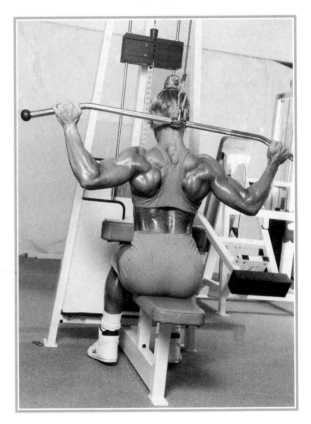

Starting Position

1. Stand in front of the lat pull-down machine, and grasp the bar with an overhand grip (wide).
2. Sit down with your feet flat on the floor, back straight, and thighs secured underneath the thigh pads.
3. At this point your arms are fully extended, holding the bar overhead.

Exercise Technique

1. Initiate the movement by pulling your elbows downward and backward.
2. As the bar approaches your head, lean slightly forward, allowing the bar to touch the top part of your neck.
3. Slowly bring the bar back to the starting position. Repeat the movement until you complete the desired number of repetitions.

Back Extension

Primary Muscles Worked
- Erector spinae

Secondary Muscles Worked
- Gluteals
- Trapezius (lower)

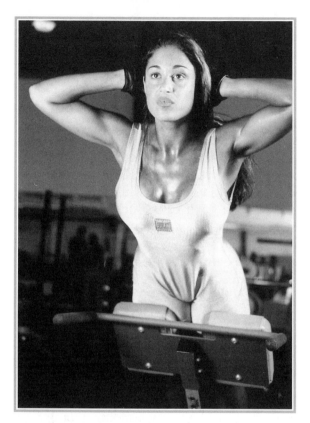

Starting Position

1. Holding the handles of the back extension machine, secure your ankles underneath the small pads and lower your hips onto the larger pads at the front of the apparatus.

2. Keep your legs straight and arms crossed behind your head throughout the entire movement.

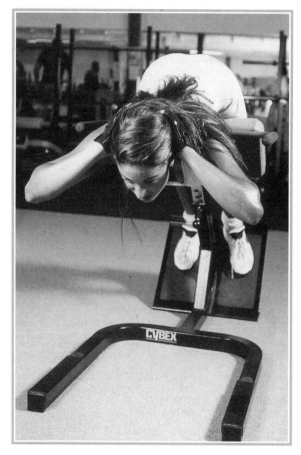

Exercise Technique

1. Lower your torso until it is almost perpendicular to the floor.

2. Slowly bring your torso back to the starting position. Repeat the movement until you complete the desired number of repetitions.

3. Remember not to arch upward excessively, for this can cause compression of the vertebrae in your spine.

DELTOIDS AND TRAPEZIUS

The whole idea behind bodybuilding is to make your physique stand out above the rest. If you combine a wide shoulder structure with well-developed deltoids and a thin waistline, you can potentially build the type of symmetry and size that wins bodybuilding titles and competitions. No one with weak deltoids has ever won a major bodybuilding title or competition. In fact, no one with even average deltoids will ever win a major bodybuilding show.

The deltoids are so important to bodybuilders because they are visible from every angle during a pose. Therefore weak deltoids can be detected from every angle. Have you ever seen a competitive bodybuilder turn to his back side to perform the back double biceps pose, and that huge mound of flesh that creates the rear deltoid is lacking? It is an unfavorable attribute. You can prevent this problem by using the exercises in this section, which starts off with exercises for each of the deltoid muscle groups. Mass exercises—such as the seated front dumbbell press or standing dumbbell side and bent laterals—will definitely put size on all three deltoid heads, especially the medial deltoids (standing dumbbell side laterals).

For teens who are starting to train, clavicle widening movements can be very effective. Your ligaments, tendons, and cartilage are still soft, and your epiphyseal plates have not yet closed (your bones have not stopped growing). Therefore, further bone growth is still possible; in fact, the skeletal frame and fascia tissues can still stretch. Although most bodybuilders are not in their teens and their bone plates have stopped growing, they can still widen their clavicles through a thickening of the cartilage. By building a lot of mass on their medial deltoids, they can give the illusion that their shoulders are wider than they really are.

Exercises such as ultra-wide chin-ups and wide-grip lat machine pull-downs can stretch the clavicles and widen the shoulder blades. Ultra-wide chin-ups must not be confused with wide-grip chin-ups for the lats. Your hands must be placed as wide as physically possible. For clavicle stretching to occur, you must perform the reps slowly and fully, and at the bottom of each rep hang and feel the stretching and widening of your shoulder blades. It is as if you were trying to dislocate your scapulae (without actually doing it). If you are not strong enough to perform the ultra-wide chin-ups, use wide-grip lat machine pull-downs for a clavicle stretch, and superset them with wide-grip chin-up hangs. Your aim in wide-grip chin-up hangs is to hold the widened position as long as you can without actually dislocating your clavicles. Remember that pain and discomfort are normal with these exercises because you are stretching and pulling the clavicles apart. Understand also that these exercises are not performed for lat development.

The trapezius muscles are large muscles in the upper back area. They form a star. The points of the star are situated at the base of the skull (upper points), near the points of the shoulders, and about halfway down the spine (lower point). The primary function of the trapezius muscles is to pull the shoulders upward and backward. They also contract to help arch the lower back. No part of the human body is more visible year-round than the neck. Because of the trapezius muscles, bodybuilders are easily visible in a large crowd. Many critics have written that bodybuilders actually "wear their sport."

Standing Dumbbell Side Lateral

Primary Muscles Worked

- Medial deltoids

Secondary Muscles Worked

- Anterior deltoids
- Trapezius (upper and lower)

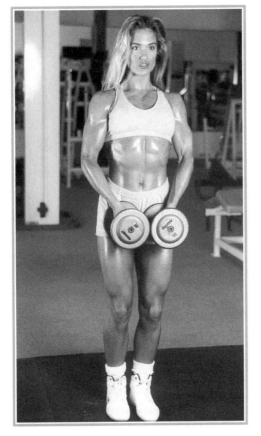

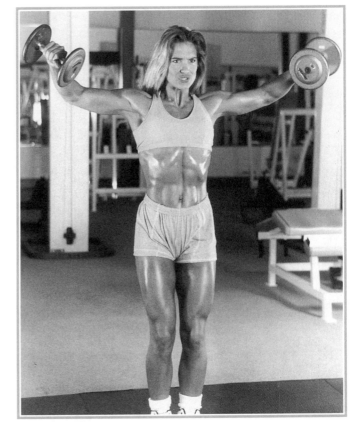

Starting Position

1. Stand with your back straight, knees slightly bent, and feet slightly less than shoulder-width apart.
2. Keep your back erect and elbows slightly flexed throughout the entire movement.
3. Grasp the dumbbells using an overhand grip with palms facing each other.
4. Press the dumbbells together approximately 4 to 6 inches (10 to 15 cm) in front of your hips.

Exercise Technique

1. Keeping your elbows slightly bent, raise the dumbbells laterally in an arc toward the ceiling until your arms are parallel to the floor; hold for 1-2 seconds.
2. Slowly lower the dumbbells to the starting position. Repeat the movement until you complete the desired number of repetitions.

Standing Dumbbell Bent Lateral

Primary Muscles Worked

- Posterior deltoids

Secondary Muscles Worked

- Medial deltoids
- Trapezius (upper)
- Teres minor
- Rhomboids
- Infraspinatus

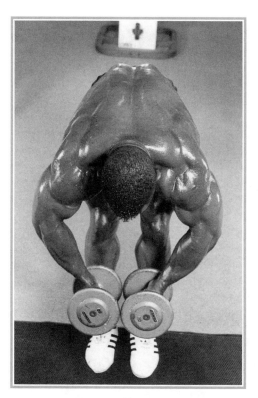

Starting Position

1. Stand with your back straight, knees bent, and feet shoulder-width apart.
2. Grasp the dumbbells using an overhand grip with palms facing each other.
3. Bend at the hips until your back is parallel to the floor and your arms are hanging down in an extended position (perpendicular to the floor).

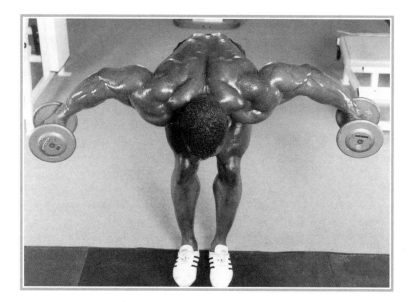

Exercise Technique

1. Keeping your elbows slightly bent, raise the dumbbells laterally in an arc-like motion until your arms are parallel to the floor.
2. Slowly lower the dumbbells to the starting position. Repeat the movement until you complete the desired number of repetitions.

Seated Front Dumbbell Press

Primary Muscles Worked

- Anterior deltoids

Secondary Muscles Worked

- Pectoralis major
- Triceps brachii
- Trapezius (upper and lower)
- Serratus anterior

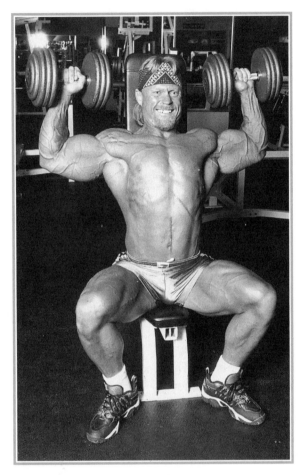

Starting Position

1. Grasp two dumbbells using an overhand grip, and sit down on an upright bench.
2. Lift the dumbbells to shoulder level.
3. Rotate your palms so they are facing forward.

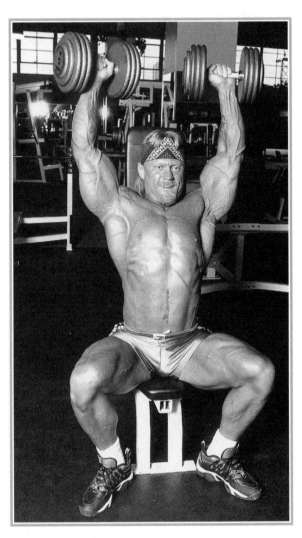

Exercise Technique

1. Slowly push the dumbbells directly upward until they touch each other at straight arms' length, and then slowly return the dumbbells to the starting position.
2. Remember never to lock your elbows at the top of the movement.
3. Repeat the movement until you complete the desired number of repetitions.

Seated Front Barbell Press

Primary Muscles Worked

- Anterior deltoids

Secondary Muscles Worked

- Pectoralis major
- Triceps brachii
- Trapezius
- Serratus anterior

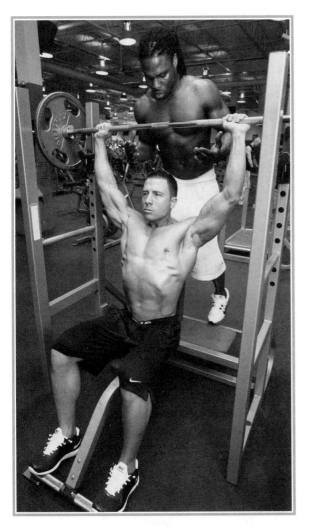

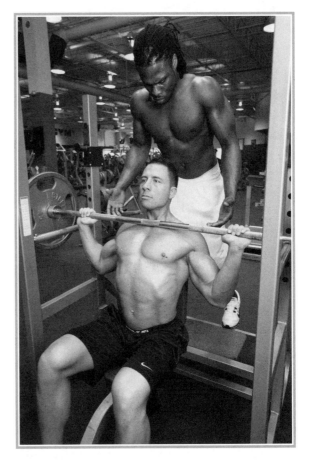

Starting Position

1. Sit on the bench with your back pressed firmly against the padding for support.
2. Grasp the barbell using an overhand grip with hands approximately 3 to 5 inches (8 to 13 cm) wider than shoulder-width apart.
3. Have a spotter help you lift the Olympic bar from the standards.
4. At this point the Olympic bar is straight above your head with your elbows slightly flexed.

Exercise Technique

1. Slowly lower the weight down to your anterior deltoids (in front of head), and without bouncing the barbell at the bottom of the movement, push it upward to the starting position.
2. Never lock your elbows at the top of the movement.
3. Repeat the movement until you complete the desired number of repetitions.

Front Barbell Shrug (Olympic Bar)

Primary Muscles Worked

- Trapezius (upper)
- Rhomboids

Secondary Muscles Worked

- Pectoralis major
- Triceps brachii
- Trapezius (lower)
- Serratus anterior

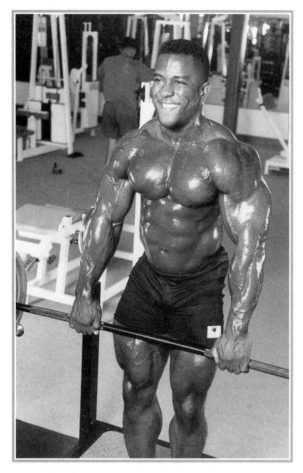

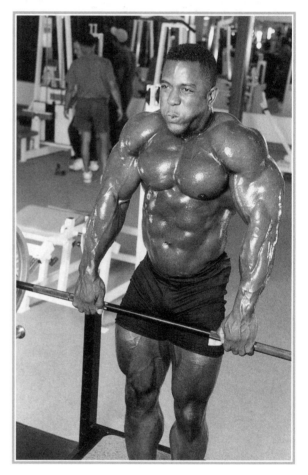

Starting Position

1. Keep your back erect, your knees slightly bent, and a shoulder-width stance throughout the movement.
2. Grasp the Olympic bar using an overhand grip with hands slightly wider than shoulder-width apart.
3. At this point the barbell is at straight arms' length with a slight bend in your elbows.
4. The Olympic bar is resting across your upper thighs.

Exercise Technique

1. To initiate the movement, lift your shoulders toward your ears, and hold the contraction for 1-2 seconds.
2. When the contraction is complete, slowly lower the bar to a point where a comfortable stretch is felt in the working muscles (facilitates maximum range of motion).
3. Repeat the movement until you complete the desired number of repetitions.

Primary Muscles Worked	Secondary Muscles Worked
• Anterior deltoids	• Forearm extensors • Medial and posterior deltoids • Rhomboids • Pectoralis major

Standing Front Dumbbell Raise

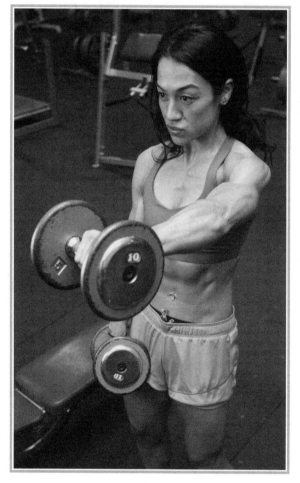

Starting Position

1. Stand with your back straight, knees slightly bent, and feet slightly less than shoulder-width apart.

2. Grasp the dumbbells using an overhand grip with palms facing downward.

3. Let your arms hang straight down at your sides, holding the dumbbells approximately 2 to 4 inches (5 to 10 cm) from upper thigh level.

Exercise Technique

1. Keeping your elbows slightly bent throughout the entire movement, raise the right dumbbell from upper thigh level to eye level, and slowly lower the dumbbell to starting position.

2. Repeat the movement with the left dumbbell; continue alternating right and left until you complete the desired number of repetitions.

Upright Row (Olympic Bar)

Primary Muscles Worked

- Trapezius
- Deltoids (anterior and medial)

Secondary Muscles Worked

- Biceps brachii
- Brachialis
- Forearm flexors

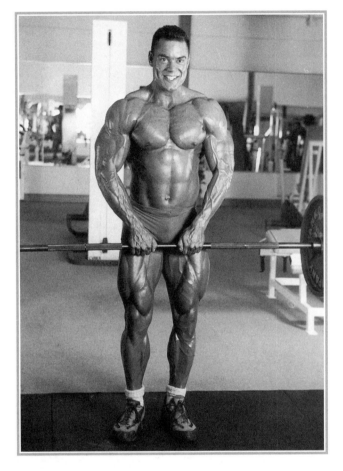

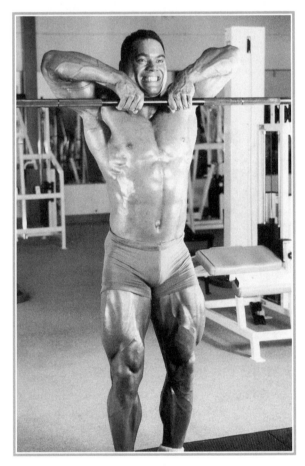

Starting Position

1. Keep your back erect, your knees slightly bent, and a shoulder-width stance throughout the movement.
2. Grasp the barbell with an overhand grip with hands approximately two thumb-widths apart.
3. At this point the barbell is at straight arms' length with a slight bend in your elbows.
4. The Olympic bar is resting across the upper thighs.

Exercise Technique

1. Raise the bar from the extended position to the point where it reaches your chin (raise elbows high), and slowly lower the bar to the starting position.
2. Repeat the movement until you complete the desired number of repetitions.

Press Behind the Neck (Olympic bar)

Primary Muscles Worked

- Posterior deltoids
- Trapezius (upper)
- Triceps brachii

Secondary Muscles Worked

- Trapezius (lower)
- Rhomboids
- Infraspinatus
- Teres major and minor
- Latissimus dorsi

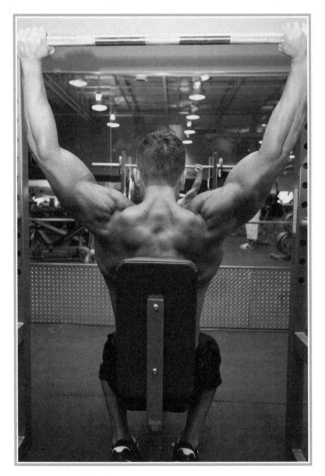

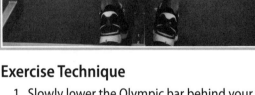

Starting Position

1. Sit on the bench with your back pressed firmly against the padding for support.
2. Grasp the Olympic bar using an overhand grip with hands placed 3 to 5 inches (8 to 13 cm) wider than shoulder-width apart.
3. Lift the Olympic bar from the standards, and hold it directly above your head with elbows slightly flexed.

Exercise Technique

1. Slowly lower the Olympic bar behind your head to a level slightly below your ears.
2. Without bouncing at the bottom of the movement, push the bar upward to the starting position.
3. Never lock your elbows at the top of the movement.
4. Repeat the movement until you complete the desired number of repetitions.

BICEPS

The biceps are most bodybuilders' favorite muscles to train. Despite the biceps' relatively small size compared with the muscles of the thighs, back, and chest, our love affair with the biceps no doubt arises from our culture's association of big biceps with strength and masculinity. Every great champion in the past seven decades has had huge arms and biceps.

The exercises in this section will help you build your biceps. Use biceps preacher curls, standing dumbbell curls, and incline dumbbell curls to pack mass and peak your biceps. Movements such as dumbbell or cable concentration curls are better for adding height to the peak of your biceps muscles.

Biceps Preacher Curl (Olympic Bar)

Primary Muscles Worked
- Biceps brachii
- Brachialis

Secondary Muscles Worked
- Forearm flexors

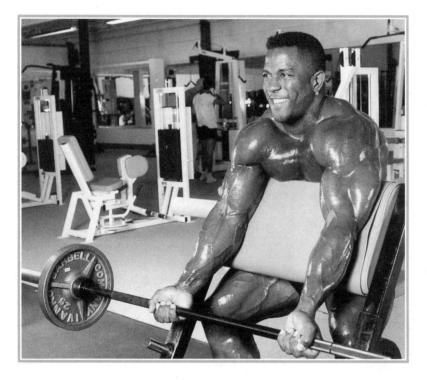

Starting Position
1. Sit on the preacher curl bench.
2. Grasp the Olympic bar using an underhand grip (palms facing upward) with hands shoulder-width apart.
3. Arms are extended (not locked) with your triceps resting over the angled surface of the preacher bench.

Exercise Technique
1. Initiate the movement by flexing at the elbow and curling the bar upward toward the shoulders.
2. Your triceps always maintain direct contact with the angled surface of the preacher bench.
3. Slowly lower the bar to the starting position. Repeat the movement until you complete the desired number of repetitions.

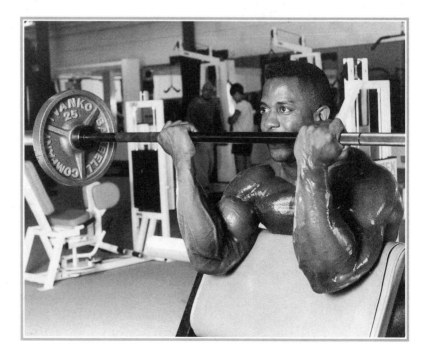

Incline Seated Dumbbell Curl (Alternate Arms)

Primary Muscles Worked
- Biceps brachii

Secondary Muscles Worked
- Forearm flexors

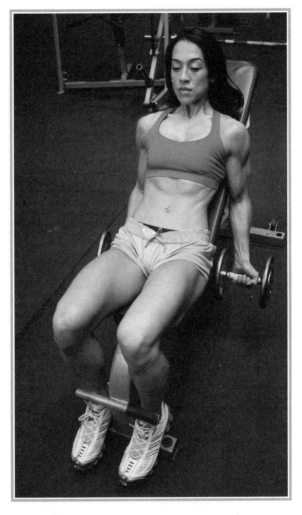

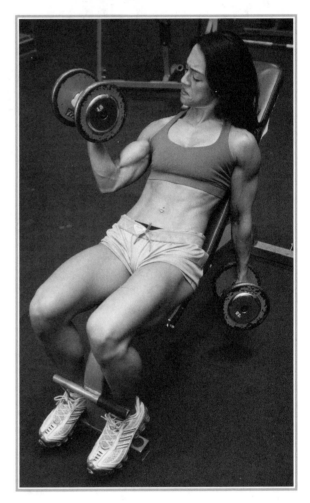

Starting Position

1. Lie on an incline bench with your back pressed firmly against the padding and feet flat on the floor.
2. Hang your arms down at your sides, holding the dumbbells with an underhand grip (palms facing upward).

Exercise Technique

1. Slowly curl the right dumbbell toward your right shoulder.
2. When maximal biceps contraction occurs, slowly lower the dumbbell to the starting position, and repeat the movement with the left arm.
3. Continue alternating right and left arms until you complete the desired number of repetitions.

Standing Biceps Curl (Olympic Bar, Narrow Grip)

Primary Muscles Worked
- Biceps brachii
- Brachialis

Secondary Muscles Worked
- Forearm flexors
- Pronator teres
- Wrist flexors (flexor pollicis longus, flexor digitorum superficialis)

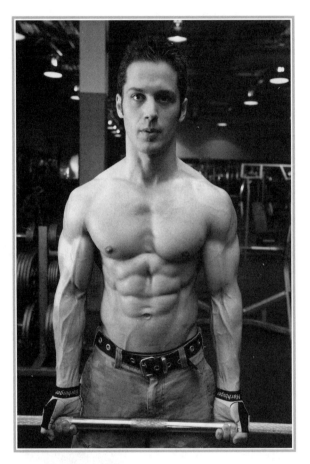

Starting Position

1. Grasp the barbell using an underhand grip (palms facing forward) with hands slightly less than shoulder-width apart.
2. Stand with your back erect, knees slightly bent, and feet shoulder-width apart throughout the movement.
3. Arms are fully extended and pressed firmly against your torso.
4. At this point the bar is resting across your upper thighs.

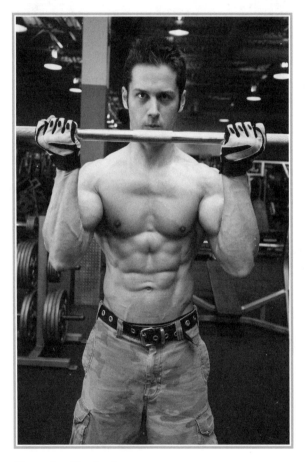

Exercise Technique

1. Initiate the movement by flexing at the elbows, curling the bar toward your shoulders.
2. When your biceps are maximally contracted, slowly lower the bar to the starting position. Repeat the movement until you complete the desired number of repetitions.

Standing Dumbbell Curl (Alternate Arms)

Primary Muscles Worked

- Biceps brachii

Secondary Muscles Worked

- Forearm flexors
- Pronator teres
- Wrist flexors (flexor pollicis longus, flexor digitorum superficialis)

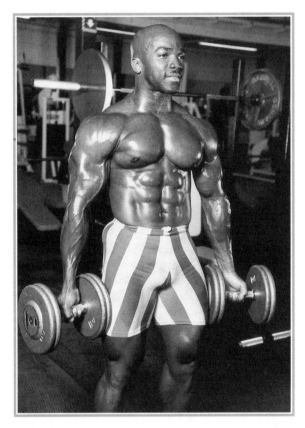

Starting Position

1. Grasp the dumbbells using an underhand grip (palms facing forward).
2. Stand with your back erect, knees slightly bent, and feet shoulder-width apart throughout the movement.
3. Arms are fully extended, and the dumbbells are hanging straight down at your sides.

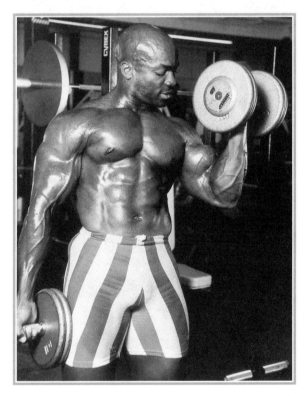

Exercise Technique

1. Initiate the movement by flexing at the elbow, curling the left dumbbell up toward your shoulder.
2. Slowly lower the dumbbell to the starting position, and repeat the movement with the right arm.
3. Continue alternating arms until you complete the desired number of repetitions.

Concentration Dumbbell Curl

Primary Muscles Worked	Secondary Muscles Worked
• Biceps brachii	• Forearm flexors
	• Brachialis

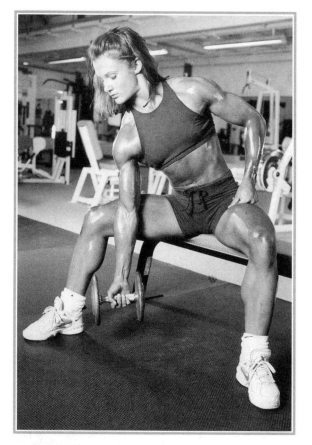

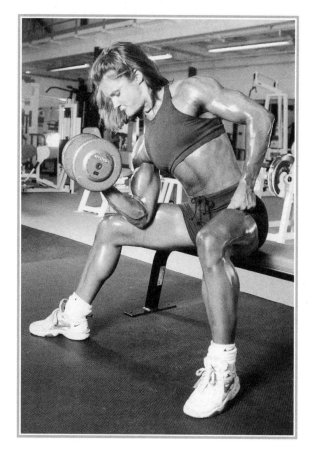

Starting Position

1. Grasp the dumbbell with your right hand, using an underhand grip (palms facing upward), and sit on a flat bench.

2. Legs are spread wide apart.

3. Lean forward at the waist, and rest your right elbow on the inside of your right thigh with your arm in full extension.

Exercise Technique

1. With your elbow resting on the inside of your thigh, slowly curl the dumbbell toward your shoulder.

2. When maximal biceps contraction occurs, slowly lower the dumbbell to the starting position. Repeat the movement until you complete the desired number of repetitions.

3. Repeat for the left hand.

Standing Biceps Curl (Olympic Bar, Wide Grip)

Primary Muscles Worked	Secondary Muscles Worked
• Biceps brachii (short head) • Brachialis	• Biceps brachii (long head) • Forearm flexors • Wrist flexors

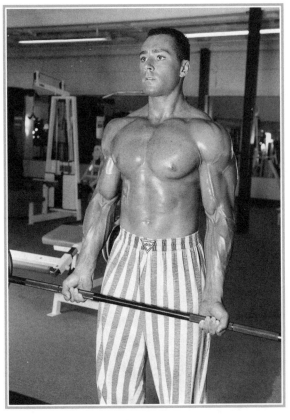

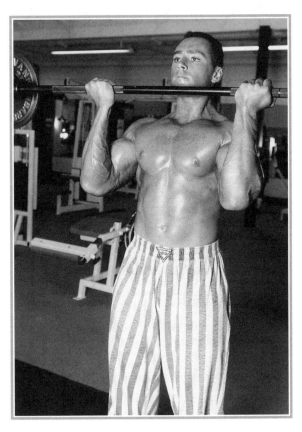

Starting Position

1. Grasp the barbell using an underhand grip (palms facing upward) with hands 2 to 3 inches (5 to 8 cm) wider than shoulder-width apart.
2. Stand with your back erect, knees slightly bent, and feet slightly wider than shoulder-width apart throughout the movement.
3. At this point your arms are fully extended with the bar resting across your upper thighs.

Exercise Technique

1. Initiate the movement by flexing at the elbow, curling the bar up toward your shoulder.
2. When the biceps are maximally contracted, slowly lower the bar to the starting position. Repeat the movement until you complete the desired number of repetitions.

Standing EZ Biceps Curl (Wide Grip)

Primary Muscles Worked

- Biceps brachii (short head)
- Brachialis

Secondary Muscles Worked

- Biceps brachii (long head)
- Forearm flexors

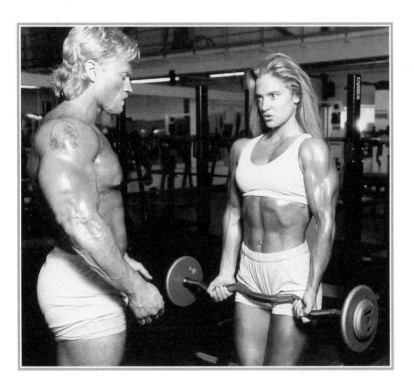

Starting Position

1. Stand with your back straight, knees slightly bent, and feet slightly less than shoulder-width apart throughout the entire movement.
2. Grasp the EZ curl bar using an underhand grip (palms facing forward) with hands slightly wider than shoulder-width apart.
3. Arms are fully extended and pressed against the sides of your torso.

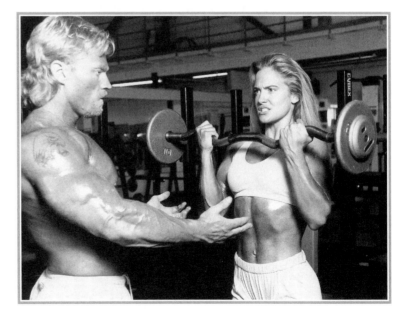

Exercise Technique

1. Initiate the movement by flexing at the elbows and curling the bar up toward your shoulders.
2. When your biceps are maximally contracted, slowly lower the bar to the starting position. Repeat the movement until you complete the desired number of repetitions.

TRICEPS

Although today's bodybuilders do plenty of isolation exercises in their triceps work-outs, much of triceps mass development comes from pressing exercises. Whenever bodybuilders do bench presses for the pectorals—whether incline or decline and dips—they also place serious stress on the triceps. By performing overhead presses for the deltoids, you are also placing intense stress on the triceps muscles. As a result, the potential for overtraining the triceps muscles is high.

How many sets of triceps work should you be doing in a workout? At the beginner level, do no more than 3 to 5 sets of total triceps train-ing. With 3 to 6 months of steady training, you can probably increase this total to 5 to 7 sets. An advanced bodybuilder will probably need 8 to 12 sets for the triceps.

Decline Triceps Extension (Olympic Bar)

Primary Muscles Worked

- Triceps (outer and medial heads)

Secondary Muscles Worked

- Forearm extensors

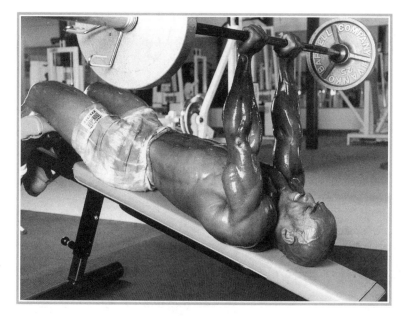

Starting Position

1. Grasp the Olympic bar using an overhand grip (palms facing downward) with hands less than shoulder-width apart.
2. Sit on the edge of the decline bench, and secure your feet and ankles underneath the pads.
3. Lie on the decline bench, simultaneously bringing the Olympic bar to a position where you simulate a bench press movement.
4. Once your arms are extended and palms are facing upward, the Olympic bar is directly over eye level.

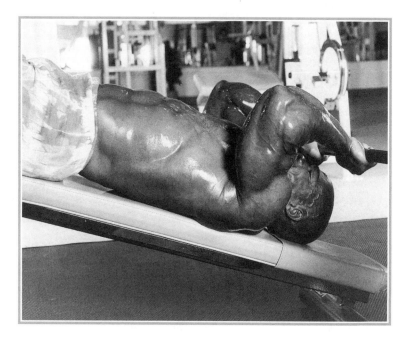

Exercise Technique

1. Keeping your upper arms fixed, slowly flex your elbows and lower the bar to your forehead.
2. Once the bar almost touches your forehead, use your triceps muscles to push your arms back to full extension.
3. Repeat the movement until you complete the desired number of repetitions.

Triceps Press-Down (Angled Bar)

Primary Muscles Worked
- Triceps (outer and medial heads)
- Anconeus

Secondary Muscles Worked
- Forearm extensors

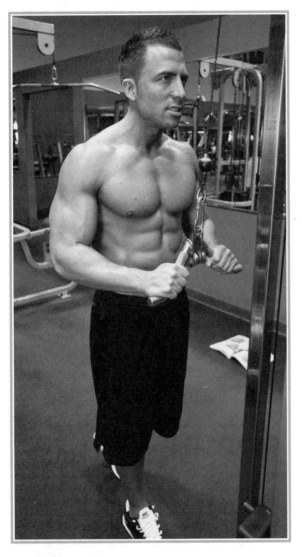

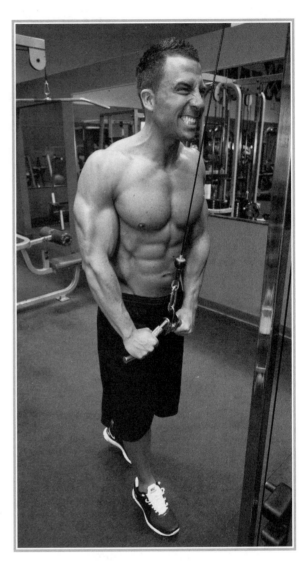

Starting Position

1. Attach the angled bar to the overhead pulley.
2. Keep your knees slightly bent, back erect, and feet shoulder-width apart or in a staggered stance.
3. Facing the overhead pulley, grasp the angled bar using an overhand grip.
4. Pull the bar down far enough to allow your upper arms to rest against the sides of your torso.
5. Your elbows should be flexed.

Exercise Technique

1. Moving only your lower arms, slowly press down on the bar until your arms are fully extended.
2. Hold the extended position for 1 to 2 seconds, and then resist as your lower arms return to the starting position.
3. Repeat the movement until you complete the desired number of repetitions.

Triceps Dip Between Benches

Primary Muscles Worked

- Triceps (outer and medial heads)

Secondary Muscles Worked

- Anterior deltoids
- Pectoralis major (lower)

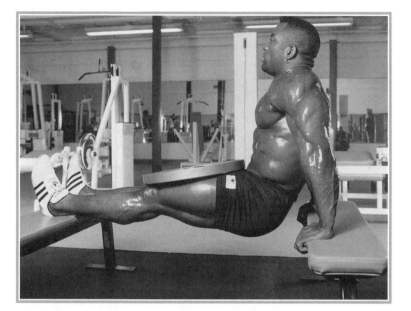

Starting Position

1. Stand between two flat benches that are approximately 3 feet (.9 m) apart (varies depending on the size of the person).
2. Place your hands on the edge of one bench, shoulder-width apart, and place your heels on the other bench.
3. Extend your arms completely, and hold this position.
4. Add a weight plate to the top of your thighs for an extra challenge.

Exercise Technique

1. Initiate the movement by slowly bending your arms until your body is lowered between the benches.
2. Slowly push back up to the starting position by straightening your arms, and repeat the movement until you complete the desired number of repetitions.

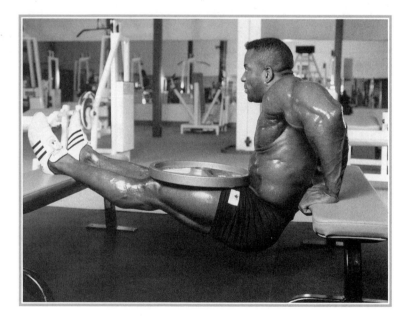

One-Arm Cable Triceps Extension (Reverse Grip)

Primary Muscles Worked
- Triceps (outer and medial heads)

Secondary Muscles Worked
- Forearm extensors

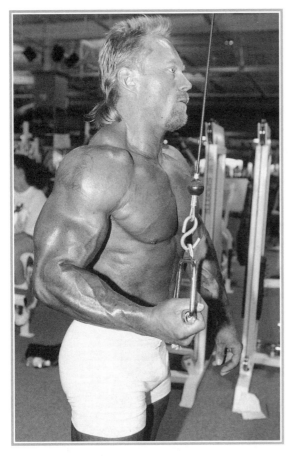

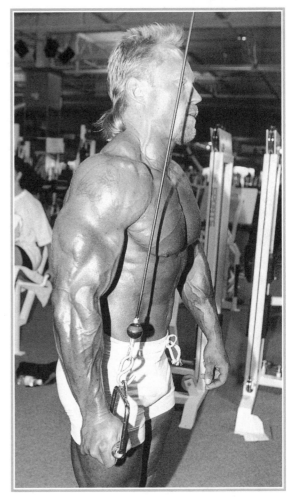

Starting Position

1. Attach a loop handle to the overhead cable pulley.
2. Facing the pulley, grasp the loop handle in your right hand with an underhand grip, and step approximately 1 foot (.3 m) back from the pulley.
3. Pull the handle down far enough to allow your upper arm to rest firmly against the side of your torso.
4. Your elbows should be flexed.

Exercise Technique

1. Moving only your lower arm, slowly pull the handle back and downward until your arm is fully extended.
2. Hold the position in full extension for 1 to 2 seconds, and then resist as your lower arm returns to the starting position.
3. Repeat the movement until you complete the desired number of repetitions.
4. Repeat for the other hand.

Overhead Rope Triceps Extension

Primary Muscles Worked	Secondary Muscles Worked
• Triceps (all heads)	• Forearm extensors

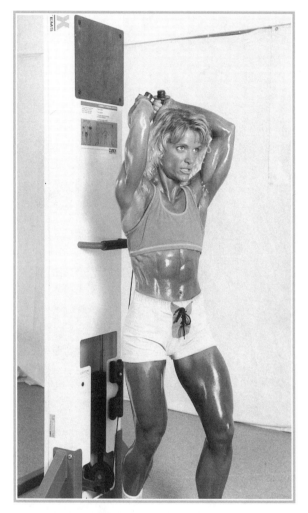

Starting Position

1. Attach the rope to the overhead pulley.
2. Stand with your back facing the pulley machine.
3. With feet staggered (one leg in front of the other), place your forward foot flat on the floor. Flex your back foot, with only the ball of your foot touching the ground.
4. Grasp the rope with an overhand grip (palms facing each other), and bend slightly forward at the waist.
5. In the starting position, your upper arms follow your ear line.
6. Your elbows are completely flexed, and the rope is behind your neck.

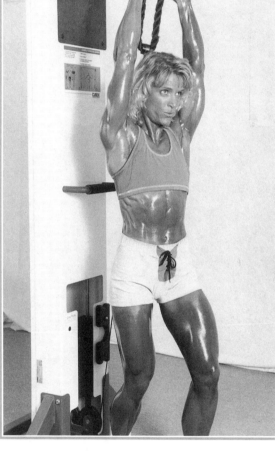

Exercise Technique

1. Initiate the movement by slowly extending the lower part of your arms.
2. Hold the fully extended position for 1 to 2 seconds.
3. Slowly bring your arms back to the starting position.
4. Repeat the movement until you complete the desired number of repetitions.
5. Bending occurs only at your elbows—your upper arms remain motionless.

Seated One-Arm Dumbbell Triceps Extension (Neutral Grip)

Primary Muscles Worked
- Triceps (inner and medial heads)
- Anconeus

Secondary Muscles Worked
- Forearm extensors
- Posterior deltoids

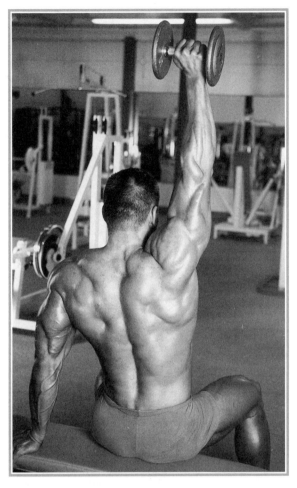

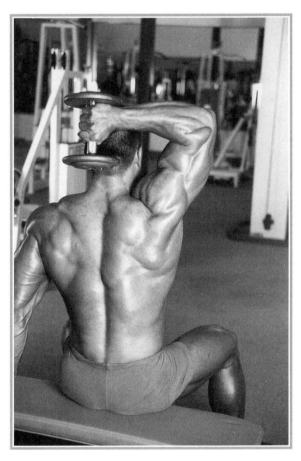

Starting Position
1. Sit on a flat bench with your feet flat on the floor.
2. Grasp a dumbbell with an overhand grip (palm faces forward throughout the movement).
3. Hold the dumbbell overhead with your arm fully extended.

Exercise Technique
1. Lower the dumbbell until your forearm is parallel to the floor.
2. At this point the dumbbell is behind your neck (finish of movement).
3. Without bouncing the weight at the bottom of the movement, slowly extend the dumbbell to the starting position. Repeat the movement until you complete the desired number of repetitions.
4. Repeat for the other hand.

Close-Grip Bench Press (Olympic bar)

Primary Muscles Worked	Secondary Muscles Worked
• Triceps (all heads)	• Latissimus dorsi
• Pectoralis major (middle and lower)	• Anterior deltoids

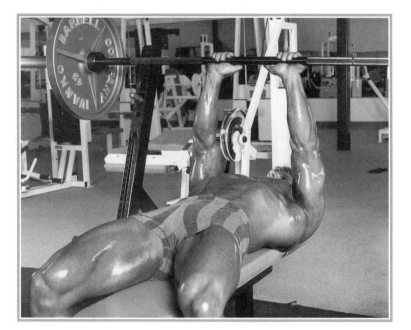

Starting Position

1. Lie on a flat bench with your back pressed firmly against the padding and feet on the floor.
2. Grasp the bar using an overhand grip with hands approximately two thumb-widths apart, and lift the bar from the standards.
3. Arms should be fully extended (not locked) with palms facing forward as you hold the bar.

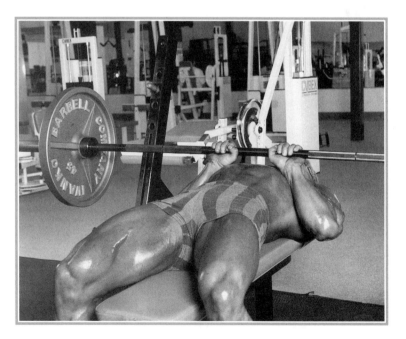

Exercise Technique

1. Bend at the elbows, lowering the bar to the midpoint of your chest.
2. Without bouncing the weight off your chest, use your triceps muscles to press it back to the starting position.
3. Repeat the movement until you complete the desired number of repetitions.

FOREARMS

Some bodybuilders have genetically gifted forearms without even directly training the muscle group. Others are less fortunate: Regardless of how hard they work, they never have fantastic forearms. Now all great pro and amateur bodybuilders at the national and international levels have exceptional forearms. If you are lucky enough to have optimal genetics for fabulous forearm development, good for you. If you are average or below average in forearm development, here are some pointers: Save your forearms for the end of your workout; train your forearms two or three times a week; and finally, train them hard and do not get discouraged—gains are slow in coming, but they will come.

Wrist Curl (Olympic Bar)

Primary Muscles Worked	Secondary Muscles Worked
• Forearm flexors	• Wrist flexors

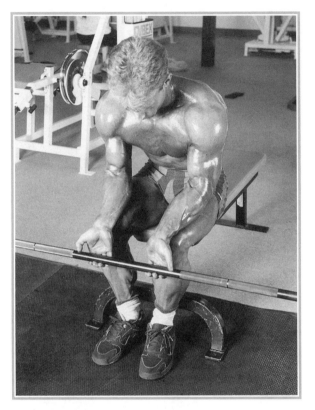

Starting Position

1. Grasp the bar with an underhand grip (palms facing upward), and sit on the end of a flat bench.
2. Place your feet flat on the floor, about shoulder-width apart or slightly wider.
3. Leaning your torso forward, run your forearms down your thighs until your wrists and hands hang over the ends of your knees.
4. Allow the weight to lower until the bar rolls onto your fingers.

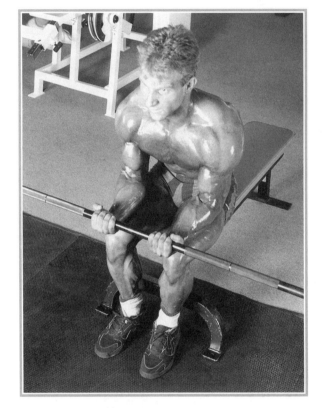

Exercise Technique

1. Using your forearm muscles, raise the bar by flexing your fingers and curling your wrists to as high a position as possible.
2. Slowly lower the weight to the starting position. Repeat the movement until you complete the desired number of repetitions.

Wrist Extension (Olympic Bar)

Primary Muscles Worked
- Forearm extensors

Secondary Muscles Worked
- Wrist extensors

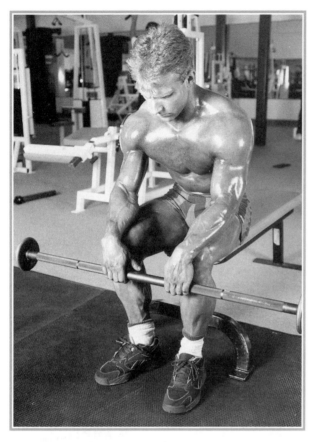

Starting Position

1. Grasp the bar with an overhand grip (palms facing downward), and sit on the end of a flat bench.
2. Place your feet flat on the floor, slightly closer than shoulder-width apart.
3. Leaning your torso forward, run your forearms down your thighs until your wrists and hands hang over the ends of your knees.
4. Allow the weight to lower until the barbell rolls onto your fingers.

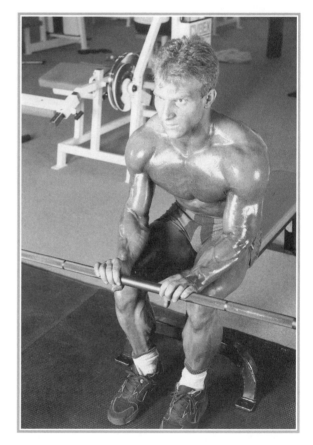

Exercise Technique

1. Using your forearm muscles, raise the bar by extending your wrists to as high a position as possible.
2. Slowly lower the weight to the starting position. Repeat the movement until you complete the desired number of repetitions.

PART FOUR

SIX PHASES of TRAINING

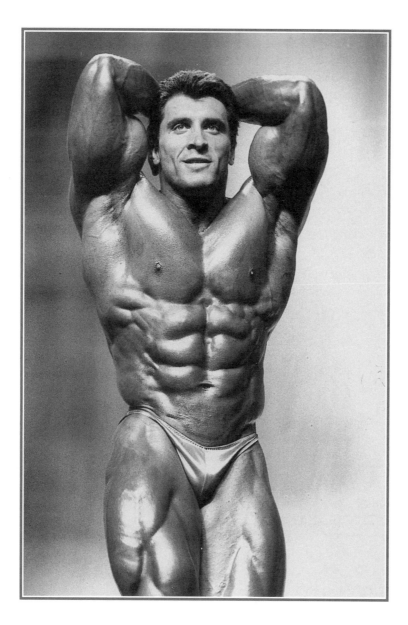

chapter 12

Anatomical Adaptation (AA)

Most entry-level bodybuilders and strength trainers start rigorous training programs without preparing the body for the high-intensity workload demands. Many times such rigorous programs immediately focus either on increasing muscle size (hypertrophy) or on increasing muscle density and strength through use of heavy loads. For the first few weeks, however, we recommend incorporating exercises that use your own body weight. Exercises such as standard push-ups, push-ups between benches, parallel bar dips (no weight), front chin-ups, reverse-grip shoulder-width pull-ups, triceps dips between benches (no weight), hanging leg raises, abdominal crunches, standing wall squats, and lunges help athletes adapt to future workload demands and improve their lifting techniques before heavy training phases are introduced.

Athletes need time to progressively adapt to a new and more demanding training stimulus without incurring injury along the way. They must develop anatomical readiness (muscles, ligaments, and tendons) for strenuous training; and they must understand that vigorous training places high stress on muscles, ligaments, and

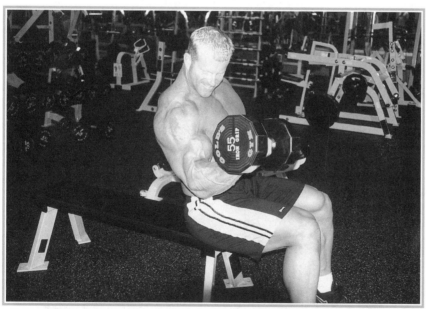

Engaging in AA training progressively adapts muscles, ligaments, and tendons to handle the workload demands placed on the body during the high-intensity training phases.

tendons, potentially leading to injury. Training programs that follow long interruptions, therefore, must begin with anatomical adaptation (AA). Between 6 and 12 weeks of progressive training can activate the main parts of the body, helping to create a foundation for more difficult programs to follow.

The following characteristics describe the scope of AA training:

- It activates all the muscles, ligaments, and tendons of the body so they will better cope with the heavy loads of subsequent training phases.
- It brings all the body parts into balance—that is, it begins to develop previously neglected muscles or body parts and to restore symmetry.
- It prevents injuries through progressive adaptation to heavy loads.
- It progressively increases an athlete's cardiorespiratory endurance.

DURATION AND FREQUENCY

Entry-level bodybuilders and strength trainers need 6 to 12 weeks to progressively adapt their muscles, ligaments, and tendons. Although the AA program is not a stressful one, some beginners might experience an increase in muscle size. A 6- to 12-week AA phase gives beginners the time to incorporate exercises that use their own body weight. After completing this period, the entry-level bodybuilder and strength trainer may proceed with the exercises listed in the design phase later in this chapter.

For recreational bodybuilders and strength trainers with 2 to 3 years of training, 6 weeks of AA training is sufficient. Advanced bodybuilders and strength trainers can incorporate a 3- to 6-week AA training phase and be well prepared for the upcoming high-intensity training demands. The key element at all levels is to complete the AA phase and enter the high-intensity training phases (hypertrophy and maximum strength) both mentally and physically prepared.

Training frequency depends on a lifter's training background and overall commitment to training. Two or three sessions per week are expected for entry-level and recreational bodybuilders, while four or five sessions per week are appropriate for advanced and elite bodybuilders.

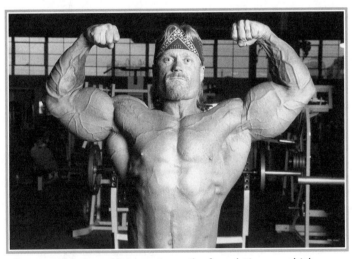

Strong tendons and ligaments are the foundation on which phenomenal amounts of muscle mass are built.

TRAINING METHODS

As previously mentioned, the purpose of the AA phase is to progressively adapt the body to work—to develop the muscles as well as their attachments to the bones. The best training method for the AA phase is circuit training (CT), mainly because it alternates muscle groups and involves most or all of the body parts and muscles.

The first variant of circuit training was proposed by Morgan and Adamson (1959) from Leeds University and was used as a method of developing general fitness. Initially, CT used several stations arranged in a circle, hence the name *circuit training*. The exercises were organized so that the muscle groups used were constantly alternating from station to station.

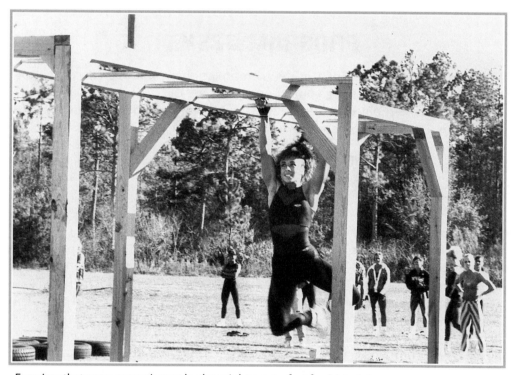

Exercises that use a person's own body weight are perfect for AA training.

A variety of exercises are appropriate for CT programs, including those that use a person's own body weight (such as dips and pull-ups) and those that require dumbbells, barbells, or strength training machines (such as leg extensions and bench presses). Select CT exercises that alternate muscle groups, thus facilitating a better and faster recovery between stations. The rest interval (RI) should be 60 to 90 seconds between stations and 1 to 3 minutes between circuits.

A circuit may be repeated several times—depending on the number of exercises involved, the number of repetitions per station, the load used, and the person's work tolerance and fitness level. Most gyms offer many different apparatuses, making it possible to create circuits that involve most or all of the muscle groups and that continually challenge athletes' skills and maintain their interest.

For people whose goal is both strength training for a better AA phase and creation of a good cardiorespiratory base, we offer the following combination:

1. 10 to 15 minutes of cardiorespiratory exercise
2. Three or four strength training exercises
3. 10 minutes of cardiorespiratory exercise
4. Three or four strength training exercises
5. 10 minutes of cardiorespiratory exercise

Such a program can last 45 to 60 minutes. To make it longer, you can either repeat the circuit or add another segment of three or four exercises, ending with more cardiorespiratory work.

PROGRAM DESIGN

From the first week of training, athletes must plan their workouts based on objective data. This means testing your 1RM for at least the main exercises or prime movers so you can objectively calculate your training loads as a percentage of maximum. (See chapter 3 and appendix C for more information.)

During the first 1 or 2 weeks, it is normal to experience some muscle soreness and fatigue—especially in people who have not been very active in the past. Once your muscles become accustomed to working again, these problems quickly disappear. As the program continues, you will begin to feel good, and the program will seem easy! The best thing you can do for yourself is continue to train as per the original plan.

The guidelines in table 12.1 can help you create your own AA phase. The total physical demand per circuit must be progressively and individually increased. Figure 12.1 demonstrates how load patterns differ between novice and experienced bodybuilders. Since novice bodybuilders need a more gradual adaptation, their load remains the same for 2 weeks (two microcycles) before increasing the demand. Experienced bodybuilders can change their load every microcycle. Use these guidelines when creating your own plan. To better monitor improvements in training and to be constantly able to calculate the load, we suggest testing for

> ## ADAPTATION CUE
>
> Resist the temptation to increase the load. There will be plenty of time to do that in the next phase. Remember that even though your muscles feel as if they have adapted, your tendons and ligaments need more time.

TABLE 12.1 **Training Guidelines for the AA Phase**

	BODYBUILDER'S CLASSIFICATION		
	Entry level	Recreational	Advanced
Duration of AA phase (weeks)	6-12	6	3-6
Number of stations	9-12	9	9
Number of sets or training sessions	2	3	3-4
RI between sets (min)	2-3	2	2
Frequency/week	2-3	3-4	3-5
Aerobic training sessions/week	1	1-2	2

Reprinted from Bompa 1996.

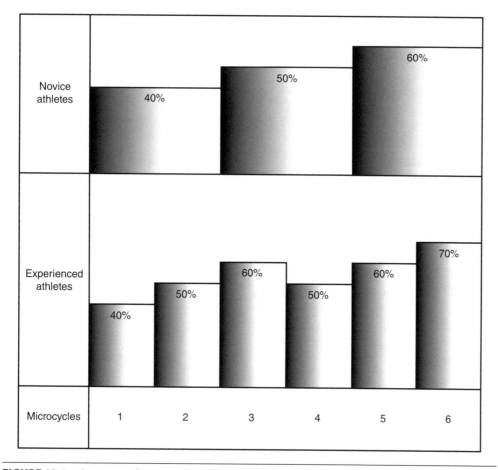

FIGURE 12.1   A suggested pattern of load increments for circuit training for novice and experienced bodybuilders and strength trainers.

Reprinted from Bompa 1996.

1RM at the beginning of weeks 1 and 4 and also at the beginning of week 1 of the next training phase. At the end of the AA phase, the load reaches a percentage of maximum that allows you to immediately make the transition to the hypertrophy phase (see chapter 13).

Tables 12.2 through 12.5 provide several types of AA training programs. To perform the circuit in each, follow the exercises from the top down, performing only one set before moving to the next station. This approach facilitates recovery for each muscle group, since the groups are constantly alternated. If too many bodybuilders are competing for the same equipment, however, or you have to wait too long between sets, then perform all the sets at one station before moving to the next. If you are doing a large number of exercises per session, you can follow a split routine in which you train the same muscle groups every second day. If you are doing a small number of exercises, you can perform all of them in one day and repeat them as many times as you train per week.

The following tips will help you properly execute your AA phase:

- Based on your level as a bodybuilder or strength trainer, create an AA plan using the guidelines, such as the number of sets or training sessions, load incrementation, rest interval between sets, the frequency of training sessions per week, and overall duration of the AA phase.

- Listen to your body so you can be both mentally and physically prepared to enter high-intensity training and avoid unnecessary injuries.
- Choose a variety of exercises that will work each body part as per the exercise program examples listed in tables 12.2 through 12.5.
- Do 20 to 25 minutes of aerobic work as part of your warm-up.
- Test for 1RM early in week 1 and at the end of weeks 4 and 7 (first week of the next phase).
- Increase the load over the 6 weeks by increasing load and adding more sets and repetitions.
- Start with a lower load and use a slower progression for the hamstring muscles because these muscles are easier to injure. Go slowly on the hamstrings!

TABLE 12.2   Six-Week AA Phase for Recreational Bodybuilders and Strength Trainers

No.	Exercise	Week 1	Week 2	Week 3	Week 4	Week 5	Week 6
1	Leg extension	40/15 × 3	50/12 × 3	60/8 × 3	50/15 × 4	60/12 × 4	70/10 × 4
2	Flat bench press	40/15 × 3	50/12 × 3	60/8 × 3	50/15 × 4	60/12 × 4	70/10 × 4
3	Seated pulley row	40/15 × 3	50/12 × 3	60/8 × 3	50/15 × 4	60/12 × 4	70/10 × 4
4	Back extension	40/15 × 3	50/12 × 3	60/8 × 3	50/15 × 4	60/12 × 4	70/10 × 4
5	Standing leg curl	40/12 × 3	40/15 × 3	50/12 × 3	40/15 × 3	50/12 × 4	50/12 × 4
6	Donkey calf raise	40/15 × 3	50/12 × 3	60/8 × 3	50/15 × 4	60/12 × 4	70/10 × 4
7	Nautilus crunch	3 × 12	3 × 15	3 × 15	4 × 12	4 × 15	4 × 15

Note: You may select exercises other than the above, as per your needs, individual development, and desire to balance muscles or parts of your body. Information is provided as load/# of repetitions × sets. So, 40/15 × 3 refers to 3 sets of 15 repetitions at a load equal to 40% of 1RM.

TABLE 12.3   Three-Week AA Phase for Advanced and Recreational Bodybuilders and Strength Trainers

No.	Exercise	Week 1	Week 2	Week 3
1	Bench press	50/15 × 3	60/12 × 4	70/10 × 4
2	Leg extension	50/15 × 3	60/12 × 4	70/10 × 4
3	Leg curl	40/8 × 3	50/10 × 3	60/12 × 4
4	Standing calf raise	50/15 × 3	60/12 × 4	70/10 × 4
5	Lat pull-down	50/15 × 3	60/12 × 4	70/10 × 4
6	Preacher curl	50/15 × 3	60/12 × 4	70/10 × 4
7	Military press	50/15 × 3	60/12 × 4	70/10 × 4
8	Abdominal crunch	To maximum exhaustion		
9	Back extension	To maximum exhaustion		

Note: Add or change exercises as per your own needs. Information is provided as load/# of repetitions × sets. So, 50/15 × 3 refers to 3 sets of 15 repetitions at a load equal to 50% of 1RM.

TABLE 12.4 Six-Week AA Phase With Strength and Cardiorespiratory Components for Entry-Level or Recreational Bodybuilders and Strength Trainers

No.	Exercise	Week 1	Week 2	Week 3	Week 4	Week 5	Week 6
1	Cardio (min)	10	10	10	15	15	15
2	Leg extension	40/15	40/15	50/12	50/12	60/10	60/12
3	Flat bench press	40/15	40/15	50/12	50/12	60/10	60/12
4	Preacher curl	40/15	40/15	50/12	50/12	60/10	60/12
5	Cardio (min)	10	10	10	10	10	10
6	Back extension	To minimum exhaustion					
7	Standing calf raise	40/15	50/15	50/18	60/15	60/18	60/20
8	Leg curl	40/10	40/12	50/12	50/15	60/12	60/15
9	Cardio (min)	10	10	10	15	15	15

Note: Information is provided as load/# of repetitions. So, 40/15 refers to 15 repetitions at a load equal to 40% of 1RM. Perform the first 5 exercises nonstop. Take 1 min rest, and do the balance (exercises 6-9). As you have just finished an entire circuit, take a 2-min rest interval. Try a second circuit, especially after you have reached a decent level of adaptation.

TABLE 12.5 Three-Week AA Phase With Strength and Cardiorespiratory Components for Advanced Bodybuilders and Strength Trainers

No.	Exercise	Week 1	Week 2	Week 3
1	Cardio (min)	10	12	15
2	Bench press	50/12	60/12	70/10
3	Leg extension	50/12	60/12	70/10
4	Leg curl	50/8	60/10	60/12
5	Lat pull-down	50/10	60/12	70/8-10
6	Cardio (min)	10	10	10
7	Military press	50/12	60/12	70/12
8	Preacher curl	50/15	60/12	70/12
9	Abdominal crunch	To maximum exhaustion		
10	Back extension	To maximum exhaustion		
11	Cardio (min)	10	12	15

Note: You may change some exercises as per your needs. Information is provided as load/# of repetitions. So, 50/12 refers to 12 repetitions at a load equal to 50% of 1RM. Perform a circuit nonstop from the top to the bottom. No RI between stations. Take a 2-min RI after the circuit. Repeat circuit once.

NUTRITION

We will assume you are beginning the metabolic diet during this phase. This may not necessarily be the case, but following that plan makes the most sense for anyone wanting to follow our periodization plan.

During most of your time on the metabolic diet, you won't often find yourself restricting calories, including the AA phase. In fact, some people find they have a problem getting enough calories, especially in the hypertrophy phase. Even

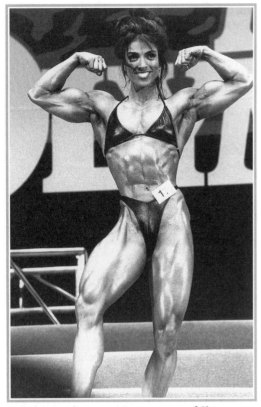

Understanding nutrition was one of Sharon Bruneau's strong points for acquiring a muscled and symmetrical physique.

in other phases, many athletes find that with increased training and exercise they can take in huge amounts of food without any negative consequences. The only phase that usually requires a gradual reduction in calories is the definition phase.

At the beginning, you should make the dietary switch gradually. Don't jump right in at a low calorie level. Often the fatigue and discomfort you may feel are simply from a lack of food rather than a lack of carbohydrate. And if some of this discomfort is from the actual metabolic switch, it is compounded if you are starving. We also don't want you to feel bloated or to suffer from the constipation and diarrhea that you may have as a result of the sometimes radical change in your macronutrient intake. Dieting per se often affects the bowels and can compound any effect that may come from starting on the metabolic diet.

Your starting point for daily calories on this diet should be 18 times your body weight. If you weigh 200 pounds (91 kg), this would call for 200 times 18, or 3,600, calories a day during the weekday portion of the diet. This intake level creates a static phase where you lose some body fat, gain some muscle mass, and maintain about the same weight. In this phase you'll be changing the ratio of internal masses to some degree, but most of what you're trying to do is allow your body its easiest path toward adapting to the diet.

As you continue in this phase, you should experiment with this formula to find your precise maintenance level for calories. This will let you know from what point you need to add or subtract calories for gains or losses in other parts of the diet. It's also not a bad idea to keep a 2- or 3-day diary of what you're eating and then have someone who has some expertise in diets look at it. That way you will get numbers and foods you can best work with and determine what you need precisely for maintenance.

One result of the metabolic diet is that the bowels must readjust to large amounts of meat; and since the fats can act as a stool softener, you may experience some diarrhea. You'll need to firm them up with a fiber supplement (see the next section on supplementation). The radical change in diet can also cause constipation. Most of the problems we've found with people initiating the diet stem from their failure to take the fiber necessary to soften stools or push processed food through the eliminative tract. Although you may be able to get away with just eating bran, there is a good chance you will need a supplement to get through this period with minimum discomfort.

Some bodybuilders have found that eating a meal high in fiber in the middle of the day provides sufficient fiber. A Caesar salad with grilled chicken, for example, provides about 8 grams of carbohydrate and 3.9 grams of fiber and, as long as you stick close to overall carbohydrate limits, should not present any problem—especially after you have been on the diet for a while.

Avoid Hidden Carbohydrate

The AA phase will run more smoothly and get you in gear more quickly if you remember that refined carbohydrates are hidden in almost everything you find on supermarket shelves. Seasoning, ketchup, mustard, salad dressings, nuts, BBQ sauce, breaded or processed meats, gourmet coffee, and sausages can all present a problem. These foods are renowned for hidden carbohydrates, and you must check the labels to know what you're getting.

Likewise, restaurants sometimes use a watery sugar on their vegetables. Our society has a sweet tooth that you will encounter at every turn. You will have to be especially careful during this start-up phase as you get used to the diet and learn where the trouble spots are.

Do Not Mix Diets

You may be strongly tempted to mix diets, combining the metabolic diet with parts of other diets such as high-carbohydrate or low-fat diets. Please resist the temptation! Many people go on the metabolic diet but try to be true to their old high-carbohydrate master. They eat meat, but it's all fish, chicken, and turkey—and while these foods may be quite nutritious and beneficial, even when used in the metabolic diet, they can't be used as a total replacement for red meat. They just don't have enough fat.

What you end up doing with the turkey, chicken, and fish approach is going on a high-protein, low-carbohydrate, *low-fat* diet. Along with being even harder to stay on than the metabolic diet, this diet will not provide the advantages you are seeking from the metabolic diet. You won't burn the fat as you should. You won't have the energy. You won't build the mass.

You need some red meat, and the more the better. You need the fat it provides. And you need to supplement your diet with other fats, such as the healthy omega3 fatty acids found in flax and fish oils. Don't shortchange yourself by trying to avoid fat (and certainly don't cut out healthy amounts of the essential fatty acids), as many do when on low-fat diets in some misled effort to stay true to forces in society who have labeled meat some kind of monster. This is simply not true.

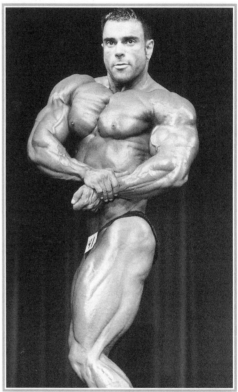

Nelson Da Silva demonstrates what happens when diet, supplements, and training come together perfectly.

SUPPLEMENTATION

In the anatomical adaptation phase you should concentrate on making the metabolic shift, keeping everything else basically the same. Besides fiber supplements and perhaps a daily vitamin and mineral tablet, you generally won't need anything else in this phase. If you are used to taking certain supplements on a regular basis, you may want to continue doing so. This phase is designed to get you into the metabolic diet and to make that all-important shift from using carbohydrates to using fats as your primary fuel—therefore it's best to concentrate on making this shift and keeping other changes to a minimum.

As noted previously, you may need a fiber supplement during the AA phase. The nutritional supplement line we formulated for the metabolic diet includes Regulate, a multi-ingredient low-carbohydrate supplement (none of the fiber is absorbed) meant to regulate the bowels and keep the whole intestinal tract healthy. Regulate is an effective blend of natural soluble and insoluble fibers formulated to deal with occasional constipation and frequent bowel movements. The various soluble fibers and other compounds contained in Regulate have also been found useful in maintaining cholesterol levels that are already within normal range, supporting a healthy heart, and increasing natural insulin sensitivity.

If you use a common commercial fiber product, check the carbohydrate count on the package before purchasing it—refined carbohydrates are often added to make such products taste better. You will probably have to take the fiber supplement for the first few weeks to a month of the diet. In most cases, your body will have fully adapted to the diet by that time or at least within a few months. If not, it's a good idea to stay on a fiber supplement on a regular or on an as-needed basis.

Other supplements you could use during the AA phase include MVM, Antiox, and EFA+. MVM is a multiple vitamin and mineral formula that provides nutritional supplementation for the body's maintenance, recuperation, and repair process. Antiox is a formula that provides antioxidant protection to all tissues in the body including the musculoskeletal system and the liver. EFA+ is essential for maximizing the fat-burning events during training and optimizing hormone production and insulin metabolism. Additionally, if you are having a hard time adjusting to the low carbohydrates, before you adjust your carbohydrate levels, try using Metabolic Diet Creatine Advantage to help get you through the rough spots.

Hypertrophy (H)

chapter 13

The standard periodization model in chapter 2 (refer to figure 2.1, page 19) calls for two 6-week hypertrophy phases (H1 and H2) to provide sufficient time for you to address your own needs for improving muscle size and refinement. Between these two H phases we recommend a 1-week transition phase during which the volume and intensity of training are significantly reduced. This week of lower-intensity training helps remove the fatigue accumulated during the first H phase and gives the body a chance to fully replenish its energy stores before commencing the next H phase. Similar short transition phases are prescribed between all the training phases of the basic model of periodization.

The following characteristics describe the scope of H training:

- It increases muscle size to the desired level by constantly taxing the ATP-PC stores.
- It refines all the muscle groups of the body.
- It improves the proportions among all the muscles of the body, especially between arms and legs, back and chest, leg flexors and extensors.

DURATION

The duration of H training depends on several factors, including the athlete's classification, training background, specific body goals (e.g., increased size vs. density, or perhaps muscle definition), and the type of periodization being followed. (Refer to chapter 3 for information on customizing your periodization plan.) To achieve substantial gains in muscle size, athletes should plan at least one or, better yet, two 6-week H phases. During this time, the athletes must apply the training methods that best suit them. They should carefully select the variations of training methods (see later in this chapter) that will achieve their planned training goals.

TRAINING METHODS

The main objective of bodybuilding is to provoke significant chemical changes in the muscles necessary for the development of mass. For some bodybuilders, unfortunately, increased muscle size often results from increased fluid and plasma within the muscles rather than enlarged contractile elements within the muscle fibers (the myosin filaments). In other words, the enlargement of the muscles may be due to a shift of body fluids to the worked muscle, as opposed to an actual increase in muscle fiber size. This is why the strength of some bodybuilders is not always proportional to their size—a problem that can be corrected by applying the periodization concept of training.

Hypertrophy training employs submaximal loads in order to avoid provoking maximum tension within the muscles. The training objective with submaximal loads is to contract muscles to exhaustion in an effort to recruit *all* the muscle fibers. As you "rep-out" to exhaustion, muscle fiber recruitment increases: As some fibers begin to fatigue, others start to function, and so on, until exhaustion is reached.

To achieve optimal training benefits, an athlete must perform the greatest number of repetitions possible during each set. Bodybuilders should always reach the state of local muscular exhaustion that prevents them from performing one more repetition, even when applying maximal force. If the individual sets are not performed to exhaustion, muscle hypertrophy will not reach the expected level because the first repetitions do not produce the stimulus necessary to increase muscle mass. *The key element in hypertrophy training is the cumulative effect of exhaustion over the total number of sets, and not just exhaustion per set.* This cumulative exhaustion stimulates the chemical reactions and protein metabolism responsible for optimal muscle hypertrophy.

Bodybuilding and hypertrophy training mostly use the fuels specific to the anaerobic system (ATP-PC). Training should be designed to exhaust or deplete these energy stores, thereby threatening the energy available for the working muscle. The RI between sets is perhaps the most important element of training if hypertrophy is to be stimulated. The RI must be implemented in such a way that the body reaches exhaustion after each set, as well as at the end of a workout. It is necessary to plan such exhaustion days mostly during the second step and especially during the third step as per the step-type loading method (refer to figures 3.5 through 3.7, pages 39 and 40).

HELPFUL TIPS FOR THE HYPERTROPHY METHOD

Even with the split-routine method, hypertrophy workouts are very exhausting to those who might perform perhaps 75 to 160 repetitions per training session. Such high muscle loading requires a long recovery period after a session. The type of training specific to this phase exhausts most if not all of the ATP-PC and glycogen stores during a demanding training session.

Remember that although ATP-PC is restored very quickly, the exhausted liver glycogen takes approximately 46 to 48 hours to replenish. It is logical, therefore, that heavy hypertrophy workouts to complete exhaustion be performed no more than three times per microcycle—preferably in the second step and especially in the third step of the four-step loading pattern.

Constant exhaustive training depletes the body's energy stores and accelerates the breakdown of contractile protein (myosin). The undesirable outcome of such overloading can be that the muscles involved no longer increase in size. Maybe we should change the old adage to "too much pain, no gain!" If you already use the overload technique, do your body a favor and try the step-type approach to loading, and watch your body evolve. In addition, be sure to alternate intensities within each microcycle. Your body will respond well to proper sequences of loading and regeneration.

This depletion can be achieved by taking shorter RIs between sets (30 to 45 seconds); when the body has only a limited amount of rest, the muscles have less time to restore the ATP-PC energy reserves. Because an exhaustive set depletes ATP-PC stores, and the short RI does not allow for its complete restoration, the body is forced to adapt by increasing its energy transport capacity, which in turn stimulates muscle growth.

Variations of Training Methods

Because repetitions to exhaustion represent the main element of success in bodybuilding and strength training, this section presents several variations of the original method. Each of the variations has the same objective—to achieve two or three more repetitions *after* you reach exhaustion. The result is increased muscle growth and hypertrophy.

Assisted Repetitions   Assisted repetitions are one way to complete additional repetitions after exhaustion. Once you have performed a set to temporary exhaustion of the neuromuscular system, a partner gives you sufficient support to enable you to perform two or three more repetitions.

Resisted Repetitions   Once you perform a set to temporary exhaustion, a partner helps you execute two or three more repetitions concentrically and provides resistance for the eccentric segments of contraction—hence the term *resisted repetitions*. During these last two or three reps, you should make the eccentric part of the contraction twice as long as the concentric part, thereby overloading the muscles beyond the standard level.

Note that the longer the active muscle fibers are held in tension, the higher the nervous tension and energy expenditure become. If a normal contraction is 2 to 4 seconds long, a repetition performed against resistance can be 6 to 8 seconds long, consuming 20 to 40 percent more energy. The longer the muscles remain in tension, the more strongly activated the muscles' metabolism becomes, stimulating muscle growth to new highs.

Cheated Repetitions   Athletes normally resort to this technique when there is no spotter available. When you are unable to perform another repetition with proper form through the entire range of motion, complement the action by jerking another segment of the body toward the performing limb. For example, perform elbow flexions to exhaustion, then jerk the trunk toward the forearm to trick, or "cheat," the body into performing additional reps. This sustains the crucial tension in the exhausted muscle. This method is limited to certain limbs and exercises and should be attempted only by athletes with a sound training base.

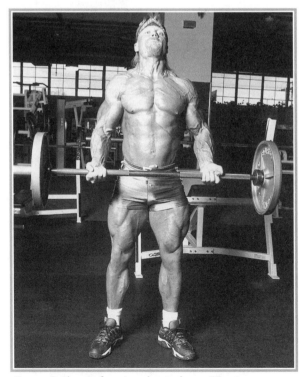

Trevor Butler performing cheated repetitions.

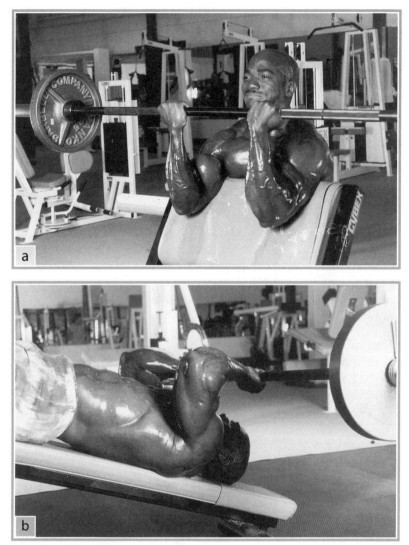

Wesley Mohammed performing a superset with *(a)* biceps preacher curls followed immediately by *(b)* decline triceps extensions.

Supersets For a superset, you perform a set for the agonistic muscles of a given joint, followed *without a rest period* by a set for the antagonistic muscles. For example, do an elbow flexion or biceps preacher curl, followed immediately by an elbow extension or decline triceps extension.

For a variation of the superset, perform a set to exhaustion, and after 20 to 30 seconds, perform another set for the same muscle group. For example, perform triceps extensions and then dips. Of course, because of exhaustion, you may not be able to perform the same number of repetitions in the second set as in the first set.

Isokinetic Method

The term *isokinetic* means "equal motion" or "same velocity of motion throughout the range of movement." Isokinetic training is performed on specially designed equipment that provides muscles with the same resistance for both the concentric and eccentric parts of the contraction. This provides maximum activation of the muscles involved. Training velocity is very important in this type of training. Training at slower speeds seems to increase contractile strength, but *only* at slow speeds, and the major gains tend to be in muscle hypertrophy.

On the other hand, training at higher speeds may allow major benefits for maximum strength. The more advanced computerized equipment allows athletes to select and set the desired training velocity. These machines are often used as strength-measuring devices.

Isokinetic equipment provides several key benefits:

- It offers a safe way to train and is therefore suitable for entry-level athletes during their early years.

- It can be used for gains in muscle hypertrophy if the exercises are performed at slower speeds to allow for maximum resistance during the concentric and eccentric parts of the contraction.

- It is well suited for the AA phase, when overall strength development and muscle attachment adaptation are the main purposes of training.
- With a higher velocity, it can result in gains in maximum strength.
- It is useful for rehabilitation of injured athletes.

Slow or Superslow Training

Although bodybuilders have successfully used the slow training system for years, proof of its effectiveness is mostly anecdotal. It is presumed that slow contraction works for the simple reason that it creates a high level of muscle tension, resulting in increased muscle hypertrophy and strength.

The proponents of slow or superslow contraction, whether using drop sets or any other variants, recommend that the duration of concentric contraction be half the length of the eccentric phase. For example: At 95 percent of 1RM, use 4 seconds for eccentric and only 2 seconds for concentric. The same ratio is suggested for lower loads: At 70 percent of 1RM, use 6 seconds for eccentric and only 3 for concentric. Some "experts," especially some self-proclaimed Internet gurus, suggest almost the opposite: 10 seconds to lift (concentric) and 5 to 10 seconds to lower the weight (eccentric).

The important thing is that the tension is high and prolonged for both the concentric and eccentric contractions. There is no magic secret regarding how many seconds one lowers or lifts the barbell, as long as the tension is consistently high and long. Note, however, that the eccentric phase creates lower tension than the concentric phase (using the same load) because the muscle needs to contract a reduced number of fibers to lower the barbell. Therefore, in order to have similar tension, the eccentric phase must be *either* longer (up to twice the length of the concentric contraction) *or* you have to increase the load to generate equal tension (i.e., add about 20 percent more weight).

Common Misconceptions

Many Internet publications, bodybuilding books, and especially some magazines are full of misconceptions, often referring to methods that promise miracles. Take care to recognize the fine line separating reality from fantasy. Here are some common misconceptions:

- *Slow movement reduces force and is the number one cause of injuries.* In reality, slow contraction increases muscle tension, keeping the myosin and actin coupling in a longer contraction and leading to increased force and muscle size. Furthermore, since exercise form, or technique, is more easily controlled during slow contraction movements, they are safer than dynamic actions. The exception to this rule is when the muscles reach a state of exhaustion. In this instance, technical control is more difficult, and athletes require a spotter's assistance to prevent problems.
- *The greater a muscle is fatigued in a limited time frame, the greater the exercise intensity.* In sport science, intensity refers to the load employed in training, which is calculated from 1RM, or 100 percent. The higher the load is, the higher the intensity is (both physiological and mental). Clearly, some of the Internet writers are confusing intensity with training demand.

- *Rest intervals between sets should be avoided.* This might be accepted with great reservation when performing drop sets, where the load decreases without rest. For example: two sets of two or three reps at 95 percent RM, then two sets of three or four reps at 90 percent RM, then two sets of 8 to 10 reps at 80 percent RM, and finally two sets of 12 to 15 reps at 70 percent RM. Considering this erroneous statement, it is easy to understand why many bodybuilders are in a constant state of overtraining. The followers of such a theory will be physically and mentally exhausted.

- *Advanced trainees often require 7 or more rest days between workouts.* First, 48 hours is sufficient to complete protein synthesis, meaning that the muscles are ready for another workout. Second, targeting a muscle group every 7 days may hamper some elements of muscle adaptation and will result in muscle damage and soreness when training is resumed.

High-Intensity Training

High-intensity training (HIT) systems follow traditional bodybuilding training principles, such as progression, overload (i.e., progressive increase of load in steps), proper technique, multijoint exercises, superslow training, preexhaustion, drop sets, using full range of motion (ROM), 8 to 12 repetitions, and no split routines. But proponents of HIT promote some misconceptions about training. For example, they suggest that training should be brief (less than an hour). This is fine for those who cannot afford a longer time, such as recreational bodybuilders or strength fitness fans, but questionable for elite athletes who often perform many sets. It is simply impossible for them to do a complete workout in less than an hour. The following are other misconceptions that exist about HIT training:

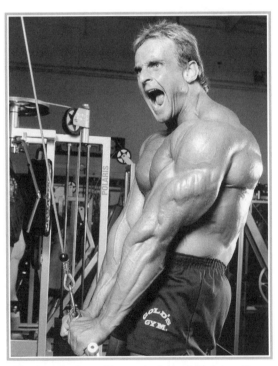

The late Andreas Munzer training with intensity.

- *As you get stronger, you are less able to tolerate high intensity.* This claim strongly contradicts sport science, which has demonstrated that highly trained athletes are well adapted to tolerate high intensity. Many bodybuilders and athletes from various other sports train daily, often two or three times, without problems. This is possible for the simple reason that they are well adapted to both high intensity and volume (quantity) of training. In some programs, especially the periodization system, training intensity is consistently alternated during the week, yet high intensity is the prevailing training standard. Consider the program followed by many Olympic weightlifters and throwers in track and field: They often train more than twice a day, 6 days a week, mostly at a high intensity.

- *Beginners should do 16 to 20 sets per workout, while advanced athletes should do only 8 to 12.* The reality is exactly the opposite. Beginners do not have the capacity and are not adapted to tolerate as much work and high intensity as advanced athletes.

Therefore, beginners should start out performing fewer repetitions but progressively work toward more repetitions with a higher intensity.

- *Beginners should train three times a week, advanced bodybuilders just once.* This is another fallacy. This theory is briefly discussed in the section describing superslow contraction training. Some HIT advocates believe the periodization system doesn't work, but the real issue may be they do not fully comprehend periodization in the first place.

Manual Resistance

Manual resistance, generally shortened simply to *manuals*, refers to use of resistance provided by a partner. This method may be advisable for children who are not yet ready for intensive training. Note, however, that the only group of muscles for which the resistance provided by a partner can match or be slightly higher than that of the performer is the deltoids. All the other muscle groups of the body will easily overcome the resistance provided by a partner. Therefore, since resistance is low, strength increases can only be minor. The manuals method was tried in Eastern Europe in the 1950s for a very short time; the conclusion was that it is most advisable for young people and entry-level bodybuilders.

PROGRAM DESIGN

As with any new training phase, H training should start with a test for 1RM. The test must be performed in the second part of the first week because this is the lowest-intensity week in the step-type loading pattern. If it is performed in the early part of the week, the athlete is slightly fatigued from the previous high-intensity week. The brief delay ensures that fatigue does not affect the accuracy of the measurement. Table 13.1 suggests training guidelines for the hypertrophy phase.

One of the main objectives of H training is to consistently train all the muscle groups in order to achieve the ultimate symmetrical shape. There are two muscle groups, however, to which additional reference should be made: hamstrings and calves.

TABLE 13.1　Training Guidelines for the H1 and H2 Phases

	BODYBUILDER'S CLASSIFICATION			
	Entry level	Recreational	Advanced	Professional
Duration of H phase (weeks)	6	3-6	3-6	12
Number of reps/set	6-12	9-12	9-12	9-12
Number of sets/exercise	2-3	4-5	4-5	3-7
RI between sets (sec)	60-120	45-60	45-60	30-45
Workouts/week	2-3	3-5	4-5	5-6
Aerobic training sessions/ week	1	1	1-2	2-3

Hamstrings   The hamstrings are often neglected and in many instances are not developed proportionately to the quadriceps muscles. When planning your own program, please keep this in mind. Furthermore, power loading is too often used for the hamstrings in the same way it is for other muscles, despite the fact that most muscle strains and injuries occur in the hamstrings. In sprinting, the hams are called "nervous" muscles since they have more nerve end plates per square inch than the quads and many other muscles. The programs we suggest often propose a 10 to 20 percent lower load for the hams than for the quads. Work slowly and carefully on the hams!

Calves   These muscles, along with the quads, support the human form in the standing or walking positions. Because of incessant low-level stimulation, they have biologically adapted by developing a higher proportion of slow twitch (76 percent) fibers than fast twitch (24 percent) fibers. As a result, it is difficult to stimulate the same growth in the calves as in most of the other muscle groups. The special physiological composition of the calves prevents them from responding well to traditional bodybuilding and strength training programs in which the same loading and RI are used for the calves as for other muscles.

Because the calves have a higher proportion of capillaries than other muscles, they are able to resupply their energy needs (ATP-PC stores) more quickly than others. To offset the energy balance of the calves, their training must be slightly different. The RI should be no longer than 45 seconds in order to inhibit immediate ATP and PC restoration. This forces the body to increase its energy transport capacity, thereby increasing the PC content of the cells and activating protein metabolism. The hypertrophy of the calves is therefore better stimulated, allowing athletes to build their calves in proportion with the rest of their bodies.

Tables 13.2 through 13.5 present suggested H-phase programs for four different classifications of bodybuilders and strength trainers. Look at table 13.1 as an example of how athletes at any level can create their own hypertrophy training programs.

The top row of each table is the date. In the examples, the 6 weeks of the program are provided, but when making your individual program, use this space to indicate the dates of the week (e.g., September 1-7). The second row in each is the step row, which contains information about the load intensity, as per the step-type loading method. The first step is low, indicating a low intensity and volume of training. Programs for the second step are of medium intensity. Finally, programs for the third step are of high intensity. The same pattern is repeated for weeks 4, 5, and 6.

The third row shows the day of training. For example, in table 13.2, days 1 and 4 consist of the top program, while days 2 and 5 consist of the bottom program. Days 3, 6, and 7 are for rest.

As you can see, all the suggested training programs are 2-day split routines, in which there are two groups of exercises, each performed twice a week. This simple split routine is superior to the traditional routines because the muscles receive more stimulation when trained twice a week than only once a week. The obvious outcome is a more dramatic increase in muscle size.

If you look at any given exercise for a single week, you can see the difference in the amount of work between the low-, medium-, and high-intensity training days, as well as the progression of expected strength gains. Changes in loading are made mostly by altering the load and number of sets.

The following tips will help you properly execute your H phase:

- Test for 1RM during week 1, during the second part of week 4, and during the first week of the next program.
- The number of exercises can be slightly increased or decreased according to your needs.
- The number of sets can be increased or decreased in response to your particular potential and needs.
- Regardless of any change made to the number of exercises or sets, always apply the suggested loading pattern.
- Decrease the load if it is too high, but maintain the same number of reps.
- Do not forget to do 5 to 10 minutes of aerobic work before your weight session.
- During the hypertrophy phase, perform all the sets per exercise before moving on to the next exercise. (This is different from the AA phase.)

TABLE 13.2 — H Phase for Entry-Level Bodybuilders and Strength Trainers

EX NO.	WEEK	1		2		3	
	STEP	LOW		MEDIUM		HIGH	
	DAY	1	4	1	4	1	
1	Leg press	40/10 × 2	40/12 × 2	40/15 × 2	40/15 × 2	50/12 × 2	
2	Seated leg curl	40/8 × 2	40/10 × 2	40/10 × 2	40/8 × 3	50/10 × 2	
3	Front dumbbell press	40/8 × 2	40/10 × 2	40/12 × 2	40/15 × 2	50/10 × 3	
4	Incline side lateral	40/8 × 2	40/8 × 2	40/10 × 2	40/8 × 3	50/10 × 2	
5	Back extension	2 × 10	2 × 12	2 × 15	2 × 15	3 × 10	
6	Diagonal curl-up	2 × 12	2 × 12	2 × 15	2 × 15	3 × 10	
	DAY	2	5	2	5	2	
1	Shrug	40/10 × 2	40/10 × 2	40/12 × 2	40/15 × 2	50/10 × 2	
2	Incline bench press	40/10 × 2	40/10 × 2	40/12 × 2	40/15 × 2	50/10 × 2	
3	Seated pulley row	40/10 × 2	40/10 × 2	40/12 × 2	40/15 × 2	50/10 × 2	
4	Triceps push-down	40/10 × 2	40/10 × 2	40/12 × 2	40/15 × 2	50/10 × 2	
5	Standing calf raise	40/10 × 2	40/12 × 2	40/15 × 2	40/15 × 2	50/12 × 2	
6	Seated calf raise	40/12 × 2	40/12 × 2	40/15 × 2	40/15 × 2	50/12 × 2	

Note: RI between sets is 1-2 min. Information is provided as load/# of repetitions × sets. So, 40/10 × 2 means 2 sets of 10 repetitions using weight equal to 40% of 1RM.

TABLE 13.3 — H Phase for Recreational Bodybuilders and Strength Trainers

EX NO.	WEEK	1		2		
	STEP	LOW		MEDIUM		
	DAY	1	4	1	4	
1	Hack squat	50/12 × 3	50/12 × 3	60/12 × 3	60/12 × 3	
2	Standing leg curl	50/10 × 3	50/10 × 3	50/12 × 3	50/12 × 3	
3	Lunge	50/12 × 3	50/12 × 3	60/12 × 3	60/12 × 3	
4	Back extension	3 × 12	3 × 12	3 × 15	3 × 15	
5	Diagonal curl-up	3 × 12	3 × 12	3 × 15	3 × 15	
6	Biceps preacher curl	50/12 × 3	50/12 × 3	60/12 × 3	60/12 × 3	
7	Triceps push-down	50/12 × 3	50/12 × 3	60/12 × 3	60/12 × 3	
	DAY	2	5	2	5	
1	Flat bench press	50/12 × 3	50/12 × 3	60/12 × 3	60/12 × 3	
2	Incline dumbbell bench press	50/12 × 3	50/12 × 3	60/12 × 3	60/12 × 3	
3	Front dumbbell press	50/12 × 3	50/12 × 3	60/12 × 3	60/12 × 3	
4	Standing dumbbell side lateral	50/10 × 3	50/10 × 3	50/12 × 3	50/12 × 3	
5	Shrug	50/12 × 3	50/12 × 3	60/12 × 3	60/12 × 3	
6	Seated pulley row	50/12 × 3	50/12 × 3	60/12 × 3	60/12 × 3	
7	Seated calf raise	50/12 × 3	50/12 × 3	60/12 × 3	60/12 × 3	
8	Standing calf raise	50/12 × 3	50/12 × 3	60/12 × 3	60/12 × 3	

Note: RI between sets is 1-2 min. Information is provided as load/# of repetitions × sets. So, 50/12 × 3 means 3 sets of 12 repetitions using weight equal to 50% of 1RM.

3 HIGH		4 LOW		5 MEDIUM		6 HIGH	
4		1	4	1	4	1	4
50/10 × 3		40/12 × 2	40/12 × 3	50/12 × 3	50/12 × 3	60/10 × 2	60/10 × 3
50/8 × 3		40/10 × 3	40/10 × 2	50/10 × 3	50/10 × 3	50/10 × 3	50/10 × 3
50/10 × 3		40/12 × 3	40/10 × 3	50/12 × 3	50/12 × 3	60/10 × 3	60/10 × 3
50/8 × 3		40/10 × 2	40/10 × 2	50/10 × 3	50/10 × 3	50/10 × 3	50/10 × 3
3 × 10		2 × 15	3 × 10	3 × 12	3 × 15	3 × 15	3 × 15
3 × 10		2 × 12	3 × 10	3 × 12	3 × 15	3 × 15	3 × 15
5		2	5	2	5	2	5
50/10 × 3		40/12 × 2	40/10 × 3	50/12 × 3	50/12 × 3	60/10 × 3	60/10 × 3
50/10 × 3		40/12 × 2	40/10 × 3	50/12 × 3	50/12 × 3	60/10 × 3	60/10 × 3
50/10 × 3		40/12 × 2	40/10 × 3	50/12 × 3	50/12 × 3	60/10 × 3	60/10 × 3
50/10 × 3		40/12 × 2	40/10 × 3	50/12 × 3	50/12 × 3	60/10 × 3	60/10 × 3
50/10 × 3		40/10 × 2	40/10 × 3	50/12 × 3	50/12 × 3	60/10 × 3	60/10 × 3
50/12 × 3		40/12 × 2	40/12 × 3	50/12× 3	50/12 × 3	60/10 × 2	60/10 × 3

3 HIGH		4 LOW		5 MEDIUM		6 HIGH	
1	4	1	4	1	4	1	4
60/15 × 3	60/12 × 4	50/12 × 3	50/12 × 3	60/12 × 4	60/12 × 4	70/10 × 4	70/10 × 4
50/10 × 4	50/10 × 4	50/10 × 3	50/10 × 3	60/10 × 3	60/10 × 3	60/8 × 4	60/8 × 4
60/15 × 3	60/12 × 4	50/12 × 3	50/12 × 3	60/12 × 4	60/12 × 4	70/10 × 4	70/10 × 4
4 × 12	4 × 15	3 × 15	3 × 15	4 × 15	4 × 15	4 × 15	4 × 15
4 × 12	4 × 15	3 × 15	3 × 15	4 × 15	4 × 15	4 × 15	4 × 15
60/15 × 3	60/12 × 4	50/12 × 3	50/12 × 3	60/12 × 4	60/12 × 4	70/10 × 4	70/10 × 4
60/15 × 3	60/12 × 4	50/12 × 3	50/12 × 3	60/12 × 4	60/10 × 3	60/8 × 4	70/10 × 4
2	5	2	5	2	5	2	5
60/15 × 3	60/12 × 4	50/12 × 3	50/12 × 3	60/12 × 4	60/10 × 3	60/8 × 4	70/10 × 4
60/15 × 3	60/12 × 4	50/12 × 3	50/12 × 3	60/12 × 4	60/10 × 3	60/8 × 4	70/10 × 4
60/15 × 3	60/12 × 4	50/12 × 3	50/12 × 3	60/12 × 4	60/12 × 4	70/10 × 4	70/10 × 4
50/10 × 4	50/10 × 4	50/10 × 3	50/10 × 3	60/10 × 3	60/10 × 3	60/8 × 4	60/8 × 4
60/15 × 3	60/12 × 4	50/12 × 3	50/12 × 3	60/12 × 4	60/12 × 4	70/10 × 4	70/10 × 4
60/15 × 3	60/12 × 4	50/12 × 3	50/12 × 3	60/12 × 4	60/10 × 3	60/8 × 4	70/10 × 4
60/15 × 3	60/12 × 4	50/12 × 3	50/12 × 3	60/12 × 4	60/12 × 4	70/10 × 4	70/10 × 4
60/15 × 3	60/12 × 4	50/12 × 3	50/12 × 3	60/12 × 4	60/12 × 4	70/10 × 4	70/10 × 4

TABLE 13.4 — H Phase for Advanced Bodybuilders and Strength Trainers

EX NO.	WEEK	1 (LOW)			2 (MEDIUM)			3 (HIGH)	
	STEP	LOW			MEDIUM			HIGH	
	DAY	1	3	5	1	3	5	1	3
1	Safety squat	60/12 × 4	Off	60/15 × 4	60/15 × 4	70/10 × 4	70/10 × 4	75/10 × 4	Off
2	Standing leg curl	60/8 × 3	Off	60/8 × 3	60/8 × 4	60/8 × 4	60/8 × 4	65/7 × 4	Off
3	Lunge	60/12 × 4	Off	60/15 × 4	60/15 × 4	70/10 × 4	70/10 × 4	75/10 × 4	Off
4	Bent-over barbell row	60/12 × 4	Off	60/15 × 4	60/15 × 4	60/15 × 4	70/10 × 4	75/10 × 4	Off
5	Back extension	3 × 15	Off	4 × 15	4 × 12	4 × 12	4 × 12	4 × 15	Off
6	Diagonal curl-up	3 × 15	Off	4 × 15	4 × 12	4 × 12	4 × 12	4 × 15	Off
7	Decline triceps extension	60/12 × 4	Off	60/15 × 4	60/15 × 4	60/15 × 4	70/10 × 4	75/10 × 4	Off
	DAY	2	4	6	2	4	6	2	4
1	Flat bench press	60/12 × 4	60/12 × 4	60/15 × 4	60/15 × 4	Off	70/10 × 4	75/10 × 4	75/10 × 4
2	Incline flys	60/12 × 4	60/12 × 4	60/15 × 4	60/15 × 4	Off	70/10 × 4	75/10 × 4	75/10 × 4
3	Front dumbbell press	60/12 × 4	60/12 × 4	60/15 × 4	60/15 × 4	Off	70/10 × 4	75/10 × 4	75/10 × 4
4	Incline side lateral	60/10 × 3	60/10 × 3	60/10 × 3	65/8 × 4	Off	65/8 × 4	70/8 × 4	70/8 × 4
5	Shrug	60/12 × 4	60/12 × 4	60/15 × 4	60/15 × 4	Off	70/10 × 4	75/10 × 4	75/10 × 4
6	Biceps preacher curl	60/12 × 4	60/12 × 4	60/15 × 4	60/15 × 4	Off	70/10 × 4	75/10 × 4	75/10 × 4
7	Donkey calf raise	60/12 × 4	60/12 × 4	60/15 × 4	60/15 × 4	Off	70/10 × 4	75/10 × 4	75/10 × 4

Note: You could decrease the number of workouts to 4, but maintain the same loading. If the number of workouts is reduced to 4, an aerobic training session should replace the 5th workout. RI between sets is 45 sec. Information is provided as load/# of repetitions × sets. So, 60/12 × 4 means 4 sets of 12 repetitions using weight equal to 60% of 1RM.

TABLE 13.5 — Three-Week H Phase for Professional Bodybuilders

EX NO.	WEEK	1 (LOW)			2 (MEDIUM)	
	STEP	LOW			MEDIUM	
	DAY	1	3	5	1	3
1	Safety squat	70/12 × 4	70/15 × 4	70/15 × 5	70/10 × 5	70/15 × 5
2	Standing leg curl	70/8 × 4	70/15 × 4	70/10 × 5	70/10 × 5	70/15 × 5
3	Lunge	70/12 × 3	70/15 × 3	70/10 × 3	70/10 × 3	70/15 × 3
4	Back extension	4 × 15	4 × 15	4 × 18	4 × 18	4 × 12
5	Biceps preacher curl	70/12 × 4	70/15 × 4	70/10 × 5	70/10 × 5	70/15 × 5
6	Decline triceps extension	70/12 × 4	70/15 × 4	70/10 × 5	70/10 × 5	70/15 × 5
	DAY	2	4	6	2	4
1	Flat bench press	70/12 × 4	70/15 × 4	75/10 × 5	75/10 × 5	70/15 × 3
2	Incline fly	70/12 × 3	70/15 × 3	75/10 × 3	75/10 × 3	70/15 × 3
3	One-arm dumbbell row	70/12 × 4	70/15 × 4	75/10 × 4	75/10 × 4	70/15 × 4
4	Incline side lateral	70/12 × 4	70/15 × 4	75/10 × 4	75/10 × 4	70/15 × 5
5	Front dumbbell press	70/12 × 3	70/15 × 3	75/10 × 3	75/10 × 3	70/15 × 4
6	Shrug	70/12 × 3	70/15 × 3	75/10 × 3	75/10 × 3	70/15 × 3
7	Two abdominal exercises	4 × 15	4 × 15	6 × 18	6 × 18	6 × 12
8	Donkey calf raise	70/12 × 4	70/15 × 4	75/10 × 5	75/10 × 5	75/15 × 5

Note: RI between sets is 30-45 sec. Information is provided as load/# of repetitions × sets. So, 70/12 × 4 means 4 sets of 12 repetitions using weight equal to 70% of 1RM.

| 3 | 4 | | | 5 | | | 6 | | |
| HIGH | LOW | | | MEDIUM | | | HIGH | | |
5	1	3	5	1	3	5	1	3	5
75/10 × 4	60/12 × 4	70/10 × 4	70/10 × 4	75/10 × 4	Off	80/8 × 4	80/8 × 5	80/8 × 5	85/5 × 5
65/7 × 4	60/10 × 3	60/10 × 3	60/10 × 4	65/7 × 4	Off	65/10 × 4	70/8 × 4	70/8 × 4	70/8 × 4
75/10 × 4	60/12 × 4	70/10 × 4	70/10 × 4	75/10 × 4	Off	80/8 × 4	80/8 × 5	80/8 × 5	85/5 × 5
75/10 × 4	60/12 × 4	60/12 × 4	70/10 × 4	75/10 × 4	Off	80/8 × 4	80/8 × 5	85/5 × 5	85/5 × 5
4 × 15	3 × 15	3 × 15	4 × 12	4 × 15	Off	4 × 15	5 × 15	5 × 15	5 × 15
4 × 15	3 × 15	3 × 15	4 × 12	4 × 15	Off	4 × 15	5 × 15	5 × 15	5 × 15
75/10 × 4	60/12 × 4	60/12 × 4	70/10 × 4	75/10 × 4	Off	80/8 × 4	80/8 × 5	85/5 × 5	85/5 × 5
6	**2**	**4**	**6**	**2**	**4**	**6**	**2**	**4**	**6**
75/10 × 4	60/12 × 4	Off	70/10 × 4	75/10 × 4	75/10 × 4	80/8 × 4	80/8 × 5	Off	85/5 × 5
75/10 × 4	60/12 × 4	Off	70/10 × 4	75/10 × 4	75/10 × 4	80/8 × 5	80/8 × 5	Off	85/5 × 5
75/10 × 4	60/12 × 4	Off	70/10 × 4	75/10 × 4	75/10 × 4	80/8 × 5	80/8 × 5	Off	85/5 × 5
70/8 × 4	60/10 × 4	Off	60/10 × 4	70/8 × 4	75/6 × 4	75/6 × 4	75/6 × 4	Off	75/6 × 4
75/10 × 4	60/12 × 4	Off	70/10 × 4	75/10 × 4	75/10 × 4	80/8 × 4	80/8 × 5	Off	85/5 × 5
75/10 × 4	60/12 × 4	Off	70/10 × 4	75/10 × 4	75/10 × 4	80/8 × 4	80/8 × 5	Off	85/5 × 5
75/10 × 4	60/12 × 4	Off	70/10 × 4	75/10 × 4	75/10 × 4	80/8 × 4	80/8 × 5	Off	85/5 × 5

| 2 | | 3 | | |
| MEDIUM | | HIGH | | |
5		1	3	5
75/8 × 3	80/7 × 3	80/7 × 6	80/6 × 4	85/4 × 7
80/7 × 5		80/6 × 5	80/6 × 4	85/4 × 6
75/8 × 1	80/7 × 2	80/7 × 3	80/6 × 3	85/4 × 3
4 × 12		4 × 15	4 × 15	4 × 15
75/8 × 3	80/7 × 3	80/7 × 4	80/7 × 3	85/4 × 6
75/8 × 3	80/7 × 3	80/7 × 4	80/7 × 3	85/4 × 6
6		**2**	**4**	**6**
75/8 × 1	80/7 × 2	80/7 × 6	80/7 × 4	85/4 × 6
75/8 × 1	80/7 × 2	80/7 × 3	80/7 × 3	85/4 × 3
75/8 × 1	80/7 × 2	80/7 × 4	80/7 × 4	85/4 × 4
75/7 × 4		80/6 × 4	80/6 × 4	80/4 × 4
75/8 × 1	80/7 × 2	80/7 × 3	80/7 × 3	85/4 × 3
75/8 × 1	80/7 × 2	80/7 × 3	80/7 × 3	85/4 × 3
6 × 12		6 × 15	6 × 15	6 × 15
75/8 × 3	80/7 × 3	80/7 × 4	80/6 × 4	85/4 × 4

NUTRITION

The H phase is similar to the bulking-up phase most bodybuilders are familiar with. As usual, you'll be increasing your caloric intake. On the metabolic diet, your goal should be to allow your body weight to increase to 15 percent above your ideal weight. By *ideal weight*, we mean what you consider to be your optimal contest weight—and you must be practical about it. If you have been competing at 200 pounds (91 kg) for 4 or 5 years but say your ideal weight is 315 pounds (143 kg), that's not practical. More reasonable would be to define your ideal weight in this phase as 215 pounds (98 kg) or so and to increase your weight to 15 percent above that—or about 250 pounds (113 kg). Throughout the phase, a gain of 2 pounds (.9 kg) per week is best.

If you go hog wild, eat like crazy, and end up going 30 percent above your ideal weight, your body will end up being 15 percent body fat or more. That's not what you want. The metabolic diet is designed to get you more muscle and limit body fat. Even though you will experience an increase in lean mass and put on less fat than you would on another diet, you still must exercise some discipline. Men's body fat should not rise above the 10 percent level and women's body fat should not rise above the 18 percent level, depending on the athletes' goals. Males end the "mass phase" when they reach their new ideal weight or rise to the 10 percent body-fat level and females when they reach their new ideal weight or rise to the 18 percent body-fat level, whichever comes first. However, whether or not you have reached your new ideal weight, the mass phase must end 12 weeks before a contest.

The specifics of the diet are the same in this phase as in the others—continue to eat a high-protein, high-fat diet on weekdays, and load up on carbohydrate foods on weekends. The only change will be in the number of calories you consume. If you want to get to a level 15 percent above your ideal weight, you obviously will have to eat more.

In this phase, bodybuilders should consume 25 calories for each pound of the targeted weight they want to achieve. For example, a bodybuilder wanting to reach 250 pounds needs to take in $25 \times 250 = 6{,}250$ calories a day. Before this phase, the bodybuilder likely would have been on a 3,600-calorie diet, so you can see the tremendous increase in calories that is required.

Such an increase in calorie consumption can present a big problem for athletes who have trouble gaining weight. They're not used to eating and don't have big appetites. They may think they're eating huge amounts but they're not. They'll find themselves at 6,000 calories one day and down to 1,500 a few days later. When asked what happened, all they say is, "I wasn't hungry." You can't do that on this diet. You have to be consistent.

If you want, you can multiply that 6,250 daily calories by 7 and make your goal 43,750 for the week. That way you can vary your caloric intake from day to day. For example, eat 7,500 calories one day and 5,000 the next—but by the end of the week you must consume 43,750 calories. Keep a written record of calories eaten to make sure you're reaching the desired levels.

Controlling Body Fat

Body fat is of critical importance. Some athletes gain more body fat than others at similar calorie levels. Depending on personal goals, moreover, some people won't mind gaining a little more fat if it means more muscle and strength. The 10 percent rule is best for competitive bodybuilders (and for any athlete who competes in a specific weight class). Other athletes, however, may be willing to go higher and find that it is acceptable if it means more hypertrophy and strength. However, we do not suggest going over a 10 percent level for men and 18 percent level for women. Just keep in mind that if your body-fat levels get too high, it will be that much harder to get the fat off.

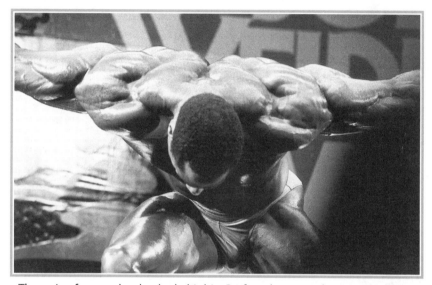

The recipe for muscles that look this big: Perform hypertrophy training, add just enough protein, and stack the proper supplements.

Since most athletes want to maximize muscle mass and strength and minimize body fat, we will use the competitive bodybuilding model to discuss reaching ideal gains in weight and muscle mass during the mass phase. Most bodybuilders can maintain a 10 percent body-fat level relatively easily if they properly use the metabolic diet. This is also a good level for keeping fat in check to prepare for competitive bodybuilding. That is why we advise those on the metabolic diet to keep close track of their body-fat level and to not let it go above 10 percent.

The goal, as noted previously, is to continue eating and gaining weight until you either reach a level 15 percent above your ideal weight or hit 10 percent body fat, whichever comes first. Chances are, no matter which comes first, you will get the mass you want on this anabolically supercharged diet. It's not like the old days with the high-carbohydrate diet when you had to gain so much weight and fat to get mass.

Hypertrophy-Phase Duration Can Vary

By always maintaining about 10 percent body fat, you can quickly get into contest shape. The amount of time before a contest along with body fat and weight are determinants of how long you will stay in this phase. If you find yourself still gaining weight but haven't reached your new ideal weight and your contest is in 12 weeks, it's time to stop the mass phase—regardless of your weight, you must begin the muscle definition phase of training to properly prepare yourself for the contest.

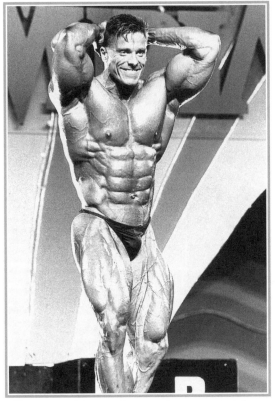

The competition-ready muscular symmetry of Achim Albrecht.

Many bodybuilders generally believe they should not gain mass quickly, but we disagree. Two pounds (.9 kg) a week is good. If you can gain 2 pounds, you won't gain a lot of fat during the week on the metabolic diet. It will be mostly muscle. Although you may vary this goal plus or minus a pound given your individual metabolism, we think 2 pounds a week is the best benchmark for bulking up.

We have seen people go through a 20-week cycle in which they bulked up for 8 weeks (3 pounds a week) and then spent 12 weeks losing 1 to 2 pounds per week in the cutting phase (i.e., muscle definition phase—*cut* is jargon that means having highly defined muscles). Although they bulked up for only 8 weeks and cut for 12, their weight for the contest was still above its previous level. And they were just as cut if not more so.

The goal is to come into a contest a little better than before you were on the diet. This may mean a net gain of only 3 or 4 pounds (1.4 to 1.8 kg). Or, in more long-term training, it could be 25 pounds (11 kg). The important point is that *everybody makes progress with this diet.* For those people who have been the same for 15 years, here is a way to break out!

Some bodybuilders prefer to aim for a big contest, such as Mr. Olympia, and take the whole year to do it. That can easily be done on this diet. You may want to mass for 30 weeks and cut for 20, gaining 60 pounds (27 kg) and losing 40 (18 kg) over the course of a year. You'll come in 20 pounds (9 kg) ahead of where you were last year and be looking great.

Keep in mind that you may also want to use the start-up or maintenance phase as you go from the mass to cutting phase. Assume you have a contest in 30 weeks. You have gained all the body mass you want in 10 weeks, but you don't want to go yet to the cutting phase. You can maintain your gains by staying on the maintenance phase for 6 to 8 weeks. Then, when you're ready, you can go into the cutting phase in preparation for the contest.

Weekly Weight Gains

You may see big fluctuations in weight, especially at the beginning of the diet, as a result of your weekly carbohydrate loads. All the extra carbohydrate and water can make for a gain of 5 to 10 pounds (2.3 to 4.5 kg) between Friday and Monday. If this happens, don't stress out. It's normal.

When you go back on the metabolic diet on Monday, you'll immediately begin shedding those pounds (which are mostly water). On Monday through Wednesday you'll be cleaning out much of what you put into your body on the weekend. By Wednesday you should be pretty well flushed out and feeling good again. Depending on what phase of the diet you are on, you can manipulate calories so that by Friday you can reach either the weekly weight gain or loss you are looking for.

SUPPLEMENTATION

In the hypertrophy phase, the increased caloric intake along with the high-fat, low-carbohydrate weekdays and carbohydrate-loading weekends should supply you with much of what you need to pack on size and muscle. However, you should use several of the more general supplements on a regular basis, including one or more of MVM, Antiox, and EFA+; use others as needed—for example, ReNew, Regulate, Joint Support, MRP LoCarb, and LoCarb sports bars. If you are running into training problems, joint pain, injuries, or overtraining, we recommend Joint Support or ReNew. MRP LoCarb and LoCarb sports bars can be extremely useful for snacks or after meals to help you reach your calorie goals in a healthy, low-carbohydrate way. Also, if you reach a plateau in this phase, especially in your training, you might want to use Exersol to maximize your training efforts.

The balanced multiple vitamin and mineral formula (MVM) meets the special needs of athletes for body maintenance, recuperation, and repair. This is important during this phase because of the rigorous, intense training schedule. The Antiox supplement during this phase is important because of the increased formation of free radicals due to the elevated mental and physical demands placed on the body during intensive training. The synergistic blend provides protection to all tissues in the body, including the musculoskeletal system and the liver.

Supplementation with EFA+ ensures the body receives essential fatty acids, such as omega-3, omega-6, EPA, DHA, CLA, GLA, and ALA, which are available to support the optimal metabolic response to intense exercise. Essential fatty acids are involved in hormone production, muscle and joint tissue repair, insulin metabolism, and fat burning. Working in concert with many ingredients, EFA+ will optimize metabolism; improve testosterone production and increase growth hormone secretion; support the body's immune system; improve natural insulin sensitivity; decrease inflammation, muscle aches, and joint pain secondary to excessive exercise; and increase the breakdown and oxidation of body fat.

During this phase if you are experiencing workout fatigue and overtraining symptoms because of the long periodization cycle, ReNew is a great advanced recovery and immune system formula. ReNew enhances the immune system by providing the necessary nutrition building blocks to boost your immunity. This is key because the immune system is the first line of defense against mental and physical stress. Use other supplementation as needed, but remember to try to eat a balanced and enriched food diet. This will aid immensely in achieving your goals and end result. For further information on Regulate, Joint Support, MRP LoCarb, and LoCarb sports bars, refer to *The Anabolic Solution* (www.metabolicdiet.com).

chapter 14

Mixed Training (M)

Before entering the maximum strength (MxS) phase described in chapter 15, athletes must gradually introduce some specific training elements for the development of maximum strength. As the name implies, mixed (M) training incorporates some workouts specific to H training and applies MxS methods for other sessions. The M phase provides a progressive transition between the H and MxS phases.

The following characteristics describe the scope of M Training:

- It continues to improve muscle hypertrophy.
- It introduces MxS methods in order to increase chronic hypertrophy, or long-term muscle tone and density.
- It uses desired proportions between the two types of training, depending on the needs of the athlete. For example, the following proportions may be used:
    - 40 percent H and 60 percent MxS
    - 50 percent H and 50 percent MxS
    - 60 percent H and 40 percent MxS

Regardless of the proportions used, M training ensures a more progressive transition into the maximum strength phase, where extremely heavy loads might challenge an athlete's ability to cope with the stress and strains of high-intensity workouts.

DURATION

The mixed phase should last for 3 to 6 weeks for entry-level and recreational bodybuilders and strength trainers and 3 weeks for advanced and professional athletes. After completing the mixed training phase, athletes, no matter what level, should determine whether they can handle the higher load increments that the MxS phase presents.

In some instances, the strength of bodybuilders' muscles are not proportionate to their size. In other words, some bodybuilding training programs are more conducive to size than to maximum strength and its benefit of increased muscle tone. The main reason: For traditional bodybuilding programs, the load is only 60 to 80 percent of 1RM. But the load necessary to increase maximum strength is much higher, often up to 95 or even 100 percent. Therefore, one of the goals of M training is a better progression from H to MxS training. This progression is ensured by employing variable proportions between the H and MxS phases.

PROGRAM DESIGN

Table 14.1 presents the proportions of an H and MxS mixed training program for four classifications of bodybuilders. The program can be repeated as many times as necessary, depending on the length of the M phase. As the table shows, MxS training is consistently recommended for the first workout of the week or after a rest day. Since MxS training employs loads that come close to maximum potential, planning for these sessions must take into account the athlete's ability to reach maximum concentration before and during training.

TABLE 14.1	M Phase: Proportions of H and MxS Training						
Classification	**Mon**	**Tues**	**Wed**	**Thurs**	**Fri**	**Sat**	**Sun**
Entry level	H	H	Off	MxS	Off	H	Off
Recreational	MxS	H	Off	MxS	Off	H	Off
Advanced	MxS	H	MxS	H	Off	H	Off
Professional	MxS	H	H	Off	MxS	H	Off

Factor in Fatigue

It is well known that fatigue affects one's ability to lift heavy loads, such as those used in MxS. If, for example, athletes perform a MxS workout after an H workout, they will have decreased lifting efficiency for the heavy loads. On the other hand, starting H training with slight residual fatigue tends to have a stimulating effect on the development of muscle. A slightly fatigued muscle seems to exhaust the ATP-PC stores more quickly, thereby stimulating muscle growth. In the case of mixed training, then, factor fatigue into the process and always plan MxS workouts before H workouts.

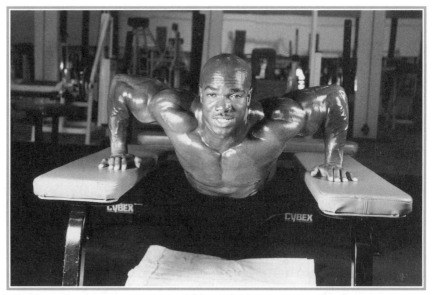

Fatigue exhausts energy stores quickly, and this appears to stimulate muscle growth.

Tables 14.2 through 14.9 provide M training programs for entry-level, recreational, advanced, and professional athletes. To follow the same sequence of H and MxS training days shown in table 14.1, you must split the plan for each level into two parts—one for the H portion and one for the MxS portion.

The suggested training program in table 14.2 shows the H portion of the M program for entry-level athletes, with 3 days planned for the development of H—days 1, 2, and 6. Table 14.3 shows the MxS portion of the M program for entry-level athletes, with only 1 day planned for MxS training. Please perform only those exercises you have chosen; do *not* complete both programs.

TABLE 14.2 **M Phase: H Training Portion for Entry-Level Bodybuilders and Strength Trainers**

EX NO.	WEEK	1			2			3		
	STEP	LOW			MEDIUM			HIGH		
	DAY	1	3	6	1	3	6	1	3	6
1	Leg extension	40/15 × 3	Off		50/12 × 3	Off		60/12 × 3	Off	
2	Leg press	40/12 × 3	Off	40/12 × 3	50/12 × 3	Off	50/12 × 3	60/10 × 3	Off	60/10 × 3
3	Lunge	40/12 × 3	Off	40/12 × 3	50/12 × 3	Off	50/12 × 3	60/10 × 3	Off	60/10 × 3
4	Standing leg curl	40/10 × 3	Off	40/10 × 3	50/10 × 3	Off	50/12 × 3	50/10 × 3	Off	50/10 × 3
5	T-bar row	40/12 × 3	Off		50/12 × 3	Off		60/10 × 3	Off	
6	Back extension	3 × 10	Off		3 × 12	Off		3 × 15	Off	
7	Seated calf raise	40/12 × 3	Off		50/12 × 3	Off		60/10 × 3	Off	
8	Flat fly	40/12 × 3	Off	40/12 × 3	50/12 × 3	Off	50/12 × 3	60/10 × 3	Off	60/10 × 3
	DAY	2	5	6	2	5	6	2	5	6
1	Front dumbbell press	40/12 × 3	Off		50/12 × 3	Off		60/10 × 3	Off	
2	Incline side lateral	40/12 × 3	Off	40/12 × 3	50/12 × 3	Off	50/12 × 3	60/10 × 3	Off	60/10 × 3
3	Upright row	40/12 × 3	Off		50/12 × 3	Off		60/10 × 3	Off	
4	Shrug	40/12 × 3	Off	40/12 × 3	50/12 × 3	Off	50/12 × 3	60/10 × 3	Off	60/10 × 3
5	Decline triceps extension	40/12 × 3	Off	40/12 × 3	50/12 × 3	Off	50/12 × 3	60/10 × 3	Off	60/10 × 3
6	Diagonal curl-up	3 × 10	Off	3 × 10	3 × 12	Off	3 × 12	3 × 15	Off	3 × 15

Note: 40/15 × 3 means load/# of repetitions × sets (in this example, 3 sets of 15 repetitions using weight equal to 40% of 1RM); RI between sets = 1-2 min.

TABLE 14.3 **M Phase: MxS Training Portion for Entry–Level Bodybuilders and Strength Trainers**

EX NO.	WEEK	1	2		3
	STEP	LOW	MEDIUM		HIGH
	DAY	4	4		5
1	Leg press	70/7 × 3	70/8 × 1	80/6 × 2	80/6 × 3
2	Flat bench press	70/7 × 3	70/8 × 1	80/6 × 2	80/6 × 3
3	Supine leg curl	50/10 × 3	60/10 × 3		70/7 × 3
4	T-bar row	50/10 × 3	60/10 × 3		70/8 × 3
5	Seated calf raise	70/7 × 3	70/8 × 1	80/6 × 2	80/6 × 3

Note: 70/7 × 3 means load/# of repetitions × sets (in this example, 3 sets of 7 repetitions using weight equal to 70% of 1RM); RI between sets = 3 min.

TABLE 14.4 **M Phase: H Training Portion for Recreational Bodybuilders and Strength Trainers**

EX NO.	WEEK	1	2	3
	STEP	LOW	MEDIUM	HIGH
	DAY	2	2	2
1	Front dumbbell press	50/12 × 3	60/12 × 3	70/8 × 4
2	Incline side lateral	50/12 × 3	60/12 × 3	70/8 × 4
3	Biceps preacher curl	50/12 × 3	60/12 × 3	70/8 × 4
4	Shrug	50/12 × 3	60/12 × 3	70/8 × 4
5	Seated calf raise	50/12 × 3	60/12 × 3	70/8 × 4
	DAY	**6**	**6**	**6**
1	Hack squat	50/12 × 3	60/12 × 3	70/8 × 4
2	Supine leg curl	50/12 × 3	60/12 × 3	70/8 × 4
3	Seated pulley row	50/12 × 3	60/12 × 3	70/8 × 4
4	Incline fly	50/10 × 3	60/10 × 3	60/8 × 4
5	Triceps push-down	50/12 × 3	60/12 × 3	70/8 × 4
6	Crunch	3 × 10	3 × 12	4 × 15

Note: 50/12 × 3 means load/# of repetitions × sets (in this example, 3 sets of 12 repetitions using weight equal to 50% of 1RM); RI between sets = 1-2 min.

TABLE 14.5 **M Phase: MxS Training Portion for Recreational Bodybuilders and Strength Trainers**

EX NO.	WEEK	1			2			3	
	STEP	LOW			MEDIUM			HIGH	
	DAY	1	4		1	4		1	4
1	Leg press	70/8 × 3	70/8 × 2	80/6 × 1	70/8 × 1	80/7 × 2	80/7 × 3	80/8 × 4	80/8 × 4
2	Flat bench press	70/8 × 3	70/8 × 2	80/6 × 1	70/8 × 1	80/7 × 2	80/7 × 3	80/8 × 4	80/8 × 4
3	Supine leg curl	60/10 × 3	60/10 × 3		70/8 × 3		70/8 × 3	70/8 × 4	70/8 × 4
4	Lat pull-down	70/8 × 3	70/8 × 2	80/6 × 1	70/8 × 1	80/7 × 2	80/7 × 3	80/8 × 4	80/8 × 4

Note: 70/8 × 3 means load/# of repetitions × sets (in this example, 3 sets of 8 repetitions using weight equal to 70% of 1RM); RI between sets = 3 min.

TABLE 14.6 — M Phase: H Training Portion for Advanced Bodybuilders and Strength Trainers

EX NO.	WEEK	1 LOW	2 MEDIUM	3 HIGH
	STEP	LOW	MEDIUM	HIGH
	DAY	6	6	6
1	Lunge	70/8 × 4	80/9 × 5	85/5 × 5
2	Diagonal curl-up	4 × 12	5 × 15	5 × 15
3	Biceps preacher curl	70/8 × 4	80/7 × 5	85/5 × 5

EX NO.	DAY	2/4 (W1)	6 (W1)	2/4 (W2)	6 (W2)	2/4 (W3)		6 (W3)	
1	Decline triceps extension	70/8 × 4	70/8 × 4	80/7 × 5	80/7 × 5	80/7 × 2	85/5 × 3	80/7 × 2	85/5 × 3
2	Pull-down behind the neck	70/8 × 4	70/8 × 4	80/7 × 5	80/7 × 5	80/7 × 2	85/5 × 3	80/7 × 2	85/5 × 3
3	Standing dumbbell bent lateral	60/10 × 4	70/8 × 4	70/7 × 5	80/7 × 5	75/6 × 5			
4	Shrug	70/8 × 4		80/7 × 5		80/7 × 2	85/5 × 3		
5	Back extension	4 × 12		4 × 15		5 × 15			

Note: 70/8 × 4 means load/# of repetitions × sets (in this example, 4 sets of 8 repetitions using weight equal to 70% of 1RM); RI between sets = 30-45 sec.

TABLE 14.7 — M Phase: MxS Training Portion for Advanced Bodybuilders and Strength Trainers

EX NO.	WEEK	1 Day 1		1 Day 3	2 Day 1		2 Day 3		3 Day 1	3 Day 3
	STEP	LOW			MEDIUM				HIGH	
	DAY	1		3	1		3		1	3
1	Safety squat	70/8 × 4	80/7 × 1	80/7 × 5	80/6 × 2	90/3 × 3	85/4 × 2	90/3 × 3	90/3 × 5	90/2 × 5
2	Standing leg curl	60/8 × 5		60/8 × 5	70/7 × 5		70/7 × 5		80/6 × 5	80/6 × 5
3	Flat bench press	70/8 × 4	80/7 × 1	80/7 × 5	80/6 × 2	90/3 × 3	85/4 × 2	90/3 × 3	90/3 × 5	90/2 × 5
4	Bent-over barbell row	70/8 × 4	80/7 × 1	80/7 × 5	80/6 × 2	90/3 × 3	85/4 × 2	90/3 × 3	90/3 × 5	90/2 × 5
5	Front dumbbell press	70/8 × 4	80/7 × 1	80/7 × 5	80/6 × 2	90/3 × 3	85/4 × 2	90/3 × 3	90/3 × 5	90/2 × 5
6	Donkey calf raise	60/8 × 5		60/8 × 5	70/7 × 5		70/7 × 5		80/6 × 5	80/6 × 5

Note: 70/8 × 4 means load/# of repetitions × sets (in this example, 4 sets of 8 repetitions, using weight equal to 70% of 1RM); RI between sets = 3-4 min.

TABLE 14.8 **M Phase: H Training Portion for Professional Bodybuilders and Strength Trainers**

	WEEK	1		2		3	
	STEP	LOW		MEDIUM		HIGH	
EX NO.	DAY	2	6	2	6	2	6
1	Front dumbbell press	60/12 × 3	60/12 × 3	70/10 × 3	75/8 × 3	80/7 × 2	80/7 × 2
2	Incline side lateral	60/12 × 4	60/12 × 4	70/10 × 4	75/8 × 4	80/7 × 3	80/7 × 3
3	Shrug	60/12 × 6	60/12 × 6	70/10 × 6	75/8 × 6	80/7 × 6	80/7 × 6
4	Decline triceps extension	60/12 × 4	60/12 × 4	70/10 × 6	75/8 × 6	80/7 × 6	80/7 × 6
5	Biceps preacher curl	60/12 × 3	60/12 × 3	70/10 × 3	70/10 × 3	80/7 × 3	80/7 × 3
	DAY	3		3		3	
1	Safety squat	60/12 × 6		70/10 × 7		80/7 × 3	
2	Standing leg curl	60/12 × 6		70/10 × 7		70/7 × 3	
3	Flat bench press	60/12 × 6		70/10 × 7		80/7 × 3	
4	Barbell bent-over row	60/12 × 6		70/10 × 7		80/7 × 3	
5	Back extension	60/12 × 3		70/10 × 3		80/7 × 3	
6	Nautilus crunch	60/12 × 3		70/10 × 3		80/7 × 3	
7	Donkey calf raise	60/12 × 6		70/10 × 7		80/7 × 3	

Note: 60/12 × 3 means load/# of repetitions × sets (in this example, 3 sets of 12 repetitions using weight equal to 60% of 1RM); RI between sets = 30-45 sec.

TABLE 14.9 **M Phase: MxS Training Portion for Professional Bodybuilders and Strength Trainers**

	WEEK	1		2		3			
	STEP	LOW		MEDIUM		HIGH			
EX NO.	DAY	1	5	1	5	1		5	
1	Safety squat	80/7 × 6	80/7 × 6	85/4 × 3	90/3 × 3	90/3 × 6	90/3 × 2	95/2 × 4	80/3 × 2	95/2 × 4
2	Standing leg curl	70/6 × 5	70/6 × 5	80/6 × 5		80/6 × 5	80/6 × 5		80/6 × 5	
3	Barbell bent-over row	80/7 × 6	80/7 × 6	85/4 × 3	90/3 × 3	90/3 × 6	90/3 × 2	95/2 × 4	80/3 × 2	95/2 × 4
4	Flat bench press	80/7 × 6	80/7 × 6	85/4 × 3	90/3 × 3	90/3 × 6	90/3 × 2	95/2 × 4	80/3 × 2	95/2 × 4

Note: 80/7 × 6 means load/# of repetitions × sets (in this example, 6 sets of 7 repetitions using weight equal to 80% of 1RM); RI between sets = 3-5 min.

The following tips can help you execute your M phase successfully:

- Test for 1RM as suggested for the other training phases.
- Do 5 to 10 minutes of aerobic work before and after the mixed training session. Be sure to include a warm-up and cool-down.
- The exercises may be substituted with similar exercises according to your needs and preferences.
- The number of sets can be increased or decreased according to your own potential.
- You may select exercises other than those suggested, but apply the same loading pattern.
- If a given load is too high for you, reduce it slightly until you can perform the recommended number of reps.
- Each recommended phase plan is 3 weeks in duration. If a longer M phase is needed, the entire program can be repeated.

Achieve Optimal Recovery

Unlike the exercise pattern for H training, where all the planned sets for one exercise are performed before moving on to the next exercise, MxS training requires that the athlete always reach optimal recovery between sets. The MxS exercise pattern is to perform one set for the first exercise, then to perform one set for the next exercise. Always work the exercises in series of twos from the top down. The rest interval should be about 5 to 6 minutes before going back to the original exercise. To enhance the recovery process further, the exercises are planned in such a way that the muscle groups are constantly being alternated.

It is extremely important to strictly observe the proposed rest intervals. Do not make the mistake of performing your sets too soon. Regardless of whether you feel ready before the RI is up, your body needs the time to recover from this type of training. Your last set should be as good as your first set.

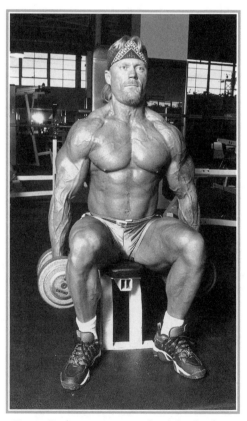

Trevor Butler preparing to finish his final set with the same high level of intensity he started with.

NUTRITION

The mixed phase and the maximum strength phase are intermediate phases between the classical hypertrophy, or bulk, phase and the definition phase. The nutrition goals in the mixed phase are at the very least to maintain the weight and muscle mass gained during the hypertrophy phase and ideally to marginally increase both while at the same time developing the strength that would normally go along with the increased weight and muscle mass. During this phase, athletes begin the process of solidifying and marginally adding to the muscle-mass gains of the hypertrophy phase; they also begin increasing their strength.

During the mixed phase, bodybuilders should daily consume between 17 and 25 calories per pound of the top body weight they attained during the hypertrophy phase. They can cut back their caloric intake by 2 calories per pound of body weight every week. Their percentage of body fat should not rise above the levels of the hypertrophy phase. Stabilize your body weight at or slightly above your weight in the hypertrophy phase, and end the calorie cutting when your weight stabilizes.

Using the example from chapter 13, the 250-pound (113 kg) bodybuilder will now cut back roughly 2 calories per pound per week. That means the first week of the mixed phase he will take in 23 calories per pound of body weight, or 23 $\times$ 250 = 5,750 calories per day. The following week he will take in 21 calories per pound of body weight, or 5,250 calories per day. The third week, he will consume 19 calories per pound of body weight, or 4,750 calories per day. The fourth week, he will consume 17 calories per pound of body weight, or 4,250 calories per day. Once his weight stabilizes so that he is no longer gaining weight, he should keep the calories at that level until beginning the definition phase.

SUPPLEMENTATION

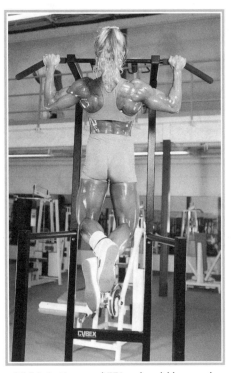

MVM, Antiox, and EFA+ should be used on a regular basis by bodybuilders who are training hard.

In the mixed phase, as in the hypertrophy phase, the food counts more than the supplements. Getting your quota of low-carbohydrate calories will supply you with much of what you need to solidify your increased muscle mass and start getting ready to decrease your body fat. However, as you drop your calories, nutritional supplements gain in importance.

You will need more than just your basic daily vitamin and mineral tablet. You should use MVM (a complete vitamin, mineral, and nutrient supplement), Antiox (an antioxidant mix), and EFA+ (an essential fatty acid formula that contains much more than just the essential fatty acids) on a regular basis. As in the hypertrophy phase, other supplements—such as Exersol (made up of Resolve, Power Drink, and Amino), ReNew, Regulate, Joint Support, MRP LoCarb, and LoCarb sports bars—can be used as needed. (For more information, see chapters 13 and 15, or refer to www.metabolicdiet.com.)

chapter 1

Maximum Strength (MxS)

Maximum strength is developed by increasing the training load and in the process increasing the contractile capability of the muscles. Training loads higher than 80 percent increase the tension in the muscle and recruit the powerful fast twitch motor units. The result is higher protein content in the muscle via increased thickness of myosin filaments. Since motor units are recruited by size, beginning with slow twitch followed by fast twitch, loads greater than 80 percent are required to recruit the powerful fast twitch motor units.

The following characteristics describe the scope of maximum strength (MxS) training:

- It increases protein content of muscle, thereby inducing chronic hypertrophy and increasing muscle tone and density.
- It increases thickness of the crossbridges and myosin filaments (this is the only way to induce chronic hypertrophy).
- It conditions muscles to recruit as many fast twitch muscle fibers as possible, through the application of heavy loads; this develops maximum strength and improves muscle tone and density.

PHYSIOLOGY BEHIND MxS TRAINING

An athlete's ability to develop maximum strength depends to a high degree on three factors.

- **The diameter, or cross-sectional area, of the muscle.** More specifically, this means the diameter of the myosin filaments, including their crossbridges. Although muscle size depends largely on the duration of the H phase, the diameter of the myosin filaments depends specifically on the volume and duration of the MxS phase. This is because MxS training is responsible for increasing the protein content of the muscles.
- **The capacity to recruit fast twitch muscle fibers.** This ability depends largely on training content. Use of maximum loads, with high application of force against resistance, is the only type of training that completely involves the powerful fast twitch motor units.

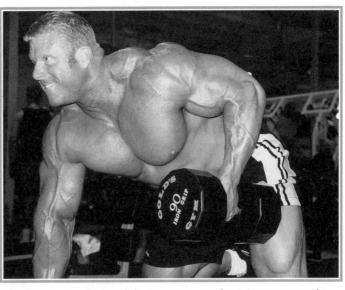

Smart lifters understand the importance of maximum strength training and muscle fiber recruitment.

- **The ability to successfully synchronize all the muscles involved in the action.** This develops over time as a function of learning, which is based on performing many repetitions of the same exercise with heavy loads. Most North American bodybuilders use only bodybuilding (i.e., hypertrophy) methods to increase muscle size. They tend to neglect training approaches that stimulate recruitment of fast twitch muscle fibers to build high-density muscle, tight muscle tone, impressive muscle separation, and more visible muscle striations. Although North American bodybuilders do increase their muscle size, the increases are usually not chronic: The growth is largely due to fluid displacement within the muscles rather than a thickening of the muscle fibers.

  The MxS phase in the periodization program can correct this deficiency. Maximum strength improves as a result of creating high tension in the muscle—and this tension can be achieved only by using loads that result in higher fast twitch muscle fiber recruitment (loads greater than 85 percent of 1RM)

DURATION AND TRAINING METHODS

We recommend that the MxS phase last 6 weeks, although other variations are possible. Exercises for the development of maximum strength must not be carried out under conditions of exhaustion, as in the H phase. During MxS training, the muscles should be allowed to recover maximally between sets. Because of its maximum activation of the central nervous system and the high levels of concentration and motivation it requires, MxS training improves the links with the central nervous system that lead to improved muscle coordination and synchronization. Strength depends not only on the size of the muscle and the total number of crossbridges but also on the central nervous system's capacity to "drive" that muscle.

High activation of the central nervous system (i.e., muscle synchronization) also results in inhibition of the antagonistic muscles. When maximum force is applied, therefore, the antagonistic muscles are coordinated in such a way that they do not contract to oppose the movement—allowing the athlete to lift even heavier weights.

Most changes in strength are said to occur at the level of muscle tissue. Little is said, however, about the involvement of the nervous system during MxS training. In fact, very little research has been conducted on the subject. The research that has been done suggests the central nervous system acts as a stimulus for gains in strength. The central nervous system normally acts as an inhibitor of motor units during contraction. Under extreme circumstances, such as a life-and-death situation, this inhibition is removed and all the motor units are activated, providing what seems to be superhuman strength. One of the main objectives of MxS training is to teach the body to eliminate central nervous system inhibition, which results in a huge improvement of strength potential.

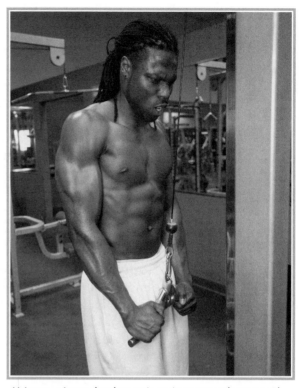

Using maximum loads to gain serious muscular strength.

Maximum Load Method (MLM)

Maximum strength improvement occurs almost solely through the maximum load method (MLM). This method should be performed only after 2 or 3 years of general bodybuilding or strength training because of the strain of training and the utilization of maximum loads. The gains are largely due to motor learning, whereby athletes learn to use and coordinate the muscles involved in training more efficiently. MLM provides the following benefits:

- It increases motor unit activation, resulting in high recruitment and firing frequency of fast twitch muscle fibers.

- It increases secretion of growth hormones and raises levels of catecholamines (compounds—primarily epinephrine and norepinephrine—that increase the strong physiological response to this type of training).

- It improves coordination and synchronization of muscle groups during performance. The better the coordination and synchronization of the muscles involved in contraction and the more they learn to recruit fast twitch muscles, the better the performance will be.

- It increases the diameter of the muscle's contractile elements.

- It raises the body's testosterone level.

The gains obtained through MLM are predominantly gains in maximum strength, with muscle hypertrophy as a secondary benefit. Large gains in muscle size through MLM are possible, but generally only in athletes who are just beginning to use MLM. For athletes with a more solid background, gains in muscle size will not be as noticeable as the gains made in maximum strength. The MxS phase sets the stage for future growth explosions through better synchronization and increased recruitment of fast twitch fibers. Highly trained athletes with 3 or 4 years of MLM training are so well adapted to such training that they are able to recruit approximately 85 percent of their fast twitch fibers. The remaining 15 percent represent a "latent reserve" that is not easily tapped through training.

Once athletes have reached such an advanced level, they may find it very difficult to further increase maximum strength. To avoid stagnating and to further improve muscle density and separation, they must use alternative methods to provide greater stimulation to the muscles. One such method is to increase the eccentric component of contractions—the increased tension helps the body to continue developing maximum strength despite an already high level of adaptation.

The most important elements to be considered in MLM training are the load used in training, the loading pattern, the rest interval, and the speed of performing the contraction. The following sections further examine each of these elements.

Load As already mentioned, maximum strength develops only when maximum tension is created in the muscle. Although lower loads stimulate the slow twitch muscle fibers, loads exceeding 85 percent 1RM are necessary if most muscle fibers, and especially fast twitch fibers, are to be recruited in contraction. Maximum loads with low repetitions result in significant nervous system adaptation, better synchronization of the muscles involved, and increased capacity to recruit fast twitch muscle fibers.

A suggestion by Goldberg et al. (1975)—that the tension developed within myofilaments is the stimulus for protein synthesis—further illustrates why training for maximum strength should be performed only with maximum loads. It is because the load for the MLM is maximum that the number of repetitions per set is low—only from one to four (or at most up to six).

Rest Interval The rest interval (RI) between sets depends partially on the athlete's fitness level and should be carefully calculated to ensure adequate recovery of the neuromuscular system. For MLM, a 3- to 5-minute RI is necessary because maximum loads involve the central nervous system (which recovers more slowly than the skeletal system). If the RI is too short, the nervous system participation—in the form of maximum concentration, motivation, and the power of the nerve impulses sent to the contracting muscle—could be less than optimal. In addition, complete restoration of the required fuel for contraction (ATP-PC) can also be jeopardized if the RI is too brief.

Speed The speed of execution plays an important role in MLM. Even when using typical maximum loads, the athlete's force against resistance must be exerted as quickly as possible. Although the magnitude of the load restricts the speed of contraction, the athlete must concentrate on activating the muscles as briskly as possible.

Eccentric Method

Strength exercises, using either free weights or most isokinetic apparatuses, involve both concentric and eccentric types of contraction. During the concentric phase, force is produced while the muscle shortens; during the eccentric segment, force is produced while the muscle lengthens, or returns to the resting position. Everyone knows the eccentric phase is easier than the concentric phase. For example, when performing the bench press, the lowering of the barbell to the chest (eccentric part of the lift) is easier than pressing the bar upward (concentric part of the lift).

Because eccentric work is easier, it allows athletes to work with heavier loads than if they were performing only concentric work, and heavier loads translate into greater strength gains. Strength training specialists and researchers have arrived at the same conclusion, which is that eccentric training creates a higher tension in the muscles than isometric or isotonic contractions. And since higher muscle tension is normally equated with greater strength development, eccentric training is a superior training method.

Some training specialists claim that the eccentric strength training method results in a 10 to 35 percent higher strength gain than other methods. The load in eccentric training is much higher than the athlete's 1RM, so the speed of performance is quite slow. Such a slow rate of contraction produces a larger stimulus for protein synthesis and therefore normally results in muscle hypertrophy and greater strength development.

During the first few days of using the eccentric method, athletes may experience muscle soreness because higher tensions provoke some minor muscle damage. As athletes adapt, the muscle soreness disappears in about 7 to 10 days. You can avoid this short-term discomfort by increasing the load progressively, using the step-type approach.

There are a number of differences in mechanical, metabolic, and neural stimuli between concentric and eccentric contractions. Although maximum concentric contractions lead to maximum muscle activation, maximum eccentric contractions do not appear to elicit complete muscle activation. In other words, a bodybuilder and strength athlete must work with heavier loads during the eccentric phase in order to develop a positive adaptation in strength. The neural command for eccentric contractions is unique in that it decides (1) which motor units should be activated, (2) how much they have to be activated, (3) when they should be activated, and (4) how the activity should be distributed within a group of muscles.

PROGRAM DESIGN

For maximum training benefits, athletes should use MLM for as long as practically possible. When they reach a plateau in which they are achieving little or no improvement, then they should begin using the eccentric method. This training approach will break through the ceiling of adaptation created by the plateau and permit achievement of new levels of strength.

Since the eccentric method employs the heaviest loads in strength training (110 to 160 percent), only athletes with a solid strength training background (i.e., 2 to 3 years of strength training or bodybuilding experience) should use it. And again, they should use it only after they are experiencing no further gains with the maximum load method (MLM).

The eccentric method can be used alone or in combination with MLM, but for only a short period of time. Eccentric training should not be abused. When overused it has limitations and can lead to a plateau that might be difficult to break. In addition, because eccentric training requires such intense mental concentration, every time maximum or supermaximum loads are used there is a great deal of psychological stress.

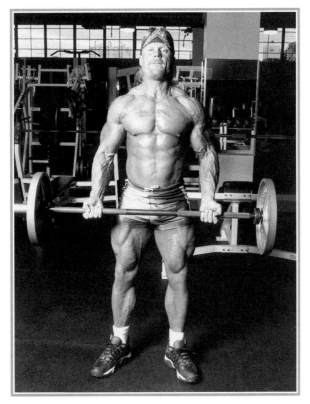

Trevor Butler's musculature shows the benefit of MxS training.

During eccentric training, which is usually performed with free weights, the assistance of two spotters is necessary because the weights are always greater than the athletes can lift concentrically by themselves. The spotters' job is to help lift the weight during the concentric portion and to watch the lifters carefully during the eccentric portion to ensure that they can handle the huge load.

Training guidelines for the eccentric method are presented in table 15.1. The load is expressed as a percentage of 1RM for the concentric contraction and is recommended to be between 110 and 160 percent. The most effective load for athletes of high caliber is around 130 to 140 percent. Less experienced athletes should use lower loads. These loads are to be used after at least two phases of MxS training in which the eccentric contraction is included. Eccentric contractions should not be used under any circumstances in the first few months of training.

Entry-level athletes must use a lower number of sets as indicated in table 15.1. Recreational athletes may need a lower number of sets than the table indicates depending on their ability and training potential. The RI is an important element in the capacity to perform highly demanding work. If, after a set, athletes have not recovered sufficiently to perform the next set at the same level, they should slightly increase the RI.

TABLE 15.1	**Training Guidelines for the MxS Phase**			
	BODYBUILDER'S CLASSIFICATION			
	Entry level	**Recreational**	**Advanced**	**Professional**
Reps/set	1-4	3-8	3-8	2-8
Sets/session	10-15	15-20	20-32	25-40
RI between sets (min)	4-5	3-5	3-5	3-5
Frequency/week: MLM	None	2-3	2-3	2-3
Eccentric	None	None	1	1-2
Rhythm, speed of contraction	Slow	Slow	Active	Active

Because eccentric contractions use extremely heavy loads, athletes must be highly motivated and have maximum concentration before performing each set. Only under such mental conditions will they be capable of effectively performing eccentric contractions. The eccentric method is rarely performed in isolation from the other maximum strength methods. Even during the MxS phase, the eccentric method is used together with MLM. We recommend only one eccentric training session. The frequency may eventually be increased for high-caliber athletes during the third step of the step-type approach to load patterning.

The following tips will help you complete a successful MxS phase:

- Test for 1RM during the second part of the first week and during the first week of the next phase.

- Since MxS training is very taxing on the neuromuscular system, reduce the number of exercises to the lowest realistic level. As much as possible, use multijoint exercises that involve several muscle groups; however, this method does not exclude the use of single-joint exercises.

- Because of the physiological and psychological stress of MxS training, the RI between sets must be 3 to 5 minutes long. Throughout the RI, relax the muscles, keep them warm with dry clothing, and do mild stretching exercises.

- If the suggested load is too high, lower it, and maintain the recommended number of repetitions.

- Adjust the program and exercises to meet your own needs and training potential.

- Do 20 to 25 minutes of aerobic exercise after training sessions.

- Advanced and professional bodybuilders and strength trainers may use more complex exercises such as deadlifts or power lifts, which involve up to six joints.

Tables 15.2 through 15.4 provide MxS programs for recreational, advanced, and professional bodybuilders and strength trainers. The load differs quite visibly among the three groups, as it must match ability and training potential.

TABLE 15.2 **MxS Phase for Recreational Bodybuilders and Strength Trainers**

	WEEK	1			2		
	STEP	LOW			MEDIUM		
EX NO.	DAY	1	3	5	1	3	
1	Leg press	70/8 × 3	75/8 × 4	75/8 × 4	80/6 × 4	80/6 × 4	
2	Supine leg curl	60/10 × 3	60/10 × 3	70/7 × 4	70/7 × 4	70/7 × 4	
3	Lat pull-down	70/8 × 3	75/8 × 4	75/8 × 4	80/6 × 4	80/6 × 4	
4	Front dumbbell press	70/8 × 3	75/8 × 4	75/8 × 4	80/6 × 4	80/6 × 4	
5	Donkey calf raise	70/8 × 3	75/8 × 4	75/8 × 4	80/6 × 4	80/6 × 4	

Note: Combinations of programs are possible. Information is provided as load/# of repetitions × sets, so 70/8 × 3 means 3 sets of 8 repetitions using weight equal to 70 percent of 1RM).

TABLE 15.3 **MxS Phase for Advanced Bodybuilders and Strength Trainers**

	WEEK	1				2		
	STEP	LOW				MEDIUM		
EX NO.	DAY	1	3	5	7	1	3	
1	Safety squat	75/8 × 4	75/8 × 4	75/8 × 4	75/8 × 4	80/6 × 5	85/5 × 5	
2	Standing leg curl	60/10 × 4	60/10 × 4	65/10 × 4	65/10 × 4	70/7 × 5	85/5 × 5	
3	Incline bench press	75/8 × 4	75/8 × 4	75/8 × 4	75/8 × 4	80/6 × 5	85/5 × 5	
4	Barbell bent-over row	75/8 × 4	75/8 × 4	75/8 × 4	75/8 × 4	80/6 × 5	85/5 × 5	
5	Donkey calf raise	75/8 × 4	75/8 × 4	75/8 × 4	75/8 × 4	80/6 × 5	85/5 × 5	
6	Nautilus crunch	60/10 × 4	60/10 × 4	65/10 × 4	65/10 × 4	70/7 × 5	85/5 × 5	

Note: In the last workout of the 3rd week, where the load is over 100 percent, the exercise is performed eccentrically. For exercises 2 and 6, use only MLM, since these exercises are inappropriate for eccentric training. Information is provided as load/# of repetitions × sets, so 75/8 × 4 means 4 sets of 8 repetitions using weight equal to 75 percent of 1RM.

TABLE 15.4 **MxS Phase for Professional Bodybuilders With a Mixture of MLM and Eccentric Method**

	WEEK	1							2			
	STEP	LOW							MEDIUM			
EX NO.	DAY	1	2	3	4		5	6	1	2	3	
1	Safety squat	70/8 × 6	70/8 × 6	Off	75/8 × 3	80/6 × 3	80/6 × 5	Off	80/6 × 6	85/4 × 6	120/4 × 6	
2	Standing leg curl	70/8 × 5	70/8 × 5	Off	75/8 × 6		75/8 × 6	Off	75/8 × 6	75/8 × 6	80/6 × 5	
3	T-bar row	70/8 × 6	70/8 × 6	Off	75/8 × 3	80/6 × 3	80/6 × 5	Off	80/6 × 6	85/4 × 6	85/4 × 6	
4	Flat bench press	70/8 × 6	70/8 × 6	Off	75/8 × 3	80/6 × 3	80/6 × 5	Off	80/6 × 6	85/4 × 6	120/4 × 6	
5	Donkey calf raise	70/8 × 6	70/8 × 5	Off	75/8 × 3	80/6 × 3	80/6 × 5	Off	80/6 × 6	85/4 × 6	120/4 × 6	
6	Nautilus crunch	70/8 × 5	70/8 × 5	Off	75/8 × 6		75/8 × 6	Off	75/8 × 6	75/8 × 6	80/6 × 5	

Note: Where the load is over 100 percent, the exercise is performed eccentrically. For exercises 2, 3, and 6, where the load is lower, use only MLM, since these exercises are inappropriate for eccentric training. Information is provided as load/# of repetitions × sets, so 75/8 × 4 means 4 sets of 8 repetitions using weight equal to 75 percent of 1RM.

| 2 | | 3 | | |
| MEDIUM | | HIGH | | |
5		1	3	5
80/6 × 3	90/3 × 1	90/3 × 4	90/3 × 4	90/3 × 4
70/7 × 4	70/7 × 4	70/7 × 4	70/7 × 4	70/7 × 4
80/6 × 3	90/3 × 1	90/3 × 4	90/3 × 4	90/3 × 4
80/6 × 3	90/3 × 1	90/3 × 4	90/3 × 4	90/3 × 4
80/6 × 3	90/3 × 1	90/3 × 4	90/3 × 4	90/3 × 4

| 2 | | 3 | | | | |
| MEDIUM | | HIGH | | | | |
5	7	1	3	5		7
90/3 × 5	90/3 × 5	90/3 × 5	95/2 × 5	95/2 × 3	100/1 × 2	120/3 × 5
90/3 × 5	90/3 × 5	80/6 × 5	80/6 × 5	80/6 × 5		80/6 × 5
90/3 × 5	90/3 × 5	90/3 × 5	95/2 × 5	95/2 × 3	100/1 × 2	120/3 × 5
90/3 × 5	90/3 × 5	90/3 × 5	95/2 × 5	95/2 × 3	100/1 × 2	120/3 × 5
90/3 × 5	90/3 × 5	90/3 × 5	95/2 × 5	95/2 × 3	100/1 × 2	120/3 × 5
90/3 × 5	90/3 × 5	80/6 × 5	80/6 × 5	80/6 × 5		80/6 × 5

| 2 | | | 3 | | | | | | |
| MEDIUM | | | HIGH | | | | | | |
4	5	6	1	2		3	4	5	6
Off	90/3 × 7	120/3 × 7	90/3 × 6	95/2 × 3	100/1 × 4	130/3 × 7	Off	95/2 × 7	130/3 × 7
Off	80/6 × 6	80/6 × 6	80/6 × 6	80/6 × 6		85/4 × 5	Off	85/4 × 5	85/4 × 5
Off	90/3 × 7	90/3 × 7	90/3 × 6	95/2 × 3	100/1 × 3	100/1 × 3	Off	95/2 × 7	95/2 × 7
Off	90/3 × 7	120/3 × 7	90/3 × 6	95/2 × 3	100/1 × 3	130/3 × 7	Off	95/2 × 7	130/3 × 7
Off	90/3 × 7	120/3 × 7	90/3 × 6	95/2 × 3	100/1 × 3	130/3 × 7	Off	95/2 × 7	130/3 × 7
Off	80/6 × 6	80/6 × 6	80/6 × 6	80/6 × 6		85/4 × 5	Off	85/4 × 5	85/4 × 5

NUTRITION

This phase, like the mixed phase, is intermediate between the classical hypertrophy (bulk) phase and the definition phase. The nutrition goals in the MxS phase are to maintain much of the weight and solidify all of the muscle mass gained during the hypertrophy phase—and ideally to increase muscle mass marginally while maximizing the strength that would normally go along with the increased weight and muscle mass.

During this phase, you want to stabilize your muscle mass gained through the hypertrophy phase and ensure that your body-fat percentage does not rise above the levels of the hypertrophy phase. Continue to consume the same number of calories as in the mixed phase—that is, the daily caloric intake that resulted in your weight being stabilized. Keep the calories at about that level until you go into the definition phase. Dietary protein intake should be at the same level and dietary fat at a lower level as compared with intakes in the hypertrophy phase.

SUPPLEMENTATION

In the MxS phase, supplements are more important than in the previous three phases. It is still important to get your quota of low-carbohydrate calories and dietary protein to supply you with much of what you need to solidify your increased muscle mass (by increasing muscle protein content and fiber density) and to start getting yourself ready to shed body fat. However, because the daily calories have decreased substantially over the hypertrophy phase, and your training intensity is increasing, supplementing your diet with some targeted supplements will allow you to make better progress.

You will need more than just your basic daily vitamin or mineral tablet. Use MVM, Antiox, and EFA+ on a regular basis. As in the hypertrophy phase, use other supplements—such as Exersol, ReNew, Regulate, Joint Support, MRP LoCarb, and LoCarb sports bars—as needed.

If you are running into training problems, joint pain, injuries, or overtraining, we recommend Joint Support or ReNew. MRP LoCarb and LoCarb sports bars can be extremely useful for snacks or after meals to help you reach your calorie goals in a healthy, low-carbohydrate way. Also, if you reach a plateau in this phase, especially in your training, you might want to use Exersol to maximize your training efforts.

In addition to the supplements already mentioned, a more sophisticated array is required during the MxS phase. At this time it's usually necessary to supplement the diet with additional lean protein and to make up the added protein calories by decreasing dietary fat. You also need to use three or four of the following formulations to maximize the anaerobic energy systems and the anabolic drive: Myosin Protein, Creatine Advantage, TestoBoost, and GHboost. Used together, TestoBoost and GHboost maximize endogenous production of testosterone, growth hormone, and IGF-1 and thus their anabolic and fat-burning effects.

Myosin Protein Complex   This supplement allows you to keep protein levels up at a time when it might be difficult to take in enough protein from foods while at the same time cutting calories. It is an advanced synergistic blend of high-quality protein powders, including a specially developed source of glutamine peptides. Myosin Protein Complex, containing both quickly and slowly absorbed proteins, is engineered to increase protein synthesis and decrease muscle breakdown. It does this by increasing the anabolic and decreasing the catabolic hormones and by providing the body with an increased immune response to combat overtraining and maximize the anabolic and fat-burning effects of exercise. Because of the gentle processes used to isolate the various proteins, the formula maintains the beneficial immune and other effects of undenatured whey, casein, and soy proteins.

Creatine Advantage This supplement keeps the energy system in high gear despite the decreased caloric intake. By increasing endogenous levels of phosphocreatine, Creatine Advantage increases the immediately available energy that is necessary to fuel the MxS phase's increased exercise intensity. Added amino acids and dipeptides allow a natural increase in the absorption and utilization of creatine and increase the volumizing, anticatabolic, and anabolic effects of the formula.

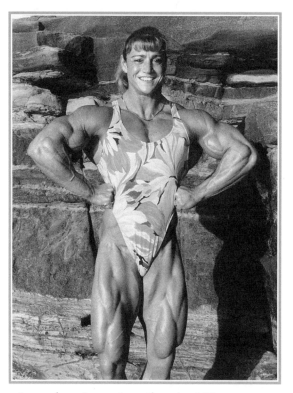

TestoBoost TestoBoost contains several natural ingredients; it is designed to improve natural testosterone formation and to decrease any potential side effects from the conversion of testosterone to estrogens and dihydrotestosterone. By boosting the body's natural testosterone levels, TestoBoost lowers body fat while increasing muscle mass.

GHboost This supplement is formulated to increase muscle mass and decrease body fat by enhancing the body's natural production of growth hormone (GH) and insulin-like growth factor 1 (IGF-1). The natural physiological increase in both GH and IGF-1, up to a level consistent with a person's genetic potential, will enhance muscle development, strength, and size while decreasing body fat.

A sound maximum strength and nutrition program have played an enormous role in the success of the sensational Laura Binetti.

Muscle Definition (MD)

During the muscle definition (MD) training phase, athletes strive to develop the most refined, polished, and visible muscles possible. This process is also known as getting ripped. Specific high-repetition training methods stimulate the body to use fatty acids as a fuel source, thus helping to burn the subcutaneous fat that is responsible for hiding those precious cuts.

The following characteristics describe the scope of MD training:

- It burns off subcutaneous fat and increases the visibility of muscle striations.

- It increases the protein content of muscles through performance of long, high-rep sets. In addition to better muscle definition, in some instances these exercises also increase muscle strength.

- It clearly increases capillary density within the muscle through increased adaptation to aerobic work, which may result in a slight increase in muscle size.

DURATION AND TRAINING METHODS

The duration of the MD phase depends on the needs of the athlete. The physiological demand of MD training can be quite severe, and as a result entry-level athletes should not perform it. For experienced athletes, the phase can be 3 weeks or 6 weeks or, as in our model (refer to figure 2.1, page 19), it can be made up of two 6-week portions. Since the latter choice ensures better achievement of muscle definition, a bodybuilder preparing for a contest would probably opt for it.

The vast majority of today's bodybuilders and strength trainers are convinced that the highest number of repetitions they ever need to perform is 15. These traditionalists believe that in order to increase muscle size a larger number of repetitions is not necessary, and this is certainly true.

The difference is that we are breaking away from the traditional approach to bodybuilding and strength training and believe that the overall body package is more important than plain mass. We want to promote better-looking bodies with higher muscle density, perfect symmetry, and increased muscle separation and striations. The type of training we promote will revolutionize the training philosophy of many bodybuilders and strength trainers. Those who use the periodization technique will never want to go back to traditional methods. The MD phase plays a very important role in sculpting the ideal body.

To maximize muscle separation, striation, and definition, you must burn off as much fat as possible. To accomplish this, the duration of nonstop muscular contraction must be increased. Bodybuilders traditionally have tried to burn off fat through aerobic work, such as running, or by using rowing machines, stationary

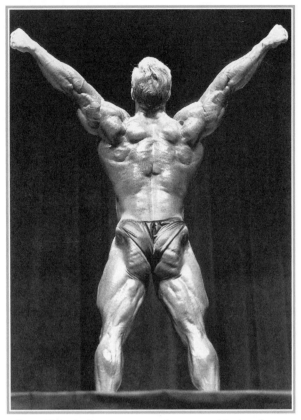

Dave Fisher's signature pose showcases his deeply striated glutes.

bikes, or stair climbers. This type of work, however, does not and should not satisfy most bodybuilders who want to become extremely lean. These activities do not entirely achieve the goal of burning off most of the body's subcutaneous fat.

The training methods promoted in the sample training programs (see the section Program Design) result in elimination of fat from the overall body and—more important—from the local muscle groups involved in the activity. The number of repetitions per muscle group and per workout must be drastically but progressively increased. It is equally important to perform the program in a nonstop fashion—to perform hundreds of repetitions per muscle group per workout. Since it is impossible to do work of such long duration nonstop for only one muscle group, the exercises must be continually alternated during the workout.

To perform extremely high repetitions per muscle group, you must decrease the load to 30 to 50 percent of 1RM. At the beginning of a high-rep, low-load set, only a limited number of muscle fibers are active. The other fibers are at rest, but they become activated as the contracting fibers become fatigued. This progressively increasing recruitment of muscle fibers allows a person to perform work for a prolonged period of time. Prolonged work exhausts the ATP-PC and glycogen energy supplies, leaving fatty acids as the only fuel available to sustain this activity. Use of this fuel source burns fat from the body, especially the subcutaneous fat. The burning off of this type of fat increases muscle striations and muscle definition.

PROGRAM DESIGN

To use fatty acids as fuel, an athlete must perform a high number of repetitions per set nonstop. Short RIs will prevent ATP-PC and glycogen from being restored, thus forcing the body to tap its fatty acid reserves. The MD program must be carefully designed. It is necessary to select exercises and workstations so that it takes only 2 or 3 seconds to move from one station to another.

Exercises are often paired together, so it is advisable to select an even number of exercises for each session, as illustrated in our sample programs. Tables 16.1 and 16.2 present MD programs for both recreational and advanced or professional athletes. The suggested exercises are for reference only, and the user has the choice of employing other exercises if needed. In the first 3 weeks, the purpose of training is to increase the number of reps to 50 or higher for each exercise. When this is accomplished, the exercises are grouped into two, then four, and so on, until eventually you can perform all eight exercises together without stopping. For maximum benefits, the ideal program is the one containing two 6-week MD phases. The longer the time spent on muscle definition, the greater the amount of fat burned, and the better the muscles will show their striations.

TABLE 16.1 **MD Phase for Recreational Bodybuilders and Strength Trainers**

No.	Exercises for all weeks	Week 1	Week 2	Week 3
1	Leg press	Increase number of reps to 30 for each exercise. RI between exercises = 1 min.	Perform 40 reps per exercise. RI between exercises = 1 min.	Perform 50 reps per exercise. RI between exercises = 1 min.
2	Front barbell press			
3	Crunch			
4	Biceps preacher curl			
		Week 4	**Week 5**	**Week 6**
5	Flat bench press	Perform 2 exercises together nonstop, or 100 reps (e.g., 50 leg presses and 50 front barbell presses). Do the same for the other 3 pairs. RI between exercises = 1 min.	Perform 4 exercises together nonstop, or 200 reps. Same for the other 4. RI between set of 4 exercises = 1 min.	Perform all 8 exercises together nonstop, or 400 reps. RI between set of 8 exercises = 1 min.
6	Leg extension			
7	Supine leg curl			
8	Lat pull-down			

For each week, complete 2 or 3 sets of 30% of 1RM.

TABLE 16.2 **MD Phase for Advanced or Professional Bodybuilders and Strength Trainers**

Weeks 1-4	Weeks 5-6	Week 7	Weeks 8-9	Weeks 10-12
Complete the first 4 weeks given in table 16.1.	Perform 4 exercises together nonstop, or 200 reps. Same for the other 4.	Perform a light week of training for regeneration.	Perform 4 exercises together nonstop, or 200 reps. Same for the other 4.	Perform 8 exercises together nonstop, or 400 reps.

Perform 3-5 sets at a load of 40-50% of 1RM, depending on your ability and work tolerance. No RI between exercises. RI between sets is 1 min. (If this is too short, increase slightly and reduce to 1 min later.)

We will use the eight exercises suggested in table 16.1 to illustrate how to apply the muscle definition training method. In the first week, the load is dropped to 30 to 50 percent 1RM, with lower loads for recreational athletes and higher loads for advanced and professional athletes. Using table 16.1 as an example, the actual program is as follows:

1. Perform 30 reps with the appropriate load on the leg press machine. Without any rest, perform 30 reps of the front barbell press.

2. Place a bar with the appropriate load on the preacher curl bench, and then perform 30 crunches followed immediately by 30 preacher curls.

3. Next, lie down on a bench and perform 30 bench presses followed by 30 leg extensions, 30 supine leg curls, and finally 30 lat pull-downs.

For the MD program, a set is the performance of all eight exercises. The suggested number of sets is not a standard or a limitation. Depending on your working potential and motivation, the number of sets can be slightly increased. You may perform a higher number of sets if the number of exercises and workstations is lower, or fewer sets if you are using 8 to 12 exercises.

The following tips will help you achieve a successful MD phase:

- MD training requires that muscle groups be constantly alternated.
- The same exercise may be performed twice per set, especially one targeting a desired muscle group.
- The number of reps may not be exactly the same for each exercise. The decision depends on your strengths and weaknesses for given muscle groups or your choice in targeting specific muscles. A very well-trained athlete may go as high as 60 or even 75.
- Speed should be moderate throughout the set. A fast lifting rhythm may produce a high level of lactic acid, which can hamper ability to finish the entire set.
- To avoid wasting time between exercises, set up all the equipment needed before the training session begins, if possible.
- The total number of MD workouts per week can be from two to four, depending on an athlete's experience—lower for recreational and higher for advanced or professional athletes. The additional one or two workouts can be divided between aerobic, H, or MxS training.

NUTRITION

The mechanics of the metabolic diet remain constant in all phases in terms of carbohydrate intake. The regimen always includes 5 high-protein days followed by 36 to 48 hours of carbohydrate loading. The only thing that changes is the number of calories consumed—and since it is important to keep protein levels high, and since carbohydrate is already low, athletes must decrease the amount of fat they eat during the low-carbohydrate phase and to a lesser extent through the higher-carbohydrate phase.

In the muscle definition phase, commonly called the "cutting" phase by bodybuilders, athletes cut calories as a way of trimming body fat. The reason for this practice is simple: After athletes have trained their bodies to burn fat as the primary fuel, lowering intake of both calories and fat primes the body to use body fat as fuel—while sparing muscle tissues.

As a rule of thumb, you should cut 500 calories per day from your diet the first week. If you were at 4,000 during the MxS phase, cut intake to 3,500 per day during the first week of your MD phase. The next week you should drop another 200 to 500 calories from the daily diet, depending on how many calories you're taking in. Someone consuming only 2,000 calories, for example, would cut down by only 200 calories. During this time you must measure body fat weekly. What you want to do is lose 1.5 to 2.0 pounds (.7 to .9 kg) of body fat each week—that way you will not lose appreciable lean mass as you cut.

If you find at the end of the second week that you have lost less than 1.5 pounds during the week, cut another 200 to 500 calories the next week, and continue cutting calories (anywhere from 100 to 500) in subsequent weeks until you are losing 1.5 pounds a week. If you are losing more than 2 pounds of body fat during the week, you have cut too many calories and will need to adjust them upward.

You don't have to make the cuts in 500-calorie increments. You can fine-tune how many calories you add or subtract. The usual progression is to make the changes 500 calories at a time at first, then perhaps 100 to 500 calories the next few weeks, and then 100 to 200 calories at a time as you get closer to your goal. The important thing to remember is that it's not calories you are really after—it's body fat. You must allow for individual variations in calorie count to get that optimal 1.5 to 2.0 pounds of fat loss per week.

You will do plenty of experimentation in this phase to find the caloric intake that is right for you. Although 500-calorie drops seem to be a good general starting point, especially for people with higher calorie intakes, you must find what works best for you. The calorie levels to which you eventually drop will vary according to your initial caloric intake and your individual metabolism. Some bodybuilders drop from 5,000 to 3,000 calories per day in the cutting phase. Others may need to drop as low as 1,500 to see what happens. If they are losing a fair amount of body fat (remember the 1.5 to 2 pounds per week guideline), and they are getting leaner and not losing significant lean body mass, they should stay at their current

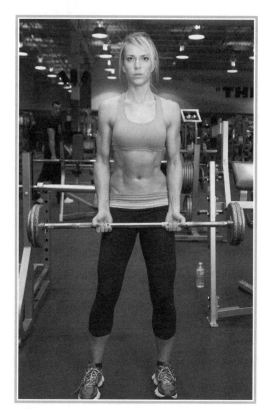

Fitness model Kasia Sitarz is focused and prepared to work hard.

level until they "lean out." At that point, they can increase calories to the point that they maintain or possibly even lose body fat while increasing lean mass again.

Bodybuilders who just want to cut up and are starting at a higher body-fat level can go directly into the definition phase. They should start at a reasonable daily calorie value, usually 15 calories per pound of body weight. Someone weighing 200 pounds (91 kg) at 17 percent body fat should start at around 3,000 calories a day and then follow the instructions on calorie adjustments to maintain optimal weekly fat loss and minimal muscle-mass loss. Don't start too low—you will have plenty of time to lose body fat in the correct way. If you start too low, the lack of food may be more of a problem than the lack of carbohydrates and may sabotage your efforts to stick to the diet through the all-important first week.

Food Choices for the MD Phase

The foods in table 16.3 are ideal for the cutting phase. In fact, you would be wise to stick to the foods in this list solely on the low-calorie, low-carbohydrate days. So if it's not here, you shouldn't eat it on those days. If needed, stick to the foods on the list when you shop to reduce the amount of off-limit foods in the house to tempt you. There'll be enough of the other foods around the house and in restaurants for the higher-carbohydrate days. The portions are small, so you'll need to use multiples depending on how many calories you're on. For example if you're on a 3,000-calorie-a-day diet, you could eat 9 ounces (275 g) of tenderloin and as such your calorie count for this would be three times the 141 calories listed in the table.

TABLE 16.3 Food Choices for Cutting

Food	Calories	Carbohydrate
MEAT		
Bacon: 3 slices	129	0
Bacon, precooked: 3 slices	80	0
Beef bologna: 2 oz (60 g)	76	.4
Beef bouillon: 1 cup	17	0
Beef broth in water: 6 oz (180 ml)	20	.6
Beef, eye of round roast: 3 oz (90 g)	143	0
Beef, lean ground: 3 oz (90 g)	218	0
Beef, rib-eye or T-bone steak: 3 oz (90 g)	188	0
Beef, tenderloin: 3 oz (90 g)	141	0
Beef, top sirloin steak: 3 oz (90 g)	176	0
Bison or buffalo, ground: 3 oz (90 g)	207	0
Corned beef, bresaola, lean prosciutto: 2 oz (60 g)	142	0
Deer, elk: 3 oz (90 g)	180	0
Kidney: 3 oz (90 g)	130	0
Lamb, lean, all cuts: 3 oz (90 g)	190	0
Pork, tenderloin/chops/ham, lean: 3 oz (90 g)	170	0
Tripe (trippa) cooked, simmered: 3 oz (90 g)	90	3
POULTRY		
Chicken (baked, broiled, or BBQ): 3 oz (90 g)	133	0
Chicken broth, low fat: 1 cup	10	1
Cornish hen: 3 oz (90 g)	160	0
Duck, meat only: 3 oz (90 g)	150	0
Pheasant or quail breast: 3 oz (90 g)	120	0
Turkey breast: 3 oz (90 g)	133	0
Turkey breast, processed: 1.5 oz (45 g)	47	0
Turkey salami: 2 oz (60 g)	111	.3
FISH AND SEAFOOD		
Fish, fresh or packed in water: 4 oz (125 g)	120	0
Oysters, 1 dozen medium: 4 oz (125 g)	130	4
Salmon, fresh or canned: 3 oz (90 g)	130	0
Shrimp, scampi, lobster, or crab: 5 oz (150 g)	125	0
Sushi/sashimi, fish only: 1 oz (30 g)	30	0
EGGS		
Egg substitute, liquid, equivalent to one large egg	45	0
Egg white from one large egg	19	0
Egg, large, hard boiled or poached	75	2
DAIRY		
Cheese (mascarpone, Parmesan): 1 oz (30 g)	110	1
Cheese, low fat: 1 oz (30 g)	60	1
Cottage cheese or plain yogurt, low fat: 1/2 cup	90	4
Skim-milk cheese: 3 oz (90 g)	80	3

Food	Calories	Carbohydrate
VEGETABLES		
Alfalfa Sprouts: 1/2 cup	5	.6
Asparagus: 1/2 cup	15	3
Beans (green, pole, snap, or wax): 1/2 cup	15	3
Brussels sprouts, cooked: 1/2 cup	25	5
Cabbage, broccoli, or cauliflower, cooked: 1/2 cup	15	3
Carrots: 1/2 cup chopped (125 g)	50	12
Celery: 1/2 cup diced	10	2.2
Coleslaw, noncalorie dressing: 2 tbsp	12	2
Cucumbers or dill pickles: 1 medium	5	1
Lettuce, loose leaf, arugula, endive: 1 cup	10	2
Lettuce greens: 2 cups plus 1 tbsp light dressing	50	3
Mushrooms: 1/2 cup	21	4
Onions, shallots, or leeks: 1/2 cup	25	6
Peppers (green, red, or yellow): 1 whole	20	4
Radishes: 1/2 cup	10	2
Rhubarb: 1 cup diced	25	5
Sauerkraut: 1/2 cup	21	4
Spinach; Swiss chard; collard, beet, turnip, or mustard greens, cooked: 1/2 cup	20	3.5
Squash (winter), zucchini: 1 cup sliced	20	4
Tomato: 1/2 cup	15	3
Watercress: 1/2 cup chopped	2	.2
FRUITS		
Apple: 1/2 apple	45	10
Lemon: 1/2 lemon	8	2.7
Orange or medium grapefruit: 1/2 orange or grapefruit	45	10
Strawberries: 1 cup	40	10
MD+ POWDER SUPPLEMENTS		
Creatine Advantage: 1 scoop (10 g)	30	3
MRP LoCarb Meal Replacement: 1 packet	250	3
Myosin Protein: 1 scoop (19 g)	70	1
Power Drink: 1 scoop (22 g)	80	2
MISCELLANEOUS		
Artificial sweeteners with no calories	0	0
Diet soda, tonic water, and other no-carbohydrate drinks	0	0
Jell-O, sugar free: 1 cup	8	0
Mustard, Dijon: 1 tbsp	15	1
Mustard, regular yellow: 1 tbsp	9	1
Mustard, regular yellow, no calorie: 1 tbsp	0	0
Oils and fats: 1 tsp (4.5 g)	40	0
Popsicles, calorie free	0	0
Salsa: 2 tbsp	14	3
Spices and herbs	0	0
Tea or coffee, black	0	0

Fish includes almost any type you can think of, such as salmon, tuna, cod, flounder, haddock, halibut, sole, eel, octopus, squid, anchovies, sardines, trout, and whiting. With fish such as eel, mackerel, and salmon, which have more body fat and therefore more calories, broil or BBQ the fish to get rid of most of the fat.

Cheeses include many of the hard cheeses and some of the soft. The low-fat variants of any of the cheeses listed are usually about half the calories of the full-fat ones. Cheeses that are OK include blue, Brie, Camembert, cheddar, Colby, Edam, goat, Gouda, Gruyère, Limburger, mascarpone, Monterey, mozzarella, Muenster, Parmesan, provolone, Roquefort, and Swiss. Pasteurized processed cheese slices are usually OK, but make sure the carbohydrate levels are less than 2 grams per 30-gram serving.

Although low-carbohydrate fruits are included on the list of allowed foods, don't overindulge on these because they will raise the daily carbohydrate intake more than any other allowed foods. It's usually a good idea to restrict your intake of fruits to the higher-carbohydrate days, at least until you reach your weight and body-composition goals. Of all the fruits, perhaps the most useful on this diet are grapefruit and strawberries, and these should be your first choices. If you need to sweeten either or both, you can use an artificial sweetener.

Grapefruit seems to encourage weight and fat loss more than most other foods, regardless of its carbohydrate content. Eating half a grapefruit (but not grapefruit pills or juice) seems to lower insulin levels (Fujioka 2004). Thus it has the opposite effect of carbohydrate on insulin and as a result doesn't act like a real carbohydrate. As well, it's been shown that the grapefruit flavanone naringenin inhibits insulin-stimulated glucose uptake in fat cells by inhibiting the activity of phosphoinositide 3-kinase (PI3K), a key regulator of insulin-induced GLUT4 translocation (Harmon and Patel 2003). This leads to a decrease in the amount of dietary carbohydrate that is stored as fat. Thus grapefruit seems to decrease the insulin response by decreasing insulin levels and by decreasing the effects of insulin on fat formation from carbohydrate. Half a medium-sized grapefruit also has 5 grams of fiber, which accounts for almost half its caloric value.

Strawberries, along with grapefruits, are an ideal fruit for those on the metabolic diet. These fruits are relatively low in carbohydrate, contain fiber, and have positive effects on health (Hannum 2004). The advantage of grapefruit is that its low sugar content affects blood sugar less. Strawberries are rich in antioxidants, which is an excellent benefit over apples and pears.

Fats include animal fats, shortening, and lard. Oils include olive, corn, vegetable, palm, peanut, soybean, walnut, coconut, flaxseed, borage seed, and fish. However, because of their high calorie content, it's wise to keep away from most extra fats and oils other than olive and fish oils when you're in the cutting phase, and even these should be used sparingly.

It's also wise in the muscle definition phase to keep to a minimum foods that, although low in carbohydrate (and thus usually allowed in the low-carbohydrate phase of the metabolic diet), are relatively high in fat. This includes sausages, salami, nuts, and peanuts. Avocado is another food that falls in the low-carbohydrate but high-calorie category, and although generally allowable in the diet, it's discouraged in the cutting phase. That's because a medium-sized avocado (about 145 grams) contains 280 calories and about 2 grams of mostly unsaturated fat (which makes up 250 of the 280 calories). It also contains about 1.5 grams of carbohydrate, 1.5 grams of protein, and 4.5 grams of dietary fiber. The mix is OK at first in the low-carbohydrate phase of the diet but does not work well for the low-carbohydrate and low-calorie requirements of the muscle definition phase.

TOP FOODS WITH FIBER FOR THE METABOLIC DIET AND MUSCLE DEFINITION

Including the following foods in your diet will ensure you're getting an optimal amount of both insoluble and soluble fiber for both bowel and overall health. These foods, because they contain more water as well as fiber, are especially useful for the cutting phase as they provide more volume, which will make you feel fuller, but fewer calories than the other foods, making it easier to stick to the diet.

Apple (with skin)	Grapefruit
Asparagus	Green beans, pole beans
Broccoli	Greens (spinach; Swiss
Brussels sprouts	chard; kale; turnip, beet,
Cabbage	and collard greens)
Carrots	Oranges
Cauliflower	Strawberries

Experimenting With Foods

On the high-calorie, higher-carbohydrate days, almost anything goes. Most people indulge in foods they're not allowed on the strict part of the diet, including breads, pasta, pizza, desserts, other fruits, and alcoholic drinks. However, you do have to watch the calorie content and keep the calorie count in a range that's appropriate for the phase you're in. In the cutting phase, you'd be wise to keep the calories low and limit the carbohydrate to 150 grams per day.

In all but the mass phase, taking in too many carbohydrate foods and calories on these reward days can set you back several days and make it more difficult to reach your body-composition and performance goals because you can take a step forward and then a step back on a weekly basis. It's OK to take two steps forward and one back week by week, as the back step can act as a strong anabolic influence and dramatically help you maximize lean body mass in the long run.

During the muscle definition phase, you should be refining contest preparation. Play with the kinds of foods you eat on the weekends to see what gives you maximum muscle size. You will know on Monday morning if what you've been eating is right for you. If it is, you will look good—your muscles will be huge, and you will be cut up with a pronounced vascularity. If you don't look good, you'll know you did something wrong. Modify your diet the next weekend to see if you can get some improvement. That's the beauty of the metabolic diet—by the time a contest approaches, you have already perfected your contest diet by practicing it during every week of the muscle definition phase. During the cutting phase, you become an expert in how to manipulate your body for a contest. (See table 16.3 for suggestions of the best foods to eat during cutting.)

Experiment with high- and low-sugar foods and with percentages of fat intake on these weekends. See what they do for you. Treat each weekend as if your contest were imminent. That way you will know what it takes to come into a contest looking your best. Your confidence will also grow because you will know what to expect from your body and how to get it contest ready.

PRECONTEST PHASE

When you get to your precontest phase, you won't have to make many changes: You will be doing the same thing you have been doing for the previous several weeks in the cutting phase. You will go off the higher-fat, high-protein diet and carb up to dramatically increase the glycogen and water inside the muscle cells. You want the cells swollen and big, but you want to cut off the carbohydrates before you begin to store extracellular water or fat and smooth out.

The metabolic diet's 5-day, 2-day week is almost like getting in shape for a contest every week. In the weekend carbohydrate-loading part of the diet, you will find out exactly how many hours you can load up on carbohydrate before you begin to smooth out and lose your contest look.

One of the many advantages of this diet is that if men or women want to enter a lot of contests, they can manipulate their diet so they never get much above their ideal body-fat percent levels during the muscle definition phase. By doing so, the athletes don't have huge gains in body fat, allowing them to drop to contest level in just 2 or 3 weeks.

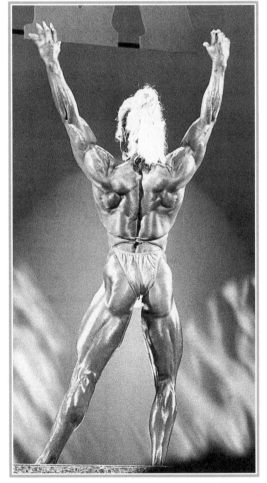

Not an ounce of body fat on this chiseled physique.

You generally want to go into the precontest phase of diet and training about 16 weeks before a major contest. Because you already know what you need to do from previous weekends on the diet, you will be doing only some fine-tuning by lowering and increasing calories a bit as needed. You shouldn't be doing anything much out of the ordinary.

By the final 6 to 8 weeks before the contest, you should look fairly close to how you want to appear on stage. With this diet you can control exactly where you're at each week. After the weekend carbohydrate-loading portion of your diet, you should be looking great on Monday—ready to hit the gym hard with the high glycogen levels, muscle swelling, and other benefits derived from a well-honed weekend diet strategy.

You can go through the precontest phase in preparation for several contests a year as long as you keep your fat levels low; yet we suggest that you go through the precontest phase no more than four times a year. That means, obviously, a maximum of four contests a year. More than this will probably prevent you from going back into the mass phase and using it properly.

You must build up lean body mass to some extent between contests, which means you will gain a bit of fat. You will still be bulking up and cutting down—but it won't be like on other diets, where you gain so much body fat that by the time you lose it you're no better off than when you started.

Be Consistent Before Competition

Two things bodybuilders do to sabotage themselves before contests is to panic or try something new. Both of these scenarios can be disastrous. Bodybuilders who find themselves too fat may begin doing aerobic exercise, thinking it will get the extra body fat off. Doing about half an hour of aerobic activity certainly will not harm you as you will burn more free fatty acids. But people sometimes begin to panic and overdo it. They start doing 3 to 4 hours a day of aerobic activity to burn off the fat; but all they do is exhaust energy stores so that their bodies start using muscle tissue for energy.

Some people start pigging out to build mass as they go into superaerobic mode, thinking that aerobics will make up for the fat buildup. It doesn't work. Increasing calories and aerobics will most probably just increase catabolic activity in your body. Aerobics, while burning fat, can also destroy muscle. Even if it doesn't do appreciable damage, it will still limit to some degree the amount of muscle you can put on. As a rule, the fewer calories you take in and the more time you allow yourself to lose the body fat, the less aerobics you will need to do, and the more lean body mass you will retain. Allow yourself time to lose extra body fat and gauge yourself effectively as you move toward a contest.

Other bodybuilders decide to try something new just before a competition, looking to get that final edge. But this is a mistake. They may start with the sodium-depletion or sodium-loading trick. They try all sorts of things they've never tried before, and all of a sudden they end up wondering how it was that they were looking so great and now look so bad. Don't shock your system before a contest. Make a smooth landing into it. Don't throw everything away by trying to get the extra edge through a crazy stunt. Do nothing out of the ordinary, and certainly do not panic.

Stop Training One to Two Weeks Out

Stop training 1 to 2 weeks before the contest. That's pretty standard wherever you go. Our advice is to do your last heavy training session 10 days before the contest to give your muscles maximum time to recuperate and achieve maximum growth. Don't worry about maintaining muscle mass and tone. Your posing will take care of that and also give you some aerobic activity. Posing should, of course, be continued throughout this entire period with the exception of the day before the contest.

But although you shut down heavy training 10 days or so before a contest, this is the only time you should back off. Cutting back in training at any other time in the process limits the effectiveness of the diet and your ultimate growth. Diet and training work hand in hand. Exercise complements the metabolic diet. Hormonal changes caused by exercise result in increased activity of the enzyme lipoprotein lipase (LPL) in the muscle, which in turn increases breakdown of free fatty acids and decreases fat buildup.

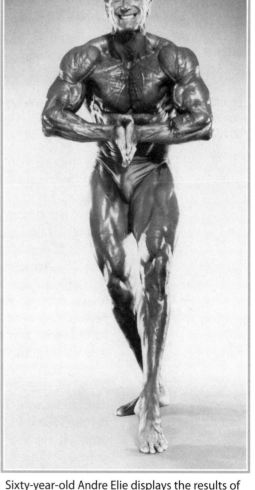

Sixty-year-old Andre Elie displays the results of dedicated contest preparation.

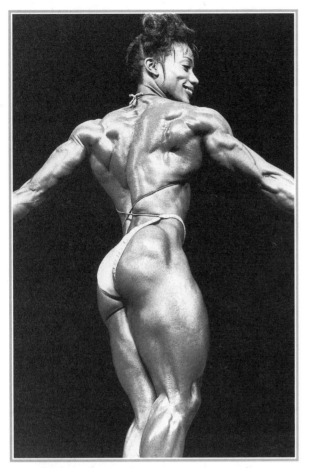

Lenda Murray's precontest preparation was always one of the best in the sport.

Identify Your Best Day

As you conduct carbohydrate loading on the weekends, you will learn how many hours into the process that you look your very best. As suggested, you can further refine that time by experimenting with the types of food you eat, allowing you to precisely dial in that time when you're at your best. This information is vital when the contest arrives because you will eventually discover a day of the week when you're in top form. All the water you gained during your carbohydrate load is gone, and you have just the right balance between muscle glycogen and water. You also feel great. Everyone's system works differently, and there are wide differences among athletes. The goal is to find the right day for you, that day each week—Monday, Tuesday, Wednesday, whatever—when you are consistently at your best.

Most contests occur on Saturday. Suppose you look your best on Wednesday of each week. Your goal then is to basically make the Saturday of your contest like a Wednesday. Because you look your best 3 days after your carbohydrate load, you should complete a carbohydrate load 3 days—in this case, on Tuesday and Wednesday—before the contest. On Saturday, 3 days later, you will look your best.

Note that the weekend before the contest, you won't carb up as usual. To carb up on the weekend and repeat the process 2 or 3 days later may well spill you back over to a carbohydrate-burning metabolism and smooth you out for that Saturday contest. Rather, skip your carbohydrate load the weekend before a contest. That way you will be on the high-protein, higher-fat part of the metabolic diet for 8 straight days, from the Monday 2 weeks before the contest to the Tuesday before the contest. Then begin your precontest carbohydrate load so you will hit the contest just right.

This is one area where the metabolic diet has a big advantage over the competition. Athletes on a high-carbohydrate diet are basically always loading up on carbohydrate foods, so it's difficult for them to manipulate their diets so their bodies respond well to carbohydrate loading before the contest. What often happens is they get off the high-carbohydrate diet for 3 days at the beginning of the week before a competition and go low carbohydrate for 72 hours; then they again load up on carbohydrate foods in an attempt to hit the contest right. The problem is, they really don't know how their bodies are going to react. Everything could work out well, or they could experience a complete disaster. With the metabolic diet, you know the exact hour when you look your best. Because your body goes through the cycle every week, it has become predictable and consistent. You know precisely what to expect since you won't be doing anything different from what you have done in the preceding months.

Prejudging

You want that exact hour when you look your best to coincide with prejudging; this is where most decisions are made. But the body is not a perfectly predictable instrument. Therefore, to be certain that you don't smooth out, give yourself 4 hours of extra time as a kind of fail-safe mechanism for prejudging. That is, if you are at your best 48 hours after carbohydrate loading, and prejudging will take place at two o'clock on Saturday, count back 48 hours. This puts you at two o'clock Thursday. Then, give yourself 4 extra hours, which means you should complete your carbohydrate loading at 6:00 p.m. on Thursday.

You also want to look good at the evening show, especially if judging is close and will be ultimately decided in the evening. Fortunately, you usually have a window of several hours during which you look good, and that window usually overlaps the evening session. Yet you still need to be careful. Some competitors look great for prejudging, then go out and eat, thinking it's all over. They come in bloated and retaining water for the evening show and in a close competition will lose because of it.

You must stay tight all day. Keep diet minimal and in the higher-fat mode. Even having food in your stomach will create a slight bulge. You want to keep everything nice and flat; so keep your regimen going through the evening contest. This, of course, is just an example. You have to work with the diet to find the best approach for you. The big difference between this diet and whatever you've been on before is the precision with which you can plan your contest regimen.

> ## FLUID RETENTION
>
> Since most people tend to retain some fluid, all bodybuilders should consider these suggestions. If you tend to retain fluid, begin to restrict yourself to distilled water and low levels of sodium 24 hours before the competition. Distilled water and low sodium levels lower the extracellular fluid. Also increase your potassium, magnesium, and calcium intake. Potassium increases the amount of fluid inside the cell. Higher potassium levels are also better for muscle contractions, though you should not create potassium levels that are too high. Calcium and magnesium help prevent cramping. You want as little extracellular fluid as possible to avoid smoothing out. On the other hand, intracellular fluid will increase cell size so you'll be bigger. It also aids vascularity.

SUPPLEMENTATION

Cycling nutritional supplements means using a different set of supplements in each phase (phase-specific supplementation). Always use supplements at the right times and for the right reasons. For example, there are vast differences in dietary needs and in the effects of various supplements between the mass and definition phases. The nutritional supplements you need on days when you train differ from what you need on rest days. Manipulating your diet and nutritional supplements in and around training increases the anabolic and fat-burning effects of the training, and it can decrease recuperation time and enhance your abilities to perform at the next training session.

Other variables that affect diet and use of nutritional supplements include bodybuilders' training backgrounds and the levels they have reached. Novice bodybuilders—in which gains come relatively easy even with simple training routines and a diet high in calories and protein—don't need the sophisticated dietary modifications and cutting-edge nutritional supplements that are necessary to improve more advanced bodybuilders.

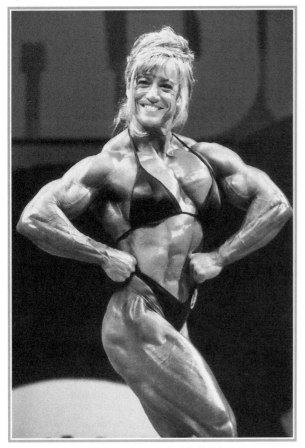

Laura Binetti displays the results of dedicated contest preparation.

Supplements come into their own in the muscle definition phase, in which they are extremely useful in maintaining and raising the anabolic and fat-burning response to the metabolic diet and training. In this phase you consistently cut calories so that your body effectively uses your body fat as fuel; yet in so doing, your system tends to change its hormones and metabolism to a survivalist mode that is counterproductive to your goals. The metabolic diet is a big help here, but the supplements are also important. The following supplements work well in this phase:

- Exersol
- MRP LoCarb and LoCarb sports bars
- TestoBoost
- GHboost
- Creatine Advantage
- Myosin Protein
- Metabolic

There is little difference between supplements used in the cutting and precontest phases. The only thing to watch out for is the effect some of the supplements may have on your definition. For example, some bodybuilders discontinue creatine a few weeks before a competition because they retain more water and are less defined if they stay on it. Also the use of certain supplements—such as Myosin Protein, Metabolic, ReNew, and Joint Support—usually should increase as the competition gets closer. (See www.metabolicdiet.com for more information.)

Transition (T)

An annual plan, as suggested in our examples, should finish with a transition (T) phase. After many months of intensive training, athletes must give their bodies a respite to allow recovery and regeneration to occur before beginning a new year of training. In addition to a year-end transition phase, we recommend employing a brief transition period between each different training phase.

The following characteristics describe the scope of T training:

- It decreases the volume and intensity of training and facilitates removal of the fatigue acquired during the previous phase or annual plan.
- It replenishes exhausted energy stores.
- It relaxes the body and the mind.

DURATION

If the year-end T phase exceeds 4 to 6 weeks the hard-sought training benefits will fade away, and the athlete will experience a detraining effect. Also, the athlete who adheres to the 4- to 6-week time frame but does no strength training during the T phase may experience a decrease in muscle size together with a considerable loss in power (Wilmore and Costill 1999).

During transition, physical activity is reduced by 60 to 70 percent. It is advisable, however, to lightly train those muscles that are or may become asymmetrically developed during a period of low-intensity training.

PROGRAM DESIGN AND DETRAINING

Improvement or maintenance of muscle size and strength is possible only if the body is constantly exposed to an adequate training stimulus. When training decreases or stops, as it does during a long transition phase, there is a disturbance in the biological state of the muscle cell and of bodily organs. Consequently, there is a marked decrease in the athlete's physiological well-being and work output (Fry, Morton, and Keast 1991; Kuipers and Keizer 1988). This state of diminished training can leave athletes vulnerable to detraining syndrome (Israel 1972) or exercise-dependency syndrome (Kuipers and Keizer 1988), the extent of which depends on the length of time away from training.

The following are effects of detraining:

- **Decrease in muscle fiber size.** A decrease in the cross-sectional area of the muscle fibers becomes visible after only a couple of weeks of inactivity. These changes result from higher rates of protein degradation (catabolism) that reverse the muscle gains made during training. Greater levels of sodium and chloride ions in the muscles also play a role in the breakdown of muscle fibers (Appell 1990).

- **Loss of strength.** Strength loss occurs during the first week of inactivity at a rate of roughly 3 to 4 percent per day (Appell 1990), largely due to the degeneration of motor units. Slow twitch fibers are usually the first to lose their force-producing capabilities, while fast twitch fibers generally take longer to be affected by inactivity. During the state of detraining, the body cannot recruit the same number of motor units that it once could, resulting in a net decrease in the amount of force that can be generated within the muscle (Hainaut and Duchatteau 1989; Houmard 1991).

- **Decrease in testosterone levels.** Detraining causes the body's natural testosterone levels to fall. And since the presence of testosterone is crucial for gains in size and strength, protein synthesis within the muscles diminishes as these levels fall (Houmard 1991). Headaches, insomnia, feelings of exhaustion, loss of appetite, increased tension, mood disturbances, and depression are among the usual symptoms associated with total abstinence from training. An athlete may develop any number of these symptoms, all of which appear to be associated with the lowered levels of testosterone and beta-endorphin, a neuroendocrine compound that is the main forerunner to euphoric postexercise feelings (Houmard 1991).

NUTRITION

We usually suggest going off the strict part of the metabolic diet during the transition phase and reintroducing a moderate amount of carbohydrate (20 to 50 percent of total caloric intake), cutting back on protein, and consuming only moderate amounts of fat—in other words, almost the normal North American diet. Don't worry about having problems getting strict with the metabolic diet when it is time to come back onto it. Your body will "remember," and it will be much easier to get back into the groove.

SUPPLEMENTATION

During the T phase, back off all your supplements except maybe MVM, the vitamin and mineral supplement. The one other supplement you may want to use during this phase is ReNew, since this supplement is meant to get your system, especially your immune system, back to normal. The immune system is the first line of defense to increase training intensity (hypertrophy, mixed training, strength training) and needs to normalize after the long periodized training cycle. ReNew is formulated not only to enhance the immune system but also to normalize the metabolism and to naturally support thyroid, testosterone, GH, insulin, and adrenergic function. It is the perfect nutritional supplement to deal with workout fatigue at the end of a long periodization session.

Understanding Food Labels

Nutrition labeling is mandatory for most packaged food in the United States and is regulated by the Food and Drug Administration (FDA) and the U.S. Department of Agriculture. The nutrition facts panel typically consists of the following components usually in this order:

- Serving size information
- Calorie information
- Amounts and percent daily values of specific nutrients
- Vitamins and minerals
- Ingredients list and information for avoiding allergies

Sounds pretty straightforward, doesn't it? Unfortunately it isn't. If you're confused by what's listed in food labels, especially the more complicated ones, you're not alone (Cowburn and Stockley 2005; Rothman et al. 2006). However, studies show that with some help in deciphering them, the nutrition facts label can be an effective educational tool to increase nutrition knowledge (Hawthorne et al. 2006).

Unfortunately, most people don't understand enough about what's on food labels to make an informed choice of what's best for them. The reason is twofold. First of all, most people don't fully understand the lingo used on the labels; and second, label information pertaining to newer low-carbohydrate products is not well regulated by the FDA and is more challenging to understand.

Most people think they understand what's important on the nutrition labels (e.g., the number of calories and maybe even the amount of carbohydrate, fat, and protein in the food or supplement). But they're wrong—labels just aren't that easy to understand and use without some guidance. The ability to read and evaluate food labels is not just a matter of choosing to eat healthy. To those of us trying to gain muscle mass and improve body composition, choosing the right mix of foods can be critical for our success. And for people trying to manage chronic disease such as a heart condition or diabetes, label reading can at times even be a lifesaving matter.

Knowing what to look for is the first step in understanding nutrition facts labels. A nutrition facts label (see figure 1) gives a lot of information, but the key is knowing how to use this information to help you make food choices that are

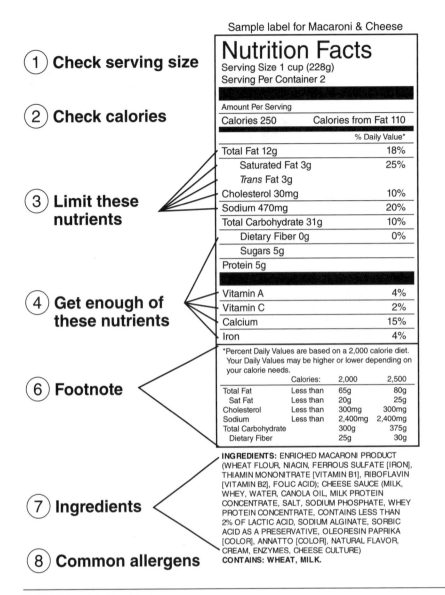

① **Check serving size**

② **Check calories**

③ **Limit these nutrients**

④ **Get enough of these nutrients**

⑥ **Footnote**

⑦ **Ingredients**

⑧ **Common allergens**

⑤ **Quick guide to % DV**

- **5% or less is low**

- **20% or more is high**

Sample label for Macaroni & Cheese

Nutrition Facts

Serving Size 1 cup (228g)
Serving Per Container 2

Amount Per Serving

Calories 250   Calories from Fat 110

% Daily Value*

Total Fat 12g	**18%**
Saturated Fat 3g	**25%**
Trans Fat 3g	
Cholesterol 30mg	**10%**
Sodium 470mg	**20%**
Total Carbohydrate 31g	**10%**
Dietary Fiber 0g	**0%**
Sugars 5g	
Protein 5g	
Vitamin A	4%
Vitamin C	2%
Calcium	15%
Iron	4%

*Percent Daily Values are based on a 2,000 calorie diet. Your Daily Values may be higher or lower depending on your calorie needs.

		Calories:	2,000	2,500
Total Fat	Less than		65g	80g
Sat Fat	Less than		20g	25g
Cholesterol	Less than		300mg	300mg
Sodium	Less than		2,400mg	2,400mg
Total Carbohydrate			300g	375g
Dietary Fiber			25g	30g

INGREDIENTS: ENRICHED MACARONI PRODUCT (WHEAT FLOUR, NIACIN, FERROUS SULFATE [IRON], THIAMIN MONONITRATE [VITAMIN B1], RIBOFLAVIN [VITAMIN B2], FOLIC ACID); CHEESE SAUCE (MILK, WHEY, WATER, CANOLA OIL, MILK PROTEIN CONCENTRATE, SALT, SODIUM PHOSPHATE, WHEY PROTEIN CONCENTRATE, CONTAINS LESS THAN 2% OF LACTIC ACID, SODIUM ALGINATE, SORBIC ACID AS A PRESERVATIVE, OLEORESIN PAPRIKA [COLOR], ANNATTO [COLOR], NATURAL FLAVOR, CREAM, ENZYMES, CHEESE CULTURE)
CONTAINS: WHEAT, MILK.

FIGURE 1   Nutrition label.

right for you. As you can see, the label is meant to give you specific information on what's in each food product, information you can use for healthy eating and achieving your goals. The nutrients on a label are ordered from what you should limit, such as fat, cholesterol, and sodium, to those nutrients you need to make sure you get enough of, such as dietary fiber, vitamins A and C, calcium, and iron. However, as you'll see, although this information is useful it does have limitations.

Serving Size Information   When you're looking at the nutrition facts label on the food product, begin reading at the top of the label with the food's recommended serving size and number of servings per package. Be sure to compare the serving size with how much you eat. For example, the serving size may be one cup, and you may eat two cups. In that case, you're eating double the serving size, so you need to double the calories and other nutrient numbers, including the percent daily value.

Calorie Information   Continue down the label to "total calories" and "calories from fat." Total calories, which includes the calories from fat, carbohydrate, and protein, is the amount of calories per recommended serving. Calories from fat is the total calories in one serving that come from fat. The reason total calories from fat is listed, and not total calories from carbohydrate or protein, is the emphasis in the last few decades on the health effects of lowering fat in the diet. Putting this information on the label allows people to easily monitor the amount of fat in their diets, with the general recommendation being that no more than 30 percent of daily calories come from fat. This translates to no more than 600 calories of an allowable 2,000 calories coming from fat.

Knowing the total calories from a portion of food allows you to compare the amount of calories in how much you will eat of the food to the total calories you need for a day. If you are trying to manage your weight, choosing foods that are lower in calories will help. Even small differences in calories per serving can add up over the course of a day. Keep the following in mind when reading the rest of the label:

- 1 gram of fat contains about 9 calories.
- 1 gram of protein contains about 4 calories.
- 1 gram of carbohydrate contains about 4 calories.

Using some simple calculations, you can figure out how much of the difference between total calories and calories from fat comes from carbohydrate and protein. You can also simply figure out the number of calories from carbohydrate and from protein by multiplying the grams of each by 4.

Amounts and Percent Daily Values of Specific Nutrients   The next section of the label lists the amounts of specific nutrients in a serving and the percentage of the daily value a serving of the food provides for each nutrient. The nutrient amounts are measured in grams or milligrams, depending on the nutrient. The percent daily values, listed in the right-hand column, are based on the recommended amount of each nutrient the average person should consume on a 2,000-calorie diet. Further down the label, a footnote of recommended daily values for standard 2,000- and 2,500-calorie diets is provided.

The percent daily values tell you if the nutrients in a serving of food contribute a lot or a little to the recommended daily intake. The goal is to eat 100 percent of each of those nutrients every day. For example, if a serving of a food is listed as 25 percent of the daily value of protein, then that food provides 25 percent of your daily protein needs based on a daily intake of 2,000 calories. Percent daily value is a useful measure of whether a food is high or low in specific nutrients. A food is considered a good source of a nutrient if the percentage is between 10 and 19 percent. If a food has 5 percent or less, it's considered to be low; if it has more than 20 percent of the percent daily value, it's considered to be high in that nutrient.

The nutrients listed first in this section of the label include those that most people should limit, including total fat, saturated fat, trans fat, cholesterol, and sodium. *Total fat* is the total amount of fat in a serving. Although it's recommended that total fat be low, today the consensus is that between 20 and 30 percent of our daily caloric intake should come from fats. However, this consensus is for ordinary people and not those who follow phase-shift diets and transform their bodies from being dependent on carbohydrates to being dependent on fats, including body fat, as their primary fuel.

Saturated fat and *trans fat* are considered bad fats because of their ability to raise cholesterol levels (as can dietary cholesterol) and increase the risk of heart disease. Saturated fat, which is found in greater amounts in butter, cheese, whole milk, whole-milk products, meat, and poultry, has in fact not been shown to raise the incidence of heart disease (Di Pasquale 2002-2008). Trans fats are used by food processors to increase the shelf life of processed food. Foods high in trans fats include stick margarine, vegetable shortening, cookies, crackers, snack foods, fried foods, and other processed foods. Since consumer awareness about trans fats has recently increased, many food manufacturers are trying to decrease or eliminate trans fats in their products.

In the United States, food manufacturers must list trans fat on all their products. If the product comes from outside the United States and the amount of trans fat is not listed, look in the ingredients list for terms such as *partially hydrogenated oils*. This indicates trans fats are probably in the product. Some dietary supplements (e.g., high-protein bars, energy bars, and meal replacements) may contain trans fat from partially hydrogenated vegetable oil as well as saturated fat and cholesterol. Because of this, the FDA requires trans fat levels to be on the label if a dietary supplement contains .5 gram or more of trans fat per serving.

The FDA does not require unsaturated fats, including polyunsaturated fat and monounsaturated fat, to be listed on the label. If they're not listed, you can estimate the total amount of unsaturated fat (although not individual amounts) in the food by subtracting the amounts of trans and saturated fats from the total fat.

Cholesterol is necessary for the endogenous production of many substances in the body, including vitamin D and some hormones. It can, of course, become a problem if it's too high.

Sodium, mainly from salt naturally present in food or, more commonly, added to food, can contribute to fluid retention and high blood pressure and thus should be limited. Knowing how much sodium is in food can be especially useful for bodybuilders looking to limit their sodium intake during contest preparation or, alternately, to sodium load.

Information on the other two macronutrients, *carbohydrate* and *protein*, are also found in this section of the label. Carbohydrate is broken down into *total carbohydrate*, *fiber*, and *sugars*. Total carbohydrate is the amount of total carbohydrate per serving measured in grams. Total carbohydrate combines the amounts of all the sources of carbohydrate in a food, including fiber, sugars, starches, sugar alcohols, and glycerin.

Dietary fiber is the amount of indigestible (insoluble fiber) or partially digestible (soluble fiber) bulk from plant foods and is measured in grams. Foods high in fiber are shown to be beneficial for weight control, diabetes, high cholesterol, and some forms of cancer. Foods with 5 grams of fiber or more are considered high-fiber foods.

Sugars are part of the total carbohydrate content and are measured in grams. These include natural sugars, normally present in the food, and added sugars. You can see which sugars have been added by looking at the ingredients list—for example, glucose, fructose, sugar, dextrose, maltose, high-fructose corn syrup, fruit juice concentrate, turbinado, maple syrup, molasses, barley, and malt. Sugar alcohols such as maltitol, xylitol, sorbitol, and glycerin should be counted as carbohydrate by those on low-carbohydrate diets. Pay close attention to labels, as manufacturers are now being regulated to account for the gram or milliliter amount per specified serving amount. These added sugars should be avoided by anyone trying to improve body composition, health, and performance. Although a case has been made for the use of sugars postexercise, simple sugars are counterproductive at any time for someone on the metabolic diet.

Protein, measured in grams, tells you how much total protein is in a single serving of a food. Although there are differences in the biological value and effects of various protein sources, there is no distinction made for the type of protein or the source. Also amino acids and peptides (including glutamine peptides from hydrolyzed wheat gluten) are not included as they're not considered whole-food proteins. In our view, this is a serious mistake because amino acids and peptides are the breakdown products of whole protein and as such should be considered in the total protein count.

Vitamins and Minerals

Vitamins and minerals are listed on food labels. Most labels, such as those for milk products, flaxseed, whole-grain breads, and yogurts, list vitamin A, vitamin C, vitamin E, calcium, iron, thiamine, magnesium, zinc, and selenium. When labels list only vitamin A, vitamin C, calcium, and iron, it's because the governing committees around the world deem these the most important for health. All are measured in percentages since the idea is to take in 100 percent of each of these nutrients daily in order to prevent deficiency diseases.

Ingredients List and Information for Avoiding Allergies

The ingredient list is another part of the nutrition label and gives you an overview of everything that's in the product. The ingredients are listed in order according to how much of the ingredient the food contains. Besides the macronutrients, other ingredients such as spices, preservatives, artificial coloring, and flavors are also listed. The ingredient list can help you determine whether the food is right for you, depending on your views on what you want and don't want to put in your body.

The FDA requires food manufacturers to list common food allergens on food labels in simple terms that adults and older children can understand. Common allergens include milk, eggs, peanuts, wheat, soy, fish, shellfish, and tree nuts. Although they are listed in the ingredients, a food label must also clearly state (after or adjacent to the list of ingredients) whether the product contains any of these allergens.

LABELING TERMS AND THEIR MEANINGS

Besides understanding the food label, consumers, especially those on special diets, need to be aware of nutrition claims posted on foods. Some labels claim that products are low in cholesterol or low in fat. But these claims have very specific meanings—which most of us aren't aware of—and can be used only if a food meets strict government definitions.

For example, the standard for *reduced* and *less* is always at least 25 percent lower than the original reference food. Although a label may say the food is reduced fat or reduced sodium, that only means the food has 25 percent less fat or sodium than the original product. So if the original product is high in fat or sodium, the reduced product will be a notch lower but will likely still be relatively high.

Even if a food is low in fat, the food may not necessarily be nutritious. A low-fat food can be high in sugar. Food companies also make claims such as "no cholesterol" (meaning there is no animal fat used in making the product), but that does not necessarily mean the product is low in fat. Table 1 provides the meanings of some terms according to government-mandated definitions.

TABLE 1	Definitions of Common Terms on Labels
Sugar free	Less than .5 g of sugar per serving
Reduced sugar	At least 25% less sugar per serving
No sugar added	No sugar added during processing or packing; can include products that already contain natural sugar such as dried fruit and juice
Calorie free	Fewer than 5 calories per serving
Low calorie	40 calories or fewer per serving
Fat free	Less than .5 g of fat per serving
Saturated fat free	Less than .5 g of saturated fat per serving, with the level of trans fatty acids no more than 1% of the total fat
Low fat	3 g or less of fat per serving, or if the serving is 30 g or less or 2 tbsp or less, per 50 g of the product
Low saturated fat	1 g or less of saturated fat per serving, with not more than 15% of the total calories from saturated fat
Reduced or less fat	At least 25% less fat per serving than the original reference food
Reduced or less saturated fat	At least 25% less saturated fat per serving than the original reference food
Light	50% less fat than the same regular product; can also be used to mean 1/3 fewer calories or 50% less sodium
Lean	Less than 10 g of fat, 4 g of saturated fat, and 95 mg of cholesterol
Extra lean	Less than 5 g of fat, 2 g of saturated fat, and 95 mg of cholesterol
Cholesterol free	Less than 2 mg of cholesterol and 2 g or less of saturated fat
Low cholesterol	20 mg or less of cholesterol and 2 g or less of saturated fat per serving, or if the serving is 30 g or less or 2 tbsp or less, per 50 g of the product
Reduced or less cholesterol	At least 25% less cholesterol and 2 g or less of saturated fat per serving than the original reference food
Sodium free	Less than 5 mg of sodium per serving
Low sodium	140 mg or less of sodium per serving
Very low sodium	35 mg or less of sodium per serving
Reduced or less sodium	At least 25% less sodium per serving than the original reference food
High fiber	At least 5 g of fiber per serving; high-fiber claims must also meet the criteria for low fat, or the level of total fat must be shown next to the high-fiber claim
Good source of fiber	2.5 to 4.9 g of fiber per serving
More added fiber	At least 2.5 g of fiber more per serving than the original reference food

Disguised Carbohydrate

If you're counting grams of carbohydrate, you need to consider most of the total carbohydrate in a product to arrive at the number you can use in your carbohydrate counting. There are a number of issues to consider, especially since many manufacturers use various tricks to significantly understate their products' carbohydrate content. Most carbohydrate foods are pretty easy to spot. Everyone knows that sugar, potatoes, rice, bread, and baked goods are mostly carbohydrate. But some carbohydrate foods or carbohydrate-like ingredients are harder to spot. And even reading the ingredients panel may not tell you much as far as how many real grams of carbohydrate are in certain foods and supplements. The confusion revolves around compounds that are sweet and have a significant calorie count but aren't technically carbohydrate foods. Neither are they fat or protein foods.

The idea of what's a carbohydrate and what's not a carbohydrate seems to be open to interpretation by just about anyone trying to prove his point or trying to deceive the public. So manufacturers who want to include some of these substances in their products—because they add the taste of carbohydrate—but don't really want to list them as carbohydrate in the nutrition panel can do so up to a point.

On the metabolic diet, the reason for low carbing is to maximize body composition. As such, you need to count grams of carbohydrate or calories from the carbohydrate. In that context, anything that disrupts fatty acid breakdown and oxidation should be considered a carbohydrate and as such can be detrimental to the diet. Whether something is technically a carbohydrate or not, what is important is how it behaves in the body as far as its impact on both endogenous and exogenous macronutrient metabolism.

For food labeling, the confusion mainly stems from the food and supplement industry. Manufacturers are a tricky bunch. First and foremost they want you to buy their products. For that to happen they have to tell you what you want to hear, whether they're bending the truth or not. The facts are that the FDA guidelines allow the use of *low carbohydrate* on a food label if that product has 3 grams or less of carbohydrate per serving. The food label terms for carbohydrate as defined by the FDA can be confusing; however, some of the definitions are straightforward, such as the following:

- Total carbohydrate is calculated by subtracting the sum of the crude protein, total fat, moisture, and ash from the total weight of the food.

- Sugars are the sum of all free monosaccharides and disaccharides (such as glucose, fructose, galactose, lactose, fructose, and sucrose).

- Sugar alcohol is the sum of saccharide derivatives in which a hydroxyl group replaces a ketone or aldehyde group whose use in the food is listed by FDA (mannitol, xylitol) or is generally recognized as safe (sorbitol).

- Other carbohydrate is the difference between total carbohydrate and the sum of dietary fiber, sugars, and sugar alcohols if present (Altman 1998).

- Glycerol and glycerin refer to the same substance. FDA nutrition labeling regulations require that when glycerin is used as a food ingredient, it must be included in the grams of total carbohydrate declared per serving. Also, when the label of a food containing glycerin has a statement regarding sugars, the glycerin content per serving must also be declared as sugar alcohol (Institute of Food Technologies 2003).

As straightforward as these definitions are, the manufactures have succeeded in muddying the waters by using some phrases to describe the carbohydrate content of their products. They know that consumers are not likely to have the time or interest in the calculations of crude protein, total fat, moisture, and ash. And if they did, they couldn't possibly come up with a really good reason to buy it. The phrases *net carbohydrate* and *impact carbohydrate* are not FDA definitions but rather terms created by companies so you'll see their product on the shelves and be attracted enough by what they're saying that you'll buy the product.

To calculate the net carbohydrate, companies subtract the grams of fiber and sugar alcohols from the total carbohydrate. The reason behind this, at least as far as these companies are concerned, is that the body does not digest fiber, so it shouldn't be counted as part of the total carbohydrate. Although what they say is true for insoluble fiber, it's not the case with either soluble fiber or sugar alcohols. Insoluble fiber, even though technically a carbohydrate, is not absorbed and is excreted unchanged. As such, it doesn't provide any calories or affect your systemic macronutrient mix. So insoluble fiber shouldn't be counted in either the carbohydrate or calorie columns.

Soluble fiber is another story and is somewhat of a gray area in the carbohydrate–calorie equation. Pectin, for example, undergoes vigorous "friendly" bacterial fermentation in the large intestine and produces high levels of short-chain fatty acids. These short-chain triglycerides are absorbed by cells in the colon and also absorbed systemically. Thus about half of soluble fiber should be counted as carbohydrate even though the calories come from short-chain fatty acids.

The bottom line is that several macronutrients and ingredients, including soluble fiber, sugar alcohols, alcohol, lactate, pyruvate, and glycerol act like carbohydrate. If they're not taken into consideration as being the equivalent of either full or partial carbohydrate, they will sabotage the effects of low-carbohydrate diets on weight loss, fat loss, and body composition.

Short-, Medium-, and Long-Chain Triglycerides

Short- and medium-chain triglycerides provide calories, but the real problem is they're used by the body preferentially over long-chain triglycerides (which make up body fat) so that like carbohydrate, they can shortchange your metabolism away from burning the fatty acids that make up body fat. Thus if you're looking to maximize body composition, short- and medium-chain fatty acids can be counterproductive.

Athletes often use medium-chain triglycerides (MCTs) to enhance body composition; however, they can be counterproductive in the low-carbohydrate phase of a phase-shift diet. Although they have a protein-sparing effect on a high-calorie diet high in complex carbohydrate, MCTs are counterproductive on a higher-fat, low-carbohydrate diet.

Instead of using the long-chain fatty acids that make up most of the body fat, the body uses the MCTs—bypassing the metabolic processes that allow the body to burn its own fat and thus decreasing the lipolytic effect of the diet on the transfer of fatty acids into the mitochondria, where they undergo beta-oxidation and are preferentially (and this is the important word for becoming fat adapted instead of carbohydrate adapted) used as fuel for the body.

The long-chain triglycerides (LCTs), found in most foods allowed in the metabolic diet and which make up body fat, have other advantages over MCTs. First of all, the LCTs have greater protein-sparing effects than do MCTs (Beaufrere et al. 1992). Unlike LCTs, MCTs have little inhibitory effect on the activity of enzymes involved in lipogenesis (increased formation of body fat) (Chanez et al. 1988; Hwang, Yano, and Kawashima 1993). Several studies show that LCTs increase lipolysis, or the breakdown of body fat (Kather et al. 1987). An overall higher level of LCTs compared with MCTs should result in decreased body-fat levels.

Sugar Alcohols   Manufacturers claim that although sugar alcohols are technically carbohydrate and a source of calories, they have a negligible effect on the blood sugar and shouldn't be counted as part of the total carbohydrate. That's not entirely true. In fact, one of the reasons for low-carbohydrate diets is so the body will become fat adapted and burn off body fat preferentially. Unfortunately, sugar alcohols act just like regular carbohydrate in short-circuiting the fat-adaption response.

The American Dietetic Association takes the middle road and looks at the calories alone by recommending that persons with diabetes managing their blood sugars by counting grams of carbohydrate should count half of the grams of sugar alcohol as carbohydrates since half of the sugar alcohol on average is digested (Powers 2003).

Hard-to-Digest Carbohydrates   Several carbohydrates are difficult for humans to digest and as such are not considered as carbohydrates by manufacturers. For example, inulin and oligofructose, storage carbohydrates that are found in some plants, have just under one-third of the effect of regular carbohydrates on metabolism and as such can be taken into account at that level—for example 3 grams of inulin would be equivalent to 1 gram of regular carbohydrate. The reason for this is that inulin and oligofructose have a beta-(2-1) bond linking the fructose molecules. These bonds render them nondigestible by human intestinal enzymes.

Thus, inulin and oligofructose pass through the mouth, stomach, and small intestine without being metabolized. As such, almost all the inulin or oligofructose ingested enters the colon, where it is totally fermented by the colonic microflora. The energy derived from fermentation is largely a result of the production of mostly short-chain fatty acids and some lactate, which are metabolized and contribute 1.5 calories per gram of useful energy for both oligofructose and inulin. Lactate and short-chain fatty acids are equivalent to carbohydrates, so this 1.5 calories per gram, out of a possible 4 calories per gram, has to be factored into your carbohydrate intake.

Food Labels and Special Interests

Most of what you've read so far will help you decide what's in the food you're eating and allow you to make healthy food choices. The information on food labels is geared mostly to the average person on an average diet. How you use the nutrition facts panel depends on the type of diet you're on and your goals. If you're looking to maximize body composition, performance, or both, or if you're following a specific diet, then you're going to use the information on the food panel a little differently from the average person.

Although it's always a good idea to minimize trans fats and sugars, the amount of other fats, protein, and carbohydrate can vary dramatically depending on what you're trying to accomplish. For example, if you're following a low-carbohydrate diet, then your total fat level will usually be high, unless you're drastically cutting back on calories. And if red meat is an important part of your diet, then your saturated fat intake will be relatively high. But that may not be a problem because when you're low carbing, saturated fat is treated differently than when you're on a high-carbohydrate diet, especially one high in sugars.

Regardless of the type of diet you're on, you should minimize your intake of sugars and trans fat and increase your intake of polyunsaturated and mono-unsaturated fats. Unfortunately, neither of the unsaturated fats is required to be listed on food labels, although some companies do. It would also be useful to have the number of calories from each macronutrient and subsections under that macronutrient. This would allow you to more accurately tailor the food for specific macronutrient requirements. For example, it would be useful to know how much of the fiber is soluble and how much is insoluble. That's because while insoluble fiber has no usable calories, soluble fiber does.

Breaking down the macronutrients into subsections allows you to see through some of the marketing ploys some manufacturers use to give a false impression of what's in their products. As you've seen, this is most needed when discussing the carbohydrate content of food and supplements, especially low-carbohydrate protein snacks, bars, and meal replacements.

Under the label's nutrition facts panel, manufacturers are required to provide information on certain nutrients; however, it would be helpful if additional information was listed. The following list provides the mandatory components, which are bolded, as well as other components that would be useful:

- **Total calories**
- **Calories from fat**
- Calories from saturated fat
- **Total fat**
- **Saturated fat**
- **Trans fat**
- Polyunsaturated fat
- Monounsaturated fat
- **Cholesterol**
- **Sodium**
- Potassium
- **Total carbohydrate**
- **Dietary fiber**
- Soluble fiber
- Insoluble fiber
- **Sugars**
- Sugar alcohols (e.g., the sugar substitutes xylitol, mannitol, and sorbitol)
- Other carbohydrates (the difference between total carbohydrate and the sum of dietary fiber, sugars, and sugar alcohol if declared)
- **Protein**
- Amino acids
- Peptides
- **Vitamin A**
- Percentage of vitamin A present as beta-carotene

- **Vitamin C**
- **Calcium**
- **Iron**
- Other essential vitamins and minerals
- Caffeine (especially in various commercial drinks such as sodas and energy drinks)

Caffeine Content of Food and Drink

Another relatively unregulated area is the caffeine content of various drinks (mostly coffee and tea, carbonated beverages, and energy drinks) and foods (mostly chocolate, especially dark chocolate, and coffee-flavored yogurt and syrup). When caffeine is added to foods and beverages, it must appear in the list of ingredients on the label. However, manufacturers aren't required to list the amount of caffeine.

Only a minority of companies voluntarily state the amount of caffeine in their products on their labels. This is a problem with carbonated beverages (Chou and Bell 2007) and especially the new crop of energy drinks, with the energy coming almost 100 percent from the caffeine content and related compounds even though the product may have several other ingredients in the mix, such as taurine, B vitamins, and sugar.

Up to 400 milligrams of caffeine per day is considered safe for healthy adults (Nawrot et al. 2003), although an upper limit of 300 milligrams is recommended for some, such as women in their childbearing years (Higdon and Frei 2006). Although these limits may seem to be high, if you look at all the sources of caffeine, reaching unhealthy levels is easier than most people think.

An average cup of brewed coffee has around 100 milligrams of caffeine. However, the caffeine content of coffee from retail outlets, including different sources of the same brands, can vary appreciably, mostly from 70 to 140 milligrams (McCusker, Goldberger, and Cone 2003; Desbrow et al. 2007). Even decaffeinated coffee contains significant amounts of caffeine (McCusker et al. 2006). Some of the energy drinks, in their bid to outdo each other, have raised caffeine levels in their products to the point where their use alone could be dangerous to health (Cohen and Townsend 2006). For example, a 20-ounce (600 ml) bottle of Fixx (enough for one training session), an energy drink aimed at those who exercise, contains 500 milligrams of caffeine. An 8-ounce (250 ml) container of Spike Shooter contains 300 milligrams of caffeine, and it wouldn't be unusual to consume more than one a day.

For a list of the levels of caffeine in foods, drinks, over-the-counter pills, and medications, go to www.erowid.org/chemicals/caffeine/caffeine_info1.shtml#1. The amount of caffeine in various beverages varies dramatically, from relatively low levels to caffeine contents equivalent to several cups of brewed coffee.

Energy drinks are an important tool in bodybuilding and strength training because exercise sessions normally exceed 30 minutes. The most effective energy drinks contain 6 percent carbohydrate (6 grams per 100 milliliters of fluid). Research shows that a 6 percent carbohydrate solution is rapidly absorbed by the intestines, delivers performance-enhancing energy, and restores electrolyte balance after sweat loss. Sports drinks with lower or higher carbohydrate formulas are unlikely to deliver on some of these attributes. The easiest way to calculate the carbohydrate percentage is by taking the total carbohydrate content of the energy drink, dividing it by the serving size in milliliters, and multiplying by 100. For example, an energy drink that has 14 grams of carbohydrate per 240-milliliter serving would have a 5.8 percent carbohydrate content:

$$14 \text{ g} \div 240 \text{ ml} \times 100 = 5.8\%$$

So this energy drink has about 6 percent when rounded to the nearest tenth. Avoid new energy drinks that are mostly high in sugars or contain just caffeine. The body will secrete water into the small intestine after being ingested. This will increase dehydration and may cause gastrointestinal discomfort. Some of the newer energy drinks contain enormous amounts of caffeine. They can give an athlete a feeling of more energy, but very high doses can lead to increased dehydration through increased urine loss (Whitney and Rolfes 2008).

Nutrition for Maximizing the Anabolic Effects of Exercise

The nutrients you take in after you exercise are almost as important as the exercise itself in deciding the effects of exercise on body composition and performance. For the metabolic diet, the ideal posttraining nutrition is different from the general consensus of carbohydrate alone or a combination of carbohydrate and protein. As such, postexercise supplements miss the mark and can actually be counterproductive for maximizing body composition (improving muscle mass and decreasing body fat), improving performance, and enhancing recovery.

There is no doubt that the timing of protein nutrition after exercise is crucial for increasing skeletal muscle protein synthesis and an overall net balance (Tipton et al. 1999). Exercise provides an adaptive response so that the body is able to make use of any nutrition supplied postexercise.

Nutrient intake on its own provides a storage response so that if someone consumes mixed amino acids after a period of fasting, protein synthesis increases, whereas protein breakdown remains the same or decreases slightly. This is different from the response after exercise.

Without nutrient intake after exercise, protein synthesis and protein breakdown increase, but the net balance does not become positive, as it does after amino acid intake after fasting. Because of the exercise stimulus, providing amino acids after exercise increases protein synthesis more than the increase that usually occurs after exercise or after consuming amino acids alone. Protein breakdown remains relatively similar postexercise without nutrient intake. Thus, consuming amino acids enhances protein synthesis and leads to a positive net protein balance and an overall increase in protein accumulation (Miller 2007).

In addition, although the increase in protein synthesis after eating is a transient storage phenomenon, physical exercise stimulates a longer-term adaptive response. Providing nutrition after physical activity takes advantage of the anabolic signaling pathways initiated by physical activity by providing amino acid building blocks and energy for protein synthesis.

OVEREMPHASIS ON POSTEXERCISE CARBOHYDRATE INTAKE

Because of the overemphasis placed on maintaining glycogen stores to maximize exercise performance, much of the research has centered around the effects of postexercise carbohydrate and of postexercise carbohydrate combined with protein (Ivy et al. 2002) on glucose transporters (GLUT1, GLUT2, GLUT4); glucose metabolism, including levels of hexokinase and glycogen synthase; and insulin (Zorzano, Palacin, and Guma 2005; Morifuji et al. 2005). There's little research dealing with just the use of protein and fat after exercise.

Muscle Glycogen and Insulin Action

It's well known that a single session of exercise increases insulin sensitivity for hours. (Cartee et al. 1989; Henriksen 2002). It's also known that bouts of resistance and endurance exercise result in a significant decrease in glycogen and that total energy content and carbohydrate content are important in the resynthesis of muscle and liver glycogen (Roy and Tarnopolsky 1998).

Glucose uptake and glycogen synthesis are enhanced in the presence of insulin after acute exercise that lowers the muscle glycogen concentration and activates glycogen synthase (Ivy and Holloszy 1981; Ren et al. 1994). Muscle glycogen concentration dictates much of this acute increase in insulin sensitivity after exercise (Derave et al. 1999). Therefore, an increased availability of dietary carbohydrate in the hours after exercise and the resultant increase in muscle glycogen resynthesis reverses the exercise-induced increase in insulin sensitivity (Kawanaka et al. 1999).

Along with glucose uptake, amino acid uptake and protein synthesis also increase after exercise. The use of fatty acids as a primary fuel also rises after exercise since glycogen resynthesis takes priority over the use of glucose for aerobic energy. But as liver and muscle glycogen levels get replenished, insulin sensitivity decreases, as does amino acid uptake, protein synthesis, and the use of fatty acids as a primary fuel. Fatty acids, preferably from the breakdown of body fat, can provide the fuel needed secondary to the prolonged increased metabolic rate that occurs after vigorous exercise, especially resistance training (Knab et al. 2011; Haden et al. 2011).

By increasing insulin levels and not providing carbohydrate, you shunt your body's metabolism to the use of more fatty acids for energy while at the same time keeping muscle glycogen levels below saturation and amino acid influx and protein synthesis elevated for a prolonged period of time postexercise. In essence, by limiting glycogen synthesis, you prolong the beneficial effects of insulin on protein synthesis and degradation and decrease the dampening effects of insulin on fatty acid breakdown and oxidation. At the same time, although you delay glycogen synthesis, you still maintain the capacity for rapidly increasing glycogen stores once you increase your carbohydrate intake.

This increased capacity for glycogen synthesis can persist for several days if the muscle glycogen concentration is maintained below normal levels by carbohydrate restriction. By keeping carbohydrate low and protein and energy high after training, you can increase protein synthesis over a prolonged period of time and get long-term anabolic effects (Cartee et al. 1989).

A recent study looked at the effects of posttraining carbohydrate deficit, while keeping calorie intake constant, on insulin action and on fat oxidation. The study showed that carbohydrate deficit postexercise resulted in increased fat oxidation and enhanced insulin action. The enhanced insulin action was proportional to the degree of carbohydrate deficit (i.e., the further the postexercise carbohydrate was decreased, the greater the insulin action) (Holtz et al. 2008).

Insulin and Nutrient Delivery to Skeletal Muscle

One of insulin's actions is to increase microvascular (nutritive) perfusion of muscle, which is enhanced by exercise (Dela et al. 1995; Hardin et al. 1995). This enhancement is crucial for maximizing the anabolic effects of exercise and targeted nutrition.

For example, Clark et al. (2003) reviewed the effects of insulin on the vascular system and on nutrient delivery to muscle, noting that there are two flow routes in muscle. One has intimate contact with the muscle cells (myocytes) and is able to exchange nutrients and hormones freely and is thus regarded as nutritive. The second has essentially no contact with myocytes and is regarded as nonnutritive. This pathway may provide blood to muscle connective tissue and adjacent fat cells, but not muscle cells.

Therefore, in the absence of increases in bulk flow to muscle, say after a training session, insulin may switch flow from the nonnutritive to the nutritive route. This capillary recruitment results in an increase in nutritive blood flow so that muscles that have been stressed and are undergoing an adaptive response will have what they need to recover and grow.

Maximum Lift Based on Repetitions

The weights provided in the chart are given in pounds. Divide the load in pounds by 2.2 to convert pounds to kilograms.

% of 1RM reps	100	95	90	85	80	75
	1	2	4	6	8	10
Pounds lifted	700.00	665.00	630.00	595.00	560.00	525.00
	695.00	660.25	625.50	590.75	556.00	521.25
	690.00	655.50	621.00	586.50	552.00	517.50
	685.00	650.75	616.50	582.25	548.00	513.75
	680.00	646.00	612.00	578.00	544.00	510.00
	675.00	641.25	607.50	573.75	540.00	507.00
	670.00	636.50	603.00	569.50	536.00	502.50
	665.00	631.75	598.50	565.25	532.00	498.75
	660.00	627.00	594.00	561.00	528.00	495.00
	655.00	622.25	589.50	556.75	524.00	491.25
	650.00	617.50	585.00	552.50	520.00	487.50
	645.00	612.76	580.50	548.25	516.00	483.75
	640.00	608.00	576.00	544.00	512.00	480.00
	635.00	603.25	571.50	539.75	508.00	476.25
	630.00	598.50	567.00	535.50	504.00	472.50
	625.00	593.75	562.50	531.25	500.00	468.75
	620.00	589.00	558.00	527.00	496.00	465.00
	615.00	584.25	553.50	522.75	492.00	461.25
	610.00	579.50	549.00	518.50	488.00	457.50
	605.00	574.75	544.50	514.25	484.00	453.75
	600.00	570.00	540.00	510.00	480.00	450.00
	595.00	565.25	535.50	505.75	476.00	446.25
	590.00	560.50	531.00	501.50	472.00	442.50
	585.00	555.75	526.50	497.25	468.00	438.75
	580.00	551.00	522.00	493.00	464.00	435.00
	575.00	546.25	517.50	488.75	460.00	431.25
	570.00	541.50	513.00	484.50	456.00	427.50
	565.00	536.75	508.50	480.25	452.00	423.75
	560.00	532.00	504.00	476.00	448.00	420.00
	555.00	527.50	499.50	471.75	444.00	416.25
	550.00	522.50	495.00	467.50	440.00	412.50
	545.00	517.75	490.50	463.25	436.00	408.75
	540.00	513.00	486.00	459.00	432.00	405.00
	535.00	508.25	481.50	454.75	428.00	401.25
	530.00	503.50	477.00	450.50	424.00	397.50
	525.00	498.75	472.50	446.25	420.00	393.75
	520.00	494.00	468.00	442.00	416.00	390.00
	515.00	489.25	463.50	437.75	412.00	386.25
	510.00	484.50	459.00	433.50	408.00	382.50
	505.00	479.75	454.50	429.25	404.00	378.75

% of 1RM reps	100	95	90	85	80	75
	1	2	4	6	8	10
Pounds lifted	500.00	475.00	450.00	425.00	400.00	375.00
	495.00	470.25	445.50	420.75	396.00	371.25
	490.00	465.50	441.00	416.50	392.00	367.50
	485.00	460.75	436.50	412.25	388.00	363.75
	480.00	456.00	432.00	408.50	384.00	360.00
	475.00	451.25	427.50	403.75	380.00	356.25
	470.00	446.50	423.00	399.50	376.00	352.50
	465.00	441.75	418.50	395.25	372.00	348.75
	460.00	437.00	414.00	391.00	368.00	345.00
	455.00	432.75	409.50	386.75	364.00	341.25
	450.00	427.50	405.00	382.50	360.00	337.50
	445.00	422.75	400.50	378.25	356.00	333.75
	440.00	418.00	396.00	374.00	352.00	330.00
	435.00	413.25	391.50	369.75	348.00	326.25
	430.00	408.50	387.00	365.50	344.00	322.50
	425.00	403.75	382.00	361.25	340.00	318.75
	420.00	399.00	378.00	357.00	336.00	315.00
	415.00	394.25	373.50	352.75	332.00	311.25
	410.00	389.50	369.00	348.50	328.00	307.50
	405.00	384.75	364.50	344.25	324.00	303.75
	400.00	380.00	360.00	340.00	320.00	300.00
	395.00	375.25	355.50	335.75	316.00	296.25
	390.00	370.50	351.00	331.50	312.00	292.50
	385.00	365.76	346.50	327.25	308.00	288.75
	380.00	361.00	342.00	323.00	304.00	285.00
	375.00	356.25	337.50	318.75	300.00	281.25
	370.00	351.50	330.00	314.50	296.00	277.50
	365.00	346.75	328.50	310.25	292.00	273.75
	360.00	342.00	324.00	306.00	288.00	270.00
	355.00	337.25	319.50	301.75	284.00	266.25
	350.00	332.50	315.00	297.50	280.00	262.50
	345.00	327.75	310.50	293.25	276.00	258.75
	340.00	323.00	306.00	289.00	272.00	255.00
	335.00	318.25	301.50	284.75	268.00	251.25
	330.00	313.50	297.00	280.50	264.00	247.50
	325.00	308.75	292.50	276.25	260.00	243.75
	320.00	304.00	288.00	272.00	256.00	240.00
	315.00	299.25	283.50	267.75	252.00	236.25
	310.00	294.50	279.00	263.50	248.00	232.50
	305.00	289.75	274.50	259.25	244.00	228.75

(continued)

% of 1RM	100	95	90	85	80	75
reps	1	2	4	6	8	10
Pounds lifted	300.00	285.00	270.00	255.00	240.00	225.00
	295.00	280.25	265.50	250.75	236.00	221.25
	290.00	275.50	261.00	246.50	232.00	217.50
	285.00	270.75	256.50	242.25	228.00	213.75
	280.00	266.00	252.00	238.00	224.00	210.00
	275.00	261.25	247.50	233.75	220.00	206.25
	270.00	256.50	243.00	229.50	216.00	202.50
	265.00	251.75	238.50	225.25	212.00	198.75
	260.00	247.00	234.00	221.00	208.00	195.00
	255.00	242.25	229.50	216.75	204.00	191.25
	250.00	237.50	225.00	212.50	200.00	187.50
	245.00	232.75	220.50	208.25	196.00	183.75
	240.00	228.00	216.00	204.00	192.00	180.00
	235.00	223.25	211.50	199.75	188.00	176.25
	230.00	218.50	207.00	195.50	184.00	172.50
	225.00	213.75	202.50	191.25	180.00	168.75
	220.00	209.00	198.00	187.00	176.00	165.00
	215.00	204.25	193.50	182.75	172.00	161.25
	210.00	199.50	189.00	178.50	168.00	157.50
	205.00	194.75	184.50	174.25	164.00	153.75
	200.00	190.00	180.00	170.00	160.00	150.00
	195.00	185.25	175.50	165.75	156.00	146.25
	190.00	180.50	171.00	161.50	152.00	142.50
	185.00	175.75	166.50	157.25	148.00	138.75
	180.00	171.00	162.00	153.00	144.00	135.00
	175.00	166.25	157.50	148.75	140.00	131.25
	170.00	161.50	153.00	144.50	136.00	127.50
	165.00	156.75	148.50	140.25	132.00	123.75
	160.00	152.00	144.00	136.00	128.00	120.00
	155.00	147.25	139.50	131.75	124.00	116.25
	150.00	142.50	135.00	127.50	120.00	112.50
	145.00	137.75	130.50	123.25	116.00	108.75
	140.00	133.00	126.00	119.00	112.00	105.00
	135.00	128.25	121.50	114.75	108.00	101.25
	130.00	123.50	117.00	110.50	104.00	97.50
	125.00	118.75	112.50	106.25	100.00	93.75
	120.00	114.00	108.00	102.00	96.00	90.00
	115.00	109.25	103.50	97.75	92.00	86.25
	110.00	104.50	99.00	93.50	88.00	82.50
	105.00	99.75	94.50	89.25	84.00	78.75

Reprinted from Bompa 1996.

Maximum Weight Chart

If for any reason (e.g., equipment) you cannot lift the load necessary to calculate 1RM, you can still determine your 1RM by lifting a lesser load (from 2RM up to 10RM). To calculate 1RM, perform the maximum number of repetitions with the load available, and then do the following:

1. From the top of the chart, choose the column head that matches the number of repetitions you did.
2. Find the row for the maximum load you had available.
3. Find the number where the selected column and row meet.
4. The number there is your 1RM at that given time.

For example, you complete four repetitions with 250 pounds. The number at the intersection of the 4 column and the 250 row is 278. This is your 1RM.

The weights provided in the chart are given in pounds. Divide the load in pounds by 2.2 to convert pounds to kilograms.

Pounds	10	9	8	7	6	5	4	3	2
5	7	6	6	6	6	6	6	5	5
10	13	13	13	12	12	11	11	11	11
15	20	19	19	18	18	17	17	16	16
20	27	26	25	24	24	23	22	22	21
25	33	32	31	30	29	29	28	27	26
30	40	39	38	36	35	34	33	32	32
35	47	45	44	42	41	40	39	38	37
40	53	52	50	48	47	46	44	43	42
45	60	58	56	55	53	51	50	49	47
50	67	65	63	61	59	57	56	54	53
55	73	71	69	67	65	63	61	59	58
60	80	77	75	73	71	69	67	65	63
65	87	84	81	79	76	74	72	70	68
70	93	90	88	85	82	80	78	76	74
75	100	97	94	91	88	86	83	81	79
80	107	103	100	97	94	91	89	86	84
85	113	110	106	103	100	97	94	92	89
90	120	116	113	109	106	103	100	97	95
95	127	123	119	115	112	109	106	103	100
100	133	129	125	121	118	114	111	108	105
105	140	135	131	127	124	120	117	114	111
110	147	142	138	133	129	126	122	119	116
115	153	148	144	139	135	131	128	124	121
120	160	155	150	145	141	137	133	130	126
125	167	161	156	152	147	143	139	135	132
130	173	168	163	158	153	149	144	141	137
135	180	174	169	164	159	154	150	146	142
140	187	181	175	170	165	160	156	151	147
145	193	187	181	176	171	166	161	157	153
150	200	194	188	182	176	171	167	162	158
155	207	200	194	188	182	177	172	168	163
160	213	206	200	194	188	183	178	173	168
165	220	213	206	200	194	189	183	178	174
170	227	219	213	206	200	194	189	184	179
175	233	226	219	212	206	200	194	189	184
180	240	232	225	218	212	206	200	195	189
185	247	239	231	224	218	211	206	200	195
190	253	245	238	230	224	217	211	205	200
195	260	252	244	236	229	223	217	211	205
200	267	258	250	242	235	229	222	216	211
205	273	265	256	248	241	234	228	222	216
210	280	271	263	255	247	240	233	227	221
215	287	277	269	261	253	246	239	232	226

Pounds	10	9	8	7	6	5	4	3	2
220	293	284	275	267	259	251	244	238	232
225	300	290	281	273	265	257	250	243	237
230	307	297	288	279	271	263	256	249	242
235	313	303	294	285	276	269	261	254	247
240	320	310	300	291	282	274	267	259	253
245	327	316	306	297	288	280	272	265	258
250	333	323	313	303	294	286	278	270	263
255	340	329	319	309	300	291	283	276	268
260	347	335	325	315	306	297	289	281	274
265	353	342	331	321	312	303	294	286	279
270	360	348	338	327	318	309	300	292	284
275	367	355	344	333	324	314	306	297	289
280	373	361	350	339	329	320	311	303	295
285	380	368	356	345	335	326	317	308	300
290	387	374	363	352	341	331	322	314	305
295	393	381	369	358	347	337	328	319	311
300	400	387	375	364	353	343	333	324	316
305	407	394	381	370	359	349	339	330	321
310	413	400	388	376	365	354	344	335	326
315	420	406	394	382	371	360	350	341	332
320	427	413	400	388	376	366	356	346	337
325	433	419	406	394	382	371	361	351	342
330	440	426	413	400	388	377	367	357	347
335	447	432	419	406	394	383	372	362	353
340	453	439	425	412	400	389	378	368	358
345	460	445	431	418	406	394	383	373	363
350	467	452	438	424	412	400	389	378	368
355	473	458	444	430	418	406	394	384	374
360	480	465	450	436	424	411	400	389	379
365	487	471	456	442	429	417	406	395	384
370	493	477	463	448	435	423	411	400	389
375	500	484	469	455	441	429	417	405	395
380	507	490	475	461	447	434	422	411	400
385	513	497	481	467	453	440	428	416	405
390	520	503	488	473	459	446	433	422	411
395	527	510	494	479	465	451	439	427	416
400	533	516	500	485	471	457	444	432	421
405	540	523	506	491	476	463	450	438	426
410	547	529	513	497	482	469	456	443	432
415	553	535	519	503	488	474	461	449	437
420	560	542	525	509	494	480	467	454	442
425	567	548	531	515	500	486	472	459	447

(continued)

Pounds	10	9	8	7	6	5	4	3	2
430	573	555	538	521	506	491	478	465	453
435	580	561	544	527	512	497	483	470	458
440	587	568	550	533	518	503	489	476	463
445	593	574	556	539	524	509	494	481	468
450	600	581	563	545	529	514	500	486	474
455	607	587	569	552	535	520	506	492	479
460	613	594	575	558	541	526	511	497	484
465	620	600	581	564	547	531	517	503	489
470	627	606	588	570	553	537	522	508	495
475	633	613	594	576	559	543	528	514	500
480	640	619	600	582	565	549	532	519	505
485	647	626	606	588	571	554	539	524	511
490	653	632	613	594	576	560	544	530	516
495	660	639	619	600	582	566	550	535	521
500	667	645	625	606	588	571	556	541	526
505	673	652	631	612	594	577	561	546	532
510	680	658	638	618	600	583	567	551	537
515	687	665	644	624	606	589	572	557	542
520	693	671	650	630	612	594	578	562	547
525	700	677	656	636	618	600	583	569	553
530	707	684	663	642	624	606	589	573	558
535	713	690	669	648	629	611	594	578	563
540	720	697	675	655	635	617	600	584	568
545	727	703	681	661	641	623	606	589	574
550	733	710	688	667	647	629	611	595	579
555	740	716	694	673	653	634	617	600	584
560	747	723	700	679	659	640	622	605	589
565	753	729	706	685	665	646	628	611	595
570	760	735	713	691	671	651	633	616	600
575	767	742	719	697	676	657	639	622	605
580	773	748	725	703	682	663	644	627	611
585	780	755	731	709	688	669	650	632	616
590	787	761	738	715	694	674	656	638	621
595	793	768	744	721	700	680	661	643	626
600	800	774	750	727	706	686	667	649	632
605	807	781	756	733	712	691	672	654	637
610	813	787	763	739	718	697	678	659	642
615	820	794	769	745	724	703	683	665	647
620	827	800	775	752	729	709	689	670	653
625	833	806	781	758	735	714	694	676	658
630	840	813	788	764	741	720	700	681	663
635	847	819	794	770	747	726	706	686	668

Pounds	10	9	8	7	6	5	4	3	2
640	853	826	800	776	753	731	711	692	674
645	860	832	806	782	759	737	717	697	679
650	867	839	813	788	765	743	722	703	684
655	873	845	819	794	771	749	728	708	689
660	880	852	825	800	776	754	733	714	695
665	887	858	831	806	782	760	739	719	700
670	893	865	838	812	788	766	644	724	705
675	900	871	844	818	794	771	750	730	711
680	907	877	850	824	800	777	756	735	716
685	913	884	856	830	806	783	761	741	721
690	920	890	863	836	812	789	767	746	726
695	927	897	869	842	818	794	772	751	732
700	933	903	875	848	824	800	778	757	737
705	940	910	881	855	829	806	783	762	742
710	947	916	888	861	835	811	789	768	747
715	953	923	894	768	841	817	794	773	753
720	960	929	900	873	847	823	800	778	758
725	967	935	906	879	853	829	806	784	763
730	973	942	913	885	859	834	811	789	768
735	980	948	919	891	865	840	817	795	774
740	987	955	925	897	871	846	822	800	779
745	993	961	931	903	876	851	828	805	784
750	1,000	968	938	909	882	857	833	811	789
755	1,107	974	944	915	888	863	839	816	795
760	1,113	981	950	921	894	869	844	822	800
765	1,120	987	956	927	900	874	850	827	805
770	1,127	994	963	933	906	880	856	832	811
775	1,133	1,000	969	939	912	886	861	838	816
780	1,140	1,006	975	945	918	891	867	843	821
785	1,147	1,013	981	952	924	897	872	849	826
790	1,153	1,019	988	958	929	903	878	854	832
795	1,160	1,026	994	964	935	908	883	859	837
800	1,167	1,032	1,000	970	941	914	889	865	842
820	1,173	1,058	1,025	994	965	937	911	886	863
840	1,180	1,084	1,050	1,018	988	960	933	908	884
860	1,187	1,110	1,075	1,042	1,012	983	956	930	905
880	1,193	1,135	1,100	1,067	1,035	1,006	978	951	926
900	1,200	1,161	1,125	1,091	1,059	1,029	1,000	973	947
920	1,207	1,187	1,150	1,115	1,082	1,051	1,022	995	968

Reprinted from Bompa 1996.

Glossary

acetylcholine—A neurotransmitter that is critical for optimal nervous system functioning; it is released at the ends of nerve fibers in the somatic and parasympathetic nervous systems.

acetyl-CoA—An intermediate in energy metabolism, produced from the breakdown of free fatty acids, glucose, and protein.

actin—A protein involved in muscle activity.

adaptation—Persistent changes in structure or function of a muscle as a direct response to progressively increased training loads.

adaptation threshold—The level of adaptation a person reaches in a given training phase. To surpass the threshold, one has to increase the stimulation (loading) level.

adenosine triphosphate (ATP)—A high-energy compound essential for the functioning of all cells in the body. ATP is very important in weightlifting, where energy for short-burst, high-intensity exercise is needed. Maximizing and replenishing ATP stores in muscle tissue is essential for optimal performance.

adipose tissue—a type of body tissue containing stored fat.

aerobic activity—A low-intensity, high-endurance activity that requires oxygen for production of energy and continuous work performed over long distances or periods of time.

aerobic endurance—The ability to maintain aerobic muscle output over long periods of time.

agonist—A muscle directly engaged in a muscle contraction and working in opposition to the action of other muscles.

all-or-none law—A stimulated muscle or nerve fiber contracts or propagates a nerve impulse either completely or not at all (i.e., a minimal stimulus causes a maximal response).

alpha-linolenic acid—An essential fatty acid.

amino acids—A group of nitrogen-based organic compounds that are the building blocks on which protein is made and muscle grown.

anabolic—The ability to produce more muscle tissue from exercise. This process involves the natural production of testosterone, growth hormone, insulin, and other hormones involved in muscle growth.

anaerobic—Exercise that occurs without oxygen.

androgenic—Possessing masculinizing properties.

antagonist—A muscle that has the opposite effect of an agonistic muscle, opposing its contraction.

anticatabolic—Preventing catabolism.

antioxidant—A compound, either naturally present in the body or taken externally, that combats free radicals produced in the body as a result of various forms of stress.

ATP deficiency theory—The theory that constant taxation of ATP (i.e., disturbance of the equilibrium between consuming and manufacturing ATP) results in increased muscle hypertrophy.

atrophy—A gradual shrinking of muscle tissue as a result of disuse or disease.

ballistic—Dynamic muscular movements.

beta-endorphin—A naturally occurring chemical substance (a peptide) produced in the brain. Endorphins produce a natural analgesic effect by binding to certain receptor sites in the body (the same sites that bind morphine). Endorphins are believed to be released during prolonged exercise.

beta-lipotropin—A trophic hormone secreted by the anterior lobe of the pituitary gland. Its physiological function is unclear, but its amino acid sequence is similar to that of endorphins and enkephalins (endogenous morphine-like substances) and hence it is also believed to produce analgesia.

beta-oxidation—The metabolic process in which fatty acids are used to generate energy.

bioelectrical impedance analysis—A method of measuring body fat. An electrical current is transmitted through the body, and the resistance or impedance to the current is measured. Because the body's fat-free mass contains much of the body's water and electrolytes and is therefore a better conductor of electrical current, impedance to the current gives information about the person's percentage of body fat.

biological value—Describes how efficiently body tissue can be created from food proteins.

branched-chain amino acids (BCAAs)—The amino acids valine, leucine, and isoleucine.

calorie—A unit of measurement used to express the energy value of food.

calorie cycling—The practice of alternating low-, medium-, and high-calorie days to prevent the body from adapting to any particular amount of food intake. Helps keep the metabolism from slowing down during periods of lower caloric intakes.

carbohydrate—Any of a group of chemical compounds, including sugars, starches, and cellulose, containing only carbon, hydrogen, and oxygen. One of the basic foodstuffs.

carbohydrate drink—A sports beverage designed to replenish the glycogen (energy) stores and provide energy substrates to exercising muscles.

carbon dioxide—A metabolic waste product from the breakdown of carbon-based molecules.

carcinogen—A substance that is either proven or suspected to cause cancer in humans or laboratory animals.

cardiac stroke volume (or stroke volume)—The amount of blood pumped out of the left ventricle per beat. The average amount is approximately 70 milliliters per beat in a resting man of average size tested in a supine position.

carnitine palmityl transferase 1 (CPT-1)—Carries free fatty acids into the mitochondria of cells for burning.

catabolic—A general term that refers to the breaking down of larger substances into smaller substances.

catabolism—The breakdown or loss of muscle tissue.

ceiling of adaptation—A certain level of adaptation a person has reached during training. The goal of training is to break through the ceiling of adaptation in order to raise it and, as a result, to improve performance.

cellular uptake—Absorption by the cells.

central nervous system (CNS)—The spinal cord and the brain.

cheat day—A planned day used during periods of dieting to help prevent the body from adapting to specific caloric intakes.

chronic hypertrophy—Long-lasting hypertrophy resulting from structural changes at the muscle level after the employment of heavy loads (greater than 80 percent 1RM).

cold therapy (cryotherapy)—A process that involves the local cooling of muscles or joints.

complete protein—Protein that contains all the nine essential amino acids. Found in animal protein sources.

complex carbohydrates—Also known as polysaccharides or starches. They are composed of many glucose units and are found in vegetables, fruits, and grains.

cortisol—A hormone secreted by the adrenal glands that stimulates catabolism.

creatine kinase—A soluble muscle protein that when found in the circulatory system is indicative of muscle damage. Specific isomers of creatine kinase are used to differentiate between damage to skeletal muscle and damage to cardiac muscle.

crossbridge—Extensions of myosin, a contractile protein. Crossbridges play a major role in muscle contraction.

de novo lipogenesis (DNL)—The formation of fat from carbohydrate and protein.

detraining—Reversal of adaptation to exercise. Effects of detraining occur more rapidly than training gains, with significant reduction of strength (and work) capacity only 2 weeks after training stops.

dipeptide—Two amino acids that are linked to form one molecule.

disaccharide—A simple sugar composed of two monosaccharides. The most common are sucrose (table sugar) and lactose (found in milk).

docosahexaenoic acid (DHA)—An omega-3 fatty acid formed in the body and found in fish oil.

dorsiflexion—Movement of the foot upward, towards the shin.

double-pyramid load pattern—Pertaining to increasing the load from the bottom up and then decreasing it again to the initial level.

dynamic flexibility—The performance of a motion requiring flexible muscles in an active manner (as opposed to static). Often called ballistic flexibility.

eccentric contraction—A muscle action that lengthens muscle fibers as it develops tension.

edema—Swelling. A local or generalized condition in which the body tissues contain an excessive amount of tissue fluid. Acute swelling, or edema, refers to the rapid buildup of tissue fluid in an area that lasts for only a short time (i.e., not chronic).

eicosapentaenoic acid (EPA)—An omega-3 fatty acid formed in the body and found in fish oil.

electromyography (EMG)—Measurement of the electrical activity of the excitable membranes of a muscle or muscle group.

endomysium—The inner layer of connective tissue surrounding a muscle fiber.

endorphin—Powerful opioid peptide manufactured in the brain that regulates pain perception. Responsible for the euphoric sensations experienced during vigorous exercise, such as the runner's high, second wind, and so on. A member of the morphine family.

end-plate potential (EPP)—Depolarization of a membrane region by a sodium influx.

energy metabolism—The processes involved in turning food into energy.

epimysium—The outer layer of connective tissue surrounding muscle.

ergogenic—Anything that increases performance.

essential amino acid—An amino acid the body cannot produce itself and that must be obtained from our diet. In some cases it also includes amino acids that cannot be produced in amounts needed under certain circumstances.

excitation—Ability to react to a stimulus.

fasciculus (pl. fasciculi)—A group or bundle of skeletal muscle fibers held together by a connective tissue called the perimysium.

fast twitch (FT) fiber—A muscle fiber characterized by fast contraction time, high anaerobic capacity, and low aerobic capacity, all making the fiber suited for high-power-output activities.

fat—A compound containing glycerol and fatty acids. One of the major basic foods.

fat-free mass—Weight of the body minus the fat.

fixators—Muscles that are stimulated to act in order to stabilize the position of a bone to perform a motion. Also know as stabilizers.

flat-pyramid load pattern—A loading pattern that after the warm-up lift stabilizes the load for the entire duration of strength training.

flexibility—Range of motion about a joint (static flexibility); opposition or resistance of a joint to motion (dynamic flexibility).

free radicals—Highly reactive molecules possessing unpaired electrons. While playing a role in the metabolism of food and energy utilization, they're also believed to contribute to molecular damage and the death of vital body cells. A prime cause of aging, disease, and, ultimately, death.

free-form amino acids—Structurally unlinked, individual amino acids.

full-spectrum amino acids—Containing all 12 of the essential amino acids.

glycemic index—A measure of how quickly a food is digested as compared with the speed of glucose digestion. Indicates whether or not a food may cause harmful insulin fluctuations. Bodybuilders have found this to be a useful tool for dieting purposes.

glycogen—The form in which carbohydrates (glucose) are stored in the muscles and liver.

glycolysis—The metabolism of glucose into pyruvic acid or lactic acid to produce ATP for energy.

growth hormone—A hormone, secreted by the anterior lobe of the pituitary gland, that stimulates growth and development.

heat therapy—A process that involves the local heating of muscles or joints.

heavy load—A load using a percentage greater than 80 to 85 percent of 1RM.

histamine—A neurotransmitter released by cells in response to injury and to allergic and inflammatory reactions, causing contraction of smooth muscle and dilation of capillaries.

homeostasis—Maintenance of a relatively stable internal physiological condition. As the stress of exercise causes changes in the internal environment, the body is constantly working to restore balance, or achieve homeostasis.

hyperemia—Increase in the quantity of blood flowing through any part of the body. This is often experienced as a "pump," or the feeling of blood-engorged muscles after weight training.

hyperplasia—Increase in the number of cells in a tissue or organ.

hypertrophy—The enlargement of the cellular components of muscle. Basically, muscle growth.

incomplete protein—A protein that is usually deficient in one or more of the essential amino acids. For example, most plant proteins are incomplete in one or more amino acids. However by combining incomplete proteins, a complete protein mix is possible.

inhibition—To repress, or slow down, the stimulating (excitation) effect of the CNS (by decreasing the electrical activity).

insulin—A hormone secreted by the pancreas that lowers blood sugar, increases fat deposits, increases protein synthesis, and decreases protein breakdown.

insulin resistance—A state where the body is resistant to normal levels of insulin.

insulin-like growth factor 1(IGF-1)—A growth factor with anabolic effects that is normally increased in the body and specifically in muscle when growth hormone levels increase.

intensity—Refers to the qualitative element of training. In bodybuilding training, intensity is expressed as a percentage of 1RM.

involution—Reduction in performance capacity.

ischemic—Lacking in blood supply. Blood starved.

isokinetic contraction—Contraction in which tension is developed but there is no change in the length of the muscle.

isotonic contraction—Contraction in which the muscle shortens while lifting a constant load. Also know as a concentric, or dynamic, contraction.

joint—Junction of two or more bones in the human body in which the bones are joined in a functional relationship.

ketones—An organic chemical compound resulting from the breakdown of triglycerides. Used as an energy source in the body and an important part of energy production in a high-fat diet.

lactic acid—Fatiguing metabolite of the glycolytic (anaerobic, or lactic acid) system resulting from the incomplete breakdown of glucose.

lactic acid system—An anaerobic energy system in which ATP is manufactured through the breakdown of glucose, in the absence of oxygen, to lactic acid. The energy is used in high-intensity work over a short duration (less than 2 minutes).

lean body mass (LBM)—All the components that make up the body except body fat.

ligament—Strong band of fibrous tissue that connects bones to each other.

limiting amino acid—The essential amino acid that is in shortest supply in the body and that is consequently responsible for the cessation of protein synthesis.

line of pull—The line of action of the tension developed by a muscle.

lipogenic—Producing body fat.

lipolysis—A process in which triglycerides (body fat) are broken down into their constituent fatty acids and glycerol.

lipolytic—Enhancing the breakdown of body fat so that ideally it can be used as an energy source.

low load—Pertaining to loads between 0 and 49 percent of 1RM.

macrocycle—A phase of training 2 to 6 weeks in duration.

macronutrient—Large food groups including carbohydrates, proteins, and fats.

macrophage—Large white blood cell that engulfs and digests antigens.

massage—A therapeutic manipulation of the soft tissues of the body with the goal of achieving normalization of those tissues.

maximum load—Refers to a load of 90 to 100 percent of 1RM.

meal replacement supplements—Any drink, powder, or other preparation used to replace or enhance a meal for purposes of weight loss, weight gain, or increasing dietary protein.

medium-chain fatty acid—Fatty acids that have 6 to 12 carbon atoms. Medium-chain triglycerides contain three medium-chain fatty acids and one glycerol.

medium load—Pertaining to loads between 50 and 89 percent of 1RM.

membrane—A structural barrier composed of lipids and proteins.

microcycle—A phase of training approximately 1 week in duration.

micronutrients—Nutrients present in the body in minute amounts in comparison to macronutrients (e.g., vitamins and minerals).

microtear—Small tear found in a muscle, ligament, or tendon.

mitochondria—A cell constituent that turns the breakdown products of food into energy, mostly in the form of ATP.

monosaccharide—Simple sugar. The two most common are glucose (blood sugar) and fructose (found in fruit).

monounsaturated fatty acid—A fatty acid that has one unsaturated carbon molecule.

motor neurons—Efferent neurons that conduct action potentials from the central nervous system to the muscles.

motor unit—An individual motor nerve and all the muscle fibers it innervates.

muscle mass—The amount of skeletal muscle in the body.

myofibril—The part of a muscle fiber containing two protein filaments: myosin and actin.

myosin—A protein involved in muscular contraction.

negative calorie balance—A state in which the body is burning more calories than it is consuming. This is necessary if weight loss is to occur.

neural adaptation—Increased nervous coordination of a group of muscles involved in contraction. Gains in strength before puberty often result from improved neural adaptation.

neuromuscular junction—Synapse between the axon terminal of a motor neuron and the motor end plate of a muscle's plasma membrane.

neuron—A nerve cell specialized to initiate, integrate, and conduct electric signals.

neutrophil—Type of white blood cell containing granules that release enzymes that help fight infection.

nonessential amino acid—An amino acid that can be synthesized by the body and therefore does not need to be supplied by the diet.

one-repetition maximum (1RM)—The maximum amount of weight a person can lift once; 100 percent of one's lifting capacity.

overcompensation—Often called supercompensation, refers to the relationship between work and regeneration as a biological base for physical and psychological arousal before a heavy workout.

overloading—An increase of work in training with the goal of improving strength.

perimysium—The connective tissue surrounding the fasciculus of skeletal muscle fibers.

periodization of bodybuilding—The methodological structure of training phases intended to bring about the best improvements in muscle size, tone, and definition.

periodization of nutrition—The structure of using nutrition and training supplements in order to match training phases.

phase-specific training—Pertaining to a particular training phase (e.g., hypertrophy phase, muscle definition phase, and so on).

phosphocreatine (PC)—A high-energy compound stored in muscles; it supplies energy for high-intensity activities that last less than 30 seconds.

placebo effect—Experiencing effects from use of an inactive, harmless substance. The effects are either imagined or result from the subject's belief that it will work.

plateau—Period during training when no observable progress is made.

PNF (proprioceptive neuromuscular facilitation)—Flexibility technique designed to enhance the relaxation and contraction of a body part, based on neurophysiological principles.

polypeptide—A chain of amino acids that contains four or more amino acids linked together.

polysaccharide—A carbohydrate that consists of many single units (monosaccharides such as glucose and fructose) linked together. Considered a complex carbohydrate in contrast to simple carbohydrates, which usually consist of one or two monosaccharides.

polyunsaturated fatty acid—A fatty acid that has more than one unsaturated carbon molecule. Polyunsaturated fatty acids tend to be liquid at room temperature.

precursor—An intermediate substance in the body's production of another substance.

prime movers—Muscles primarily responsible for performance of a technical movement.

protein—A complex molecule in the body and a macronutrient in food that is made up of amino acids linked together in various ways.

protein supplement—A supplement that supplies protein and is used to increase daily protein intake beyond the intake from food.

protein synthesis—An anabolic process in which amino acids are formed into proteins, which in muscle results in muscle hypertrophy.

proteolysis—A process in which proteins are broken down into amino acids. In skeletal muscle it is a catabolic process.

pump—The thick, full feeling during weight training that results from blood engorging the muscles being trained.

pyramid load pattern—Method of load patterning whereby the load for an exercise starts low, gradually increases with each set, and hits a high point.

RDA (recommended dietary allowance)—A guideline of food intake for the general population. RDA values may not be appropriate for serious bodybuilders because of the heightened demands placed on their bodies.

receptor—Specific protein-binding site in the plasma membrane or the interior of a target cell.

recovery—The adaptation the body uses to overcome training stress and develop a new level of conditioning that will accept the stress in the future. The time when lactic acid is removed from muscle, hormones stabilize, protein synthesis increases, and energy metabolism is restored.

sarcolemma—The cell (plasma) membrane surrounding a muscle fiber.

satellite cells—Undifferentiated cells found adjacent to skeletal muscle fibers. These cells can fuse with existing muscle fibers and contribute to muscle growth (hypertrophy). Satellite cells can possibly differentiate and form a new muscle fiber after muscle injury.

saturated fatty acid—A fatty acid that has no unsaturated carbon molecules. Saturated fatty acids are usually solid at room temperature as compared to mono- and polyunsaturated fatty acids.

sensory neuron—A nerve cell that conveys impulses from a receptor to the CNS. Examples of sensory neurons are those excited by sound, pain, light, and taste.

skewed-pyramid load pattern—A pattern in which the load is constantly increased throughout the session, with the exception of the last set, when the load is lowered.

slow twitch (ST) fiber—A muscle fiber characterized by slow contraction time, low anaerobic capacity, and high aerobic capacity, all making the fiber suited for low-power-output activities.

specificity training—Principle underlying construction of a training program for a specific activity or skill.

spotter—Person who watches and sometimes assists a lifter performing a set.

stabilizers (fixators)—Muscles that are stimulated to act on, to anchor, or to stabilize the position of a limb.

standard loading—A load that remains at the same level for a certain period of time.

static flexibility—Passively stretching an antagonistic muscle by placing it in a maximal stretch position and holding it in place.

step-loading principle—Pertaining to increasing the load from week to week, normally for 3 weeks, followed by a week of unloading so that the body can regenerate before a new increase.

stretch, or myostatic, reflex—Reflex that responds to the rate of muscle stretch. This reflex has the fastest known response to a stimulus (in this case, the rate of muscle stretch). The stretch reflex elicits a contraction of the muscle being stretched and the synergistic muscles, while inhibiting the antagonistic muscles, when it senses that a stretch is being performed too quickly or rigorously.

subcutaneous fat—Refers to fat between the skin and muscle; visible fat.

supermaximum load—A load that exceeds 100 percent of 1RM. These weights should be used only by experienced lifters, especially in the maximum strength phase of training.

synergist—A muscle that actively provides an additive contribution to the agonist muscle during a muscle contraction.

targeted supplement—A substance taken to help achieve a person's specific training goals in the areas of workload capacity, recovery, and anabolic drive.

tendon—Collagen fiber bundle that connects muscle to bone and transmits muscle contractile force to the bone.

testosterone—Male sex hormone produced in the testes; responsible for secondary male sexual characteristics.

thermogenic—Generally refers to generating heat from the oxidation of fat.

transient hypertrophy—Temporary enlargement of muscles due to water accumulation, not to permanent tissue growth. Occurs during and shortly after an intense weight-training session and subsides after a short time when the body returns to its normal state (homeostasis).

triglycerides—Fats made up of three free fatty acids and one glycerol.

twitch—A brief period of contraction followed by relaxation in the response of a motor unit to a stimulus (nerve impulse).

unloading—Decrease of load, often for the purpose of allowing the body and mind to regenerate and refresh itself before a new loading phase.

urea—Major body waste product formed from the breakdown of amino acids.

vasodilation—Expansion of the blood vessels, especially the arteries and their branches.

yo-yo dieting—The process of repeatedly gaining and losing large amounts of body weight.

References

Adam, A., and De Luca, C.J. 2005. Firing rates of motor units in human vastus lateralis muscle during fatiguing isometric contractions. *J Appl Physiol* 99:268-80.

Adams, J.S., and Hewison, M. 2008. Unexpected actions of vitamin D: New perspectives on the regulation of innate and adaptive immunity. *Nat Clin Pract Endocrinol Metab.* 4(2):80-90.

Agarwal, A., Gupta, S., and Sharma, R.K. 2005. Role of oxidative stress in female reproduction. *Reprod Biol Endocrinol* 3:28.

Aguilo, A., Tauler, P., Sureda, A., Cases, N., Tur, J., and Pons, A. 2007. Antioxidant diet supplementation enhances aerobic performance in amateur sportsmen. *J Sports Sci* 25(11):1203-10.

Allen, D., Lamb, G., and Westerblad, H. 2008. Impaired calcium release during fatigue. *J Appl Physiol* 104:296-305.

Altman, T.A. 1998. In: FDA and USDA Nutrition Labelling Guide 9. Technomic Publishing Company Inc. Lancaster, PA. pp. 15-16.

Alway, S.E. 1997. Anatomy and kinesiology of skeletal muscle: The framework for movement. *Muscle Development* 31(3):34-35, 180-81.

Amann, M., Samuele, M., Nybo, L., Duhamel, T., Noakes, T., Jaquinandi, V., Saumet, J.L., Abraham, P., Ameredes, B., Burnley, M., Jones, A., Gandevia, S., Butler, J., and Taylor, J. 2008. *J Appl Physiol* 104:1543-46.

Ameredes, B.T., Zhan, W.Z., Vanderboom, R., Prakash, Y.S., and Sieck, G.C. 2000. Power fatigue of the rat diaphragm muscle. *J Appl Physiol* 89:2215-19.

Anderson, R.A. 1986. Chromium metabolism and its role in disease processes in man. *Clin Physiol Biochem* 4(1):31-41.

Anderson, R.A., Polansky, M.M., Bryden, N.A., et al. 1982. Effect of exercise (running) on serum glucose, insulin, glucagon, and chromium excretion. *Diabetes* 31(3):212-16.

Andriamanalijaona, R., Kypriotou, M., Bauge, C., Renard, E., Legendre, F., Raoudi, M., Boumediene, K., Gatto, H., Monginoux, P., and Pujol, J.P. 2005. Comparitive effects of 2 antioxidants, selenomethionine and epigallocatechin-gallate, on catabolic and anabolic gene expression of articular chondrocytes. *J Rheumatol* 32(10):1958-67.

Appell, H.J. 1990. Muscular atrophy following immobilization: A review. *Sports Med* 10(1):42-58.

Arivazhagan, P., Ramanathan, K., and Panneerselvam, C. 2001. Effect of DL-alpha-lipoic acid on mitochondrial enzymes in aged rats. *Chem Biol Interact* 138(2):189-98.

Armstrong, R.B. 1986. Muscle damage and endurance events. *Sports Med* 3:370-81.

Arnheim, D. 1989. *Modern principles of athletic training*, 7th ed. St. Louis: Times Mirror/Mosby.

Ascherio, A., Rimm, E.B., Stampfer, M.J., Giovannucci, E.L., and Willett, W.C. 1995. Dietary intake of marine n-3 fatty acids, fish intake, and the risk of coronary disease among men. *N Engl J Med* 332(15):977-82.

Asmussen, E., and Mazin, K. 1978. A central nervous component in local muscular fatigue. *Europ J Appl Physiol* 38:9-15.

Aviram, M., and Eias, K. 1993. Dietary olive oil reduces low-density lipoprotein uptake by macrophages and decreases the susceptibility of the lipoprotein to undergo lipid peroxidation. *Ann Nutr Metab* 37(2):75-84.

Awad, A.B., and Zepp, E.A. 1979. Alteration of rat adipose tissue lipolytic response to norepinephrine by dietary fatty acid manipulation. *Biochem Biophys Res Comm* 86:138-44.

Babichev, V.N., Peryshkova, T.A., Aivazashvili, N.I., and Shishkin, I.V. 1989. Effect of alcohol on the content of sex steroid receptors in the hypothalamus and hypophysis of male rats. Biull Eksp Biol Med 107(2):204-7.

Barham, J.B., Edens, M.B., Fonteh, A.N., Johnson, M.M., Easter, L., and Chilton, F.H. 2000. Addition of eicosapentaenoic acid to gamma-linolenic acid-supplemented diets prevents serum arachidonic acid accumulation in humans. *J Nutr* 130(8):1925-31.

Barnett, G., Chiang, C.W., and Licko, V.J. 1983. Effects of marijuana on testosterone in male subjects. *Theor Biol* 104(4):685-92.

Baroga, L. 1978. Contemporary tendencies in the methodology of strength development. *Educatia Fizica si Sport* 6:22-36.

Bartoszewska, M., Kamboj, M., and Patel, D.R. 2010. Vitamin D, muscle function, and exercise performance. *Pediatr Clin North Am* 57(3):849-61.

Bartram, H.P., Gostner, A., Scheppach, W., et al. 1993. Effects of fish oil on rectal cell proliferation, mucosal fatty acids, and prostaglandin E2 release in healthy subjects. *Gastroenterology* 105(5):1317-22.

Bast, A., and Haenen, G.R. 2003. Lipoic acid: A multifunctional antioxidant. *Biofactors* 17(1-4):207-13.

Beaufrere, B., Chassard, D., Broussolle, C., Riou, J.P., and Beylot, M. 1992. Effects of D-beta-hydroxybutyrate and long- and medium-chain triglycerides on leucine metabolism in humans. *Am J Physiol (Endocrinol Metab)* 262(3 Pt. 1):E268-74.

Behm, D.G. 1995. Neuromuscular implications and applications of resistance training. *J Strength Condit Res* 9:264-74.

Belzung, F., Raclot, T., and Groscolas, R. 1993. Fish oil n-3 fatty acids selectively limit the hypertrophy of abdominal fat depots in growing rats fed high-fat diets. *Am J Physiol* 264(6 Pt 2): R1111-18.

Bendich, A. 1989. Symposium conclusions: Biological actions of carotenoids. *J Nutr* 119(1):135-36.

Bhasin, S., Woodhouse, L., Casaburi, R., Singh, A.B., Bhasin, D., Berman, N., Chen, X., Yarasheski, K.E., Magliano, L., Dzekov, C., Dzekov, J., Bross, R., Phillips, J., Sinha-Hikim, I., Shen, R., and Storer, T.W. 2001. Testosterone dose-response relationships in healthy young men. *Am J Physiol Endocrinol Metab* 281:E1172-81.

Bhathena, S.J., Berlin, E., Judd, J.T., et al. 1989. Dietary fat and menstrual-cycle effects on the erythrocyte ghost insulin receptor in premenopausal women. *Am J Clin Nutr* 50(3):460-64.

Bigland-Ritchie, B., Kakula, C., Lippold, O., and Woods, J. 1982. The absence of neuromuscular junction failure in sustained maximal voluntary contractions. *J Physiol* (Lond) 330:265-78.4

Biolo, G., Fleming, R.Y.D., and Wolfe, R.R. 1995. Physiologic hyperinsulinemia stimulates protein synthesis and enhances transport of selected amino acids in human skeletal muscle. *J Clin Invest* 95:811-19.

Blankson, H., Stakkestad, J.A., Fagertun, H., Thom, E., Wadstein, J., and Gudmundsen, O. 2000. Conjugated linoleic acid reduces body fat mass in overweight and obese humans. *J Nutr* 130(12):2943-48.

Blundell, T.L., Bedarkar, S., Rinderknecht, E., and Humbel, R.E. 1979. Insulin-like growth factors: A model for tertiary structure accounting for immunoreactivity and receptor binding. *Proc Natl Acad Sci U.S.A.* 75:180-84.

Boden, G., Jadali, F., Liang, Y., Mozzoli, M., Chen, X., Coleman, E., and Smith, C. 1991. Effects of fat metabolism on insulin-stimulated carbohydrate metabolism in normal men. *J Clin Invest* 88(3):960-66.

Bompa, T.O. 1999. *Periodization: Theory and methodology of training*. Champaign, IL: Human Kinetics.

Bompa, T.O., and Cornacchia, L.J. 1998. *Serious strength training*. Champaign, IL: Human Kinetics.

Bompa, T.O., Di Pasquale, M., and Cornacchia, L.J. 2003. *Serious strength training, second edition*. Champaign, IL: Human Kinetics.

Bond, V., Adams, R., Gresham, K., Tearney, R., Caprarola, M., Ruff, W., Gregory, H., and Stoddart, A. 2005. Human performance lab, Howard University, Washington, DC.

Bonjour, J.P., Guéguen, L., Palacios, C., Shearer, M.J., and Weaver, C.M. 2009. Minerals and vitamins in bone health: The potential value of dietary enhancement. *Br J Nutr* 101(11):1581-96. Epub 2009 Apr 1.

Booth, F., and Thomason, D. 1991. Molecular and cellular adaptation of muscle in response to exercise: Perspectives of various models. *Physiological Reviews* 71:541-85.

Booyens, J., Louwrens, C.C., and Katzeff, I.E. 1986. The Eskimo diet: Prophylactic effects ascribed to the balanced presence of natural cis unsaturated fatty acids and the absence of unnatural trans and cis isomers of unsaturated fatty acids. *Medical Hypotheses* 21(4):387-408.

Borer, K.T. 1994. Neurohumoral mediation of exercise-induced growth. *Med Sci Sport Exerc* 26(6):741-54.

Brehm, B.J., Seeley, R.J., Daniels, S.R., and D'Alessio, D.A. 2003. A randomized trial comparing a very low carbohydrate diet and a calorie-restricted low fat diet on body weight and cardiovascular risk factors in healthy women. *J Clin Endocrinol Metab* 88:1617-23.

Brilla, L.R., and Haley, T.F. 1992. Effect of magnesium supplementation on strength training in humans. *J Am Coll Nutr* 11(3):326-29.

Brown, A.D., Wallace, P., and Breachtel, G. 1987. In vivo regulation of non-insulin mediated and insulin mediated glucose uptake by cortisol. *Diabetes* 36:1230-37.

Bucci, L., Hickson, J.F., Jr., Pivarnik, J.M., et al. 1990. Ornithine ingestion and growth hormone release in bodybuilders. *Nutr Res* 10(3):239-45.

Buell, J.S., Scott, T.M., Dawson-Hughes, B., Dallal, G.E., Rosenberg, I.H., Folstein, M.F., et al. 2009. Vitamin D is associated with cognitive function in elders receiving home health services. Js Gerontol. Series A, *Biol Sci Med Sci* 64:888-895.

Burkart, V., Koike, T., Brenner, H.H., Imai, Y., and Kolb, H. 1993. Dihydrolipoic acid protects pancreatic islet cells from inflammatory attack. *Agents Actions* 38(1-2):60-65.

Butterfield, G., and Calloway, D.H. 1984. Physical activity improves protein utilization in young men. *Br J Nutr* 51:171-84.

Campbell, W.W., Barton, M.L., Jr., Cyr-Campbell, D., Davey, S.L., Beard, J.L., Parise, G., and Evans, W.J. 1999. Effects of an omnivorous diet compared with a lacto-ovo vegetarian diet on resistance-training-induced changes in body composition and skeletal muscle in older men. *Am J Clin Nutr* 70(6):1032-39.

Carey, A.L., Staudacher, H.M., Cummings, N.K., Stepto, N.K., Nikolopoulos, V., Burke, L.M., and Hawley, J.A. 2001. Effects of fat adaption and carbohydrate restoration on prolonged endurance exercise. *J Appl Physiol* 91(1):115-22.

Carrithers, J.A., Williamson, D.L., Gallagher, P.M., Godard, M.P., Schulze, K.E., and Trappe, S.W. 2000. Effects of postexercise carbohydrate-protein feedings on muscle glycogen restoration. *J Appl Physiol* 88(6):1976-82.

Cartee, G.D., Yong, D.A., Sleeper, M.D., Zierath, J., Wallberg-Henriksson, H., and Halloszy, J.O. 1989. Prolonged increase in insulin-stimulated glucose transport in muscle after exercise. *Am J Physiol Endocrinol Metab* 256:E494-99.

Ceglia, L. 2008. Vitamin D and skeletal muscle tissue and function. *Mol Aspects Med* 29(6):407-14.

Chanez, M., Bois-Joyeux, B., Arnaud, M.J., and Peret, J. 1988. Long-term consumption of a diet with moderate medium chain triglyceride content does not inhibit the activity of enzymes involved in hepatic lipogenesis in the rat. [French] Comptes Rendus de I Academie des Sciences – Serie Iii, Sciences de la vie. 307(12):685-8.

Cheung, K., Hume, P., and Maxwell, L. 2003. Delayed onset muscle soreness: Treatment strategies and performance factors. *Sports Med* 33(2):145-64.

Chou, K.H., and Bell, L.N. 2007. Caffeine content of prepackaged national-brand and private-label carbonated beverages. *J Food Sci* 72(6):C337-42.

Chung, K.W. 1989. Effect of ethanol on androgen receptors in the anterior pituitary, hypothalamus and brain cortex in rats. *Life Sci* 44(4):2273-80.

Clark, M.G., Wallis, M.G., Barrett, E.J., Vincent, M.A., Richards, S.M., Clerk, L.H., and Rattigan, S. 2003. Blood flow and muscle metabolism: A focus on insulin action. *Am J Physiol Endocrinol Metab* 284(2):E241-58.

Clifton, P.M., Noakes, M., Keogh, J., and Foster, P. 2003. Effect of an energy reduced high protein red meat diet on weight loss and metabolic parameters in obese women. *Asia Pac J Clin Nutr* 12(Suppl):S10.

Close, G.L., Ashton, T., Mcardle, A., and Maclaren, D.P. 2005. The emerging role of free radicals in delayed onset muscle soreness and contraction-induced injury. *Comp Biochem Physiol* 142:257-66.

Cohen, D.L., and Townsend, R.R. Does consumption of high-caffeine energy drinks affect blood pressure? *J Clin Hypertens* (Greenwich) 8(10):744-45.

Conley, K. 1994. Cellular energetics during exercise. *Adv Vet Sci Comp Med* 38A:1-39.

Cook, M.E., Miller, C.C., Park, Y., and Pariza, M. 1993. Immune modulation by altered nutrient metabolism: Nutritional control of immune-induced growth depression. *Poultry Sci* 72(7):1301-5.

Cordova, A., and Alvarez-Mon, M. 1995. Behaviour of zinc in physical exercise: A special reference to immunity and fatigue. *Neurosci Biobehav Rev* 19(3):439-45.

Coronado, R., Morrissette, J., Sukhareva, M., and Vaughan, D.M. 1994. Structure and function of ryanodine receptors. *Am J Physiol Cell Physiol* 266:C1485-504.

Cowburn, G., and Stockley, L. 2005. Consumer understanding and use of nutrition labeling: A systematic review. *Public Health Nutr* 8(1):21-28.

Curtis, C.L., Hughes, C.E., Flannery, C.R., Little, C.B., Harwood, J.L., and Caterson, B. 2000. N-3 fatty acids specifically modulate catabolic factors involved in articular cartilage degradation. *J Biol Chem* 275(2):721-24.

Dartnall, T., Nordstrom, M., and Semmler, J. 2008. *J Neurophysiol* 99:1008-19.

Davidson, M.H., Hunningshake, D., Maki, K.C., et al. 1999. Comparison of the effects of lean red meat vs lean white meat on serum lipid levels among free-living persons with hypercholesterolemia: A long term, randomized clinical trial. *Arch Intern Med* 159:1331-38.

Davis, J.M., Murphy, E.A., Carmichael, M.D., and Davis, B. 2009. Quercetin increases brain and muscle mitochondrial biogenesis and exercise tolerance. *Am J Physiol Regul Integr Comp Physiol*. 2009 296(4):R1071-77.

de Vogel, S., Dindore, V., van Engeland, M., Goldbohm, R.A., van den Brandt, P.A., and Weijenberg, M.P. 2008. Dietary folate, methionine, riboflavin, and vitamin B-6 and risk of sporadic colorectal cancer. *J Nutr* 138(12):2372-78.

Deitmer, J.W. 2001. Strategies for metabolic exchange between glial cells and neurons. *Respir Physiol* 129(1-2):71-81.

Dela, F., Larsen, J.J., Mikines, K.J., Ploug, T., Petersen, L.N., and Galbo, H. 1995. Insulin-stimulated muscle glucose clearance in patients with NIDDM: Effects of one-legged physical training. *Diabetes* 44:1010-20.

DeLuca, C.J., and Forrest, W.J. 1973. Some properties of motor unit action potential trains recorded during constant force isometric contractions in man. *Kybernetik* 12:160-68.

DeLuca, C.J., LeFever, R.S., McCue, M.P., and Xenakis, A.P. 1982. Behaviour of human motor units in different muscles during linearly varying contractions. *J Physiol* (Lond) 329:113-28.

Denke, M.A., and Grundy, S.M. 1991. Effects of fats high in stearic acid on lipid and lipoprotein concentrations in men. *Am J Clin Nutr* 54(6):1036-40.

Derave, W., Lund, S., Holman, G., Wojtaszewski, J., Pedersen, O., and Richter, E.A. 1999. Contraction-stimulated muscle glucose transport and GLUT-4 surface content are dependent on glycogen content. *Am J Physiol Endocrinol Metab* 277:E1103-10.

Desbrow, B., Hughes, R., Leveritt, M., and Scheelings, P. 2007. An examination of consumer exposure to caffeine from retail coffee outlets. *Food Chem Toxicol* 45(9):1588-92. Epub 2007 Feb 23.

Deschenes, M.R., Kraemer, W.J., Maresh, C.M., and Crivello, J.F. 1991. Exercise-induced hormonal changes and their effects upon skeletal muscle tissue. *Sports Med* 12:80-93.

Di Pasquale, M. 1997. *Amino acids and proteins for the athlete: The anabolic edge.* Boca Raton, FL: CRC Press.

Di Pasquale, M. 2002-2008. *The Anabolic Solution.* MetabolicDiet.com Books, MD+ Press.

Di Pasquale, M.G. 2000. *The Metabolic Diet.* Austin, TX: Allprotraining.com Books.

Diamond, F., Ringenberg, L., MacDonald, D., et al. 1986. Effects of drug and alcohol abuse upon pituitary-testicular function in adolescent males. *Adol Health Care* 7(1):28-33.

Dinan, T.G., Thakore, J., and O'Keane, V. 1994. Lowering cortisol enhances growth hormone response to growth hormone releasing hormone in healthy subjects. *Acta Physiol Scand* 151:413-16.

Dinneen, S., Alzaid, A., Miles, J., and Rizza, R. 1993. Metabolic effects of the nocturnal rise in cortisol on carbohydrate metabolism in normal humans. *J Clin Invest* 92(5):2283-90.

Dodd, S.L., Herb, R.A., and Powers, S.K. 1993. Caffeine and exercise performance: An update. *Sports Med* 15(1):14-23.

Dorgan, J.F., Judd, J.T., Longcope, C., Brown, C., Schatzkin, A., Clevidence, B.A., Campbell, W.S., Nair, P.P., Franz, C., Kahle, L., and Taylor, P.R. 1996. Effects of dietary fat and fiber on plasma and urine androgens in men: A controlled feeding study. *Am J Clin Nutr* 64:850-55.

Dorup, I., Flyvbjerg, A., Everts, M.E., and Clausen. T. 1991. Role of insulin-like growth factor-1 and growth hormone in growth inhibition induced by magnesium and zinc deficiencies. *Brit J Nutr* 66(3):505-21.

Dragan, G.I., Vasiliu, A., and Georgescu, E. 1985. Research concerning the effects of Refit on elite weightlifters. *J Sports Med Physical Fitness* 25(4):246-50.

Dragan, G.I., Wagner, W., and Ploesteanu, E. 1988. Studies concerning the ergogenic value of protein supply and l-carnitine in elite junior cyclists. *Physiologie* 25(3):129-32.

Dray, F., Kouznetzova, B., Harris, D., and Brazeau, P. 1980. Role of prostaglandins on growth hormone secretion: PGE2 a physiological stimulator. *Adv Prostagl Thrombox Res* 8:1321-28.

Duhamel, T., Stewart, R., Tupling, A., Ouyang, J., and Green, H. 2007. *J Appl Physiol* 103:1212-20.

Duntas, L.H. 2009. Selenium and inflammation: Underlying anti-inflammatory mechanisms. *Horm Metab Res* 41(6):443-47.

Durnin, J.V. 1982. Muscle in sports medicine: Nutrition and muscular performance. *Int J Sports Med* 3(Suppl 1):52-57.

Ebbing, C., and P. Clarkson. 1989. Exercise-induced muscle damage and adaptation. *Sports Med* 7:207-34.

Enoka, R. 1996. Eccentric contractions require unique activation strategies by the nervous system. *J Appl Physiol* 81:2339-46.

Eritsland, J., Arnesen, H., Seljeflot, I., and Hostmark, A.T. 1995. Long-term metabolic effects of n-3 polyunsaturated fatty acids in patients with coronary artery disease. *Am J Clin Nutr* 61(4):831-36.

Evans, J.R. 2006. Antioxidant vitamin and mineral supplements for slowing the progression of age-related macular degeneration. *Cochrane Database Syst Rev* 19(2):CD000254.

Evans, W.J. 1987. Exercise-induced skeletal muscle damage. *Phys Sports Med* 15(1):89-100.

Evans, W.J., and Cannon, J.G. 1991. The metabolic effects of exercise-induced muscle damage. *Exerc Sport Sci Rev* 19:99-125.

Eyjolfson, V., Spriet, L.L., and Dyck, D.J. 2004. Conjugated linoleic acid improves insulin sensitivity in young sedentary humans. *Med Sci Sports Exerc* 36(5):814-20.

Fahey, TD. How to cope with muscle soreness. *Powerlifting USA.* 15 (7): 10-11, 1992.

Faust, A., Burkart, V., Ulrich, H., Weischer, C.H., and Kolb, H. 1994. Effect of lipoic acid on cyclophosphamide-induced diabetes and insulitis in non-obese diabetic mice. *Int J Immunopharmacol* 16(1):61-66.

Flatt, J.P. 1995. Use and storage of carbohydrate and fat. *Am J Clin Nutr* 61(Suppl 4):S952-59.

Fossati, P., and Fontaine, P. 1993. Endocrine and metabolic consequences of massive obesity. *Rev Praticien* 43(15):1935-39.

Fox, E.L., Bowes, R.W., and Foss, M.L. 1989. *The physiological basis of physical education and athletics.* Dubuque, IA: Brown.

Frederick, A., and Frederick, C. 2006. *Stretch to win.* Champaign, IL: Human Kinetics.

Fry, R.W., Morton, R., and Keast, D. 1991. Overtraining in athletics. *Sports Med* 2(1):32-65.

Fryburg, D.A. 1994. Insulin-like growth factor-1 exerts growth hormone- and insulin-like actions on human muscle protein metabolism. *Am J Physiol* 267:E331-36.

Fujioka, K., Greenway, F., Sheard, J., Ying, Y. 2006.The effects of grapefruit on weight and insulin resistance: relationship to the metabolic syndrome. *J Med. Food.* 9(1):49-54.

Ganong, W.F. 1988. The stress response: A dynamic overview. *Hosp Pract* 23:155-71.

Garcia-Roves, P.M., Han, D.H., Song, Z., Jones, T.E., Hucker, K.A., and Holloszy, J.O. Prevention of glycogen supercompensation prolongs the increase in muscle GLUT4 after exercise. *Am J Physiol Endocrinol Metab* 285:E729-36.

Garland, S.J., Enoka, R.M., Serrano, L.P., and Robinson, G.A. Behavior of motor units in human biceps brachii during a submaximal fatiguing contraction. *J Appl Physiol* 76:2411-19.

Garg, M.L., Wierzbicki, A., Keelan, M., Thomson, A.B., and Clandinin, M.T. 1989. Fish oil prevents change in arachidonic acid and cholesterol content in rats caused by dietary cholesterol. *Lipids* 24(4):266-70.

Garrandes, F., Colson, S., Pensini, M., Seynnes, O., and Legros, P. 2007. Neuromuscular fatigue profile in endurance-trained and power-trained athletes. *Med Sci Sports Exerc* 39(1):149-58.

Gaullier, J.M., Halse, J., Hoye, K., Kristiansen, K., Fagertun, H., Vik, H., and Gudmundsen, O. 2004. Conjugated linoleic acid supplementation for 1 year reduces body fat mass in healthy overweight humans. *Am J Clin Nutr* 79(6):1118-25.

Ghavami-Maibodi, S.Z., Collipp, P.J., Castro-Magana, M., Stewart, C., and Chen, S.Y. 1983. Effect of oral zinc supplements on growth, hormonal levels and zinc in healthy short children. *Ann Nutr Metab* 273:214-19.

Gohil, K., Rothfuss, L., Lang, J., and Packer, L. 1987. Effect of exercise training on tissue vitamin E and ubiquinone content. *J Appl Physiol* 63(4):1638-41.

Goldberg, A.L., Etlinger, J.D., Goldspink, D.F., and Jablecki, C. 1975. Mechanism of work-induced hypertrophy of skeletal muscles. *Med Sci Sports Exerc* 7:185-98.

Goldin, B.R., Woods, M.N., Spiegelman, D.L., et al. 1994. The effect of dietary fat and fiber on serum estrogen concentrations in premenopausal women under controlled dietary conditions. *Cancer* 74(Suppl 3):1125-31.

Goodman, M.N., Lowell, B., Belur, E., and Ruderman, N.B. 1984. Sites of protein conservation and loss during starvation: Influence of adiposity. *Am J Physiol* 246(5 Pt 1):E383-90.

Grandjean, A.C. 1983. Vitamins, diet, and the athlete. *Clin Sports Med* 2(1):105-14.

Grimby, G. 1992. *Strength and power in sport*, ed. P.V. Komi. Oxford: Blackwell Scientific.

Habito, R.C., Montalto, J., Leslie, E., and Ball, M.J. 2000. Effects of replacing meat with soybean in the diet on sex hormone concentrations in healthy adult males. *Br J Nutr* 84(4):557-63.

Haden, T., Lox, C., Rose, P., Reid, S., and Kirk, E.P. 2011. One-set resistance training elevates energy expenditure for 72 h similar to three sets. *Eur J Appl Physiol* 111(3):477-84.

Hainaut, K., and Duchatteau, J. 1989. Muscle fatigue: Effects of training and disuse. *Muscle and Nerve* 12:660-69.

Hamalainen, E.K., Adlercreutz, H., Puska, P., et al. 1983. Decrease of serum total and free testosterone during a low-fat high-fiber diet. *J Steroid Biochem* 18(3):369-70.

Hamalainen, E.K., Adlercreutz, H., Puska, P., et al. 1984. Diet and serum sex hormones in healthy men. *J Steroid Biochem* 20(1):459-64.

Hamilton, B. 2010. Vitamin D and human skeletal muscle. *Scand J Med Sci Sports* 20(2):182-90.

Han, Y.S., Proctor, D.N., Geiger, P.C., and Sieck, G.C. 2001. Reserve capacity for ATP consumption during isometric contraction in human skeletal muscle fibers. *J Appl Physiol* 90(2):657-64.

Hannum, S.M. 2004. Potential impact of strawberries on human health: A review of the science. *Crit Rev Food Sci Nutr* 44(1):1-17.

Hansen, J.C., Pedersen, H.S., and Mulvad, G. 1994. Fatty acids and antioxidants in the Inuit diet. Their role in ischemic heart disease (IHD) and possible interactions with other dietary factors: A review. *Arctic Med Res* 53(1):4-17.

Hardin, D.S., Azzarelli, B., Edwards, J., Wigglesworth, J., Maianu, L., Brechtel, G., Johnson, A., Baron, A., and Garvey, W.T. 1995. Mechanisms of enhanced insulin sensitivity in endurance-trained athletes: Effects on blood flow and differential expression of GLUT4 in skeletal muscles. *J Clin EndocrinolMetab* 80:2437-46.

Harmon, A.W., and Patel, Y.M. 2003. Naringenin inhibits phosphoinositide 3-kinase activity and glucose uptake in 3T3-L1 adipocytes. *Biochem Biophys Res Commun* 305(2):229-34.

Harris, D.B., Harris, R.C., Wilson, A.M., and Goodship, A. 1997. ATP loss with exercise in muscle fibres of the gluteus medius of the thoroughbred horse. *Res Vet Sci* 63(3):231-37.

Harris, W.S. and Bulchandani, D. 2006. Why do omega-3 fatty acids lower serum triglycerides? *Curr Opin Lipid* 17(4):387-93.

Hartman, J.H., and Tünneman, H. 1988. *Fitness and strength training.* Berlin: Sportsverlag.

Hartoma, T.R., Nahoul, K., and Netter, A. 1977. Zinc, plasma androgens and male sterility. *Lancet* 2:1125-26.

Hawthorne, K.M., Moreland, K., Griffin, I.J., and Abrams, S.A. 2006. An educational program enhances food label understanding of young adolescents. *J Am Diet Assoc* 106(6):913-16.

Head, S. 2010. Branched fibres in old dystrophic mdx muscle are associated with mechanical weakening of the sarcolemma, abnormal Ca2+ transients and a breakdown of Ca2+ homeostasis during fatigue. *Exp Physiol* 95(5):641-56.

Heden, T., Lox, C., Rose, P., Reid, S., and Kirk, E.P. 2011. One-set resistance training elevates energy expenditure for 72 h similar to three sets. *Eur J Appl Physiol* 111(3):477-84.

Helge, J.W. 2000. Adaption to a fat-rich diet: Effects on endurance performance in humans. *Sports Med* 30(5):347-57.

Henriksen, E.J. 2002. Effects of acute exercise and exercise training on insulin resistance. *J Appl Physiol* 93:788-96.

Henzen, C. 1995. Fish oil-healing principle in the Eskimo Diet? *Schweizerische Rundschau für Medicine Praxis* 84(1):11-15.

Hickson, R.C., Czerwinski, S.M., Falduto, M.T., and Young, A.P. 1990. Glucocorticoid antagonism by exercise and androgenic-anabolic steroids. *Med Sci Sports Exerc* 22:331-40.

Hickson, R.C., Czerwinski, S.M., and Wegrzyn, L.E. 1995. Glutamine prevents downregulation of myosin heavy chain synthesis and muscle atrophy from glucocorticoids. *Am J Physiol* 268(4 Pt 1):E730-34.

Hickson, R.C., Kurowski, T.T., Andrews, G.H., et al. 1986. Glucocorticoid cytosol binding in exercise-induced sparing of muscle atrophy. *J Appl Physiol* 60:1413-19.

Higdon, J.V., and Frei, B. 2006. Coffee and health: A review of recent human research. *Crit Rev Food Sci Nutrition* 46(2):101-23.

Hodgson, J.M., Wahlqvist, M.L., Boxall, J.A., and Lalazs, N.D. 1993. Can linoleic acid contribute to coronary artery disease? *Am J Clin Nutr* 58(2):228-34.

Hodgson, J.M., Ward, N.C., Burke, V., Beilin, L.J., and Puddy, I.B. 2007. Increased lean red meat intake does not elevate markers of oxidative stress and inflammation in humans. *J Nutr* 137(2):363-67.

Holtz, K.A., Stephens, B.R., Sharoff, C.G., Chipkin, S.R., and Braun, B. 2008. The effect of carbohydrate availability following exercise on whole-body insulin action. *Appl Physiol Nutr Metab* 33(5):946-56.

Horber, F.F., and Haymond, M.W. 1990. Human growth hormone prevents the protein catabolic side effects of prednisone in humans. *J Clin Invest* 86:265-72.

Houmard, J.A. 1991. Impact of reduced training of performance in endurance athletes. *Sports Med* 12(6):380-93.

Howarth, K.R., Moreau, N.A., Phillips, S.M., and Gibala, M.J. 2009. Coingestion of protein with carbohydrate during recovery from endurance exercise stimulates skeletal muscle protein synthesis in humans. *J Appl Physiol* 106(4):1394-402. Epub 2008 Nov 26.

Howatson, G., and Someren, K. 2008. The prevention and treatment of exercise-induced muscle damage. *Sports Med* 38(6):483-503.

Howell, J., Chleboun, G., and Conatser, R. 1993. Muscle stiffness, strength loss, swelling and soreness following exercise-induced injury in humans. *J Phys* 464:183-96.

Hsu, J.M. 1977. Zinc deficiency and alterations of free amino acid levels in plasma, urine and skin extract. *Progr Clin Biol Res* 14:73-86.

Hubal, M., Rubinstein, S., and Clarkson, P. 2007. Mechanisms of variability in strength loss after muscle-lengthening actions. *Med Sci Sports Exerc* 39(3):461-68.

Hunt, C.D., Johnson, P.E., Herbel, J., and Mullen, L.K. 1992. Effects of dietary zinc depletion on seminal volume of zinc loss, serum testosterone concentrations and sperm morphology in young men. *Am J Clin Nutr* 56(1):148-57.

Hwang, S.G., Yano, H., and Kawashima, R. 1993. Institution department of animal science, faculty of agriculture, Kyoto University, Japan. Influence of dietary medium- and long-chain triglycerides on fat deposition and lipogenic enzymes activities in rats. *J Am Coll Nutr* 12(6):643-50.

Ingram, D.M., Bennett, F.C., Willcox, D., and de Klerk, N. 1987. Effect of low-fat diet on female sex hormone levels. *J Mat Cancer Inst* 79(6):1225-29.

Institute of Food Technologists. 2003. Food laws and regulations division, Newsletter Vol. 9, No. 1. Available at: www.ift.org .

Ip, C., Scimeca, J.A., and Thompson, H.J. 1994. Conjugated linoleic acid: A powerful anticarcinogen from animal fat sources. *Cancer* 74(Suppl 3):1050-54.

Ip, C., Singh, M., Thompson, H.J., and Scimeca, J.A. 1994. Conjugated linoleic acid suppresses mammary carcinogenesis and proliferative activity of the mammary gland in the rat. *Cancer Res* 54(5):1212-15.

Israel, S. 1972. The acute syndrome of detraining. *GDR National Olympic Committee* 2:30-35.

Ivy, J.L., and Holloszy, J.O. 1981. Persistent increase in glucose uptake by rat skeletal muscle following exercise. *Am J Physiol* 241:C200-203.

Ivy, J.L., Goforth, H.W., Jr., Damon, B.M., McCauley, T.R., Parsons, E.C., and Price, T.B. 2002. Early postexercise muscle glycogen recovery is enhanced with a carbohydrate-protein supplement. *J Appl Physiol* 93(4):1337-44.

Iwasaki, K., Mano, K., Ishihara, M., et al. 1987. Effects of ornithine or arginine administration on serum amino acid levels. *Biochem Int* 14(5):971-76.

Jacobson, B.H., Weber, M.D., Claypool, L., and Hunt, L.E. 1992. Effect of caffeine on maximal strength and power in elite male athletes. *Br J Sports Med* 26(4):276-80.

Jenkins, D.J.A. 1982. Lente carbohydrate: A newer approach to the management of diabetes. *Diabetes Care* 5:634-39.

Jenkins, D.J.A., Wolever, T.M.S., Collier, G.R., Ocana, A., Rao, A.V., Buckley, G., Lam, Y., Mayer, A., and Thompson, L.U. 1987. Metabolic effects of a low-glycemic-index diet. *Am J Clin Nutr* 46:968.

Jones, W., Li, X., Qu, Z.C., et al. 2002. Uptake, recycling, and antioxidant actions of alpha-lipoic acid in endothelial cells. *Free Radic Biol Med* 33:83-93.

Kara, E., Gunay, M., Cicioglu, I., Ozal, M., Kilic, M., Mogulkoc, R., and Baltaci A.K. 2010. Effect of zinc supplementation on antioxidant activity in young wrestlers. *Biol Trace Elem Res* 134(1):55-63.

Katan, M.B., Zock, P.L., and Mensink, R.P. 1994. Effects of fats and fatty acids on blood lipids in humans: An overview. *Am J Clin Nutr* 60(Suppl 6):S1017-22.

Kather, H., Wieland, E., Scheurer, A., Vogel, G., Wildenberg, U., and Joost, C. 1987. Influences of variation in total energy intake and dietary composition in regulation of fat cell lipolysis in ideal-weight subjects. *J Clin Inv* 80(2):566-72.

Katsouyanni, K., Skalkidis, Y., Petridou, E., et al. 1991. Diet and peripheral arterial occlusive disease: The role of poly-, mono-, and saturated fatty acids. *Am J Epidemiol* 133(1):24-31.

Kawanaka, K., Han, D., Nolte, L.A., Hansen, P.A., Nakatani, A., and Holloszy, J.O. 1999. Decreased insulin-stimulated GLUT-4 translocation in glycogen-super compensated muscles of exercised rats. *AmJ Physiol Endocrinol Metab* 276:E907-12.

Kerksick, C., Harvey, T., Stout, J., Campbell, B., Wilborn, C., Kreider, R., Kalman, D., Ziegenfuss, T., Lopez, H., Landis, J., Ivy, J.L., and Antonio, J. 2008. International Society of Sports Nutrition position stand: Nutrient timing. *J Int Soc Sports Nutr* 5:17.

Keys, A., Menotti, A., Karvonen, J., et al. 1986. The diet and 15-year-death rate in seven countries study. *Am J Epidemiol* 124(6):903-15.

Kieffer, F. 1986. [Trace elements: Their importance for health and physical performance.] *Deut Zeit Sportmed* 37(4):118-23.

Kinnunen, S., Hyyppa, S., Oksala, N., Laaksonen, D.E., Hannila, M.L., Sen, C.K., and Atalay, M. 2009. Alpha-lipoic acid supplementation enhances heat shock protein production and decreases postexercise lactic acid concentrations in exercised standardbred trotters. *Res Vet Sci* May 7.

Kirkendall, D.T. 1990. Mechanisms of peripheral fatigue. *Med Sci Sports Exerc* 22(4):444-49.

Kleiner, S., and Greenwood-Robinson, M. 2007. *Power eating*, 3rd ed. Champaign, IL: Human Kinetics.

Knab, A.M., Shanely, R.A., Corbin, K., Jin, F., Sha, W., and Nieman. D.C. 2011. A 45-minute vigorous exercise bout increased metabolic rate for 14 hours. *Med Sci Sports Exerc* 43(9):1643-48. Epub 2011 Feb 8.

Kobayashi, J., Yokoyama, S., and Kitamura, S. 1995. Eicosapentaenoic acid modulates arachidonic acid metabolism in rat alveolar macrophages. *Prostaglandins Leukot Essent Fatty Acids* 52(4):259-62.

Kobayashi Matsui, H. 1983. Analysis of myoelectric signals during dynamic and isometric contraction. *Electromyog Clin Neurophysiol* 26:147-60.

Kruger, M.C. 1995. Eicosapentaenoic acid and docosahexaenoic acid supplementation increases calcium balance. *Nutr Res* 5:211-19.

Kuipers, H., and Keizer, H.A. 1988. Overtraining in elite athletes: Review and directions for the future. *Sports Med* 6:79-92.

Laires, M.J., and Monterio, C. 2008. Exercise, magnesium and immune function. *Magnes Res* 21(2):92-96.

Lamb, G.D., and Stephenson, D.G.; Bangsbo, J., and Juel, C.J. 2006. Point:Counterpoint: Lactic acid accumulation is an advantage/disadvantage during muscle activity. *J Appl Physiol* 100:1410-14.

Lambert, E.V., Hawley, J.A., Goedecke, J., Noakes, T.D., and Dennis, S.C. 1997. Nutritional strategies for promoting fat utilization and delaying the onset of fatigue during prolonged exercise. *J Sports Sci* 15(3):315-24.

Lapachet, R.A., Miller, W.C., and Arnall, D.A. 1996. Body fat and exercise endurance in trained rats adapted to a high-fat and/or high-carbohydrate diet. *J Appl Physiol* 80(4):1173-79.

Laricheva, K.A., Ialovaia, N.I., Shubin, V.I., Smirnov, P.V., and Beliaev, V.S. 1977. Use of the specialized protein product, SP-11, in the nutrition of highly trained sportsmen in heavy athletics. *Vopr Pitan* Jul-Aug(4):47-51.

Lateef, H., Aslam, M.N., Stevens, M.J., and Varani, J. 2005. Pretreatment of diabetic rats with lipoic acid improves healing of subsequently-induced abrasion wounds. *Arch Dermatol Res* 297(2):75-83.

Lavoie, J.M., Helie, R., Peronnet, F., Cousineau, D., and Provencher, P.J. 1985. Effects of muscle CHO-loading manipulations on hormonal responses during prolonged exercise. *Int J Sports Med* 6(2):95-99.

Lavy, A., Ben-Amotz, A., and Aviram, M. 1993. Preferential inhibition of LDL oxidation by the all-trans isomer of beta-carotene in comparison with 9-cis beta-carotene. *Eur J Clin Chem Clin Biochem* 31(2):83-90.

Lee, H.A., and Hughes, D.A. 2002. Alpha-lipoic acid modulates NF-kappaB activity in human monocytic cells by direct interaction with DNA. *Exp Gerontol* 37(2-3):401-10.

Leenen, R., Roodenburg, A.J., Vissers, M.N., Schuurbiers, J.A., van Putte, K.P., Wieman, S.A., and van de Put, F.H. 2002. Supplementation of plasma with olive oil phenols and extracts: Influence on LDL oxidation. *J Agric Food Chem* 50(5):1290-97.

Lefavi, R.G., Anderson, R.A., Keith, R.E., et al. 1992. Efficacy of chromium supplementation in athletes: Emphasis on anabolism. *Int J Sport Nutr* 2(2):111-22.

Lefebvre, P.J., and Scheen, A.J. 1995. Improving the action of insulin. *Medecine Clinique et Experimentale[Clin Invest Med* 18(4):340-47.

Lemon, P.W. 1998. Effects of exercise on dietary protein requirements. *Int J Sport Nutr* 8(4):426-47.

Lemon, P.W. 2000. Beyond the zone: Protein needs of active individuals. *J Am Coll Nutr* Oct19(Suppl 5):S513-21.

Lichtenstein, A.H., Ausman, L.M., Carrasco, W., et al. 1993. Effects of canola, corn, and olive oils on fasting and postprandial plasma lipoproteins in humans as part of a National Cholesterol Education Program Step 2 diet. *Arterioscl Thromb* 13(10):1533-42.

Lichtenstein, A.H., Ausman, L.M., Carrasco, W., et al. 1994. Rice bran oil consumption and plasma lipid levels in moderately hypercholesterolemic humans. *Arterioscl Thromb* 14(4):549-56.

Liu, S., Baracos, V.E., Quinney, H.A., and Clandinin, M.T. 1994. Dietary omega-3 and polyunsaturated fatty acids modify fatty acyl composition and insulin binding in skeletal-muscle sarcolemma. *Biochem J* 299(Pt 3):831-37.

Lukasju, H.C.L. 2005. Low dietary zinc decreases erythrocyte carbonic anhydrase activities and impairs cardiorespiratory function in men during exercise. *Am J Clin Nutr* 81:1045-51.

Maassen, N., and Schneider, G. 1997. Mechanism of fatigue in small muscle groups. *Int J Sports Med* 18(4):S320-21.

Magistretti, P.J., and Pellerin, L. 2000. Functional brain imaging: Role metabolic coupling between astrocytes and neurons. *Rev Med Suisse Romande* 120(9):739-42.

Mai, K., Bobbert, T., Kullmann, V., Anders, J., Rochlitz, H., Osterhoff, M., Weickert, M.O., Bahr, V., Mohlig, M., Pfeiffer, A.F., Diederich, S., and Spranger, J. 2006. Free fatty acids increase androgen precursors in vivo. *J Clin Endocrinol Metab* 91(4):1501-7.

Malomsoki, J. 1983. [The improvement of sports performance by means of complementary nutrition]. *Sportorvosi szemle [Hungarian Review of Sports Medicine]* 24(4):269-82.

Manninen, A.H. 2006. Hyperinsulinaemia, hyperaminoacidaemia and post-exercise muscle anabolism: The search for the optimal recovery drink. *Br J Sports Med* 40(11):900-905.

Mantzioris, E., James, M.J., Givson, R.A., and Cleland, L.G. 1995. Differences exist in relationships between dietary linoleic and alpha-linolenic acids and their respective long-chain metabolites. *Am J Clin Nutr* 61(2):320-24.

Margaritis, I., Rousseau, A.S., Hininger, I., Palazzetti, S., Arnaud, J., and Roussel, A.M. 2005. Increase in selenium requirements with physical activity loads in well-trained athletes is not linear. *Biofactors* 23(1):45-55.

Mariotti, F., Mahe, S., Luengo, C., Benamouzig, R., and Tome, D. 2000. Postprandial modulation of dietary and whole-body nitrogen utilization by carbohydrates in humans. *Am J Clin Nutr* 72:954-62.

Marsden, C.D., Meadows, J.C., and Merton, P.A. 1971. Isolated single motor units in human muscle and their rate of discharge during maximum voluntary effort. *J Physiol* (London) 217:12P.

Massaro, M., Carluccio, M.A., and De Caterina, R. 1999. Direct vascular anti-atherogenic effects of oleic acid: A clue to the cardioprotective effects of the Mediterranean diet. *Cardiologia* 44(6):507-13.

Matsuda, J.J., Zermocle, R.F., Vailus, A.C., Perrini, V.A., Pedrini-Mille, A., and Maynard, J.A. 1986. Structural and mechanical adaptation of immature bone to strenuous exercise. *J Appl Physiol* 60(6):2028-34.

Mauras, N., and Beaufrere, B. 1995. Recombinant human insulin-like growth factor-1 enhances whole body protein anabolism and significantly diminishes the protein catabolic effects of prednisone in humans without a diabetogenic effect. *J Clin Endocrinol Metab* 80(3):869-74.

May, M.E., and Buse, M.G. 1989. Effects of branched-chain amino acids on protein turnover. *Diab Metab Rev* 5(3):227-45.

Mcbride, J.M., Kraemer, W.J., Triplett-Mcbride, T., and Sebastianelli, W. 1998. Effect of resistance exercise on free radical production. *Med Sci Sports Exerc* (3):67-72.

McCall, G.E., Byrnes, W.C., Dickinson, A., Pattany, P.M., and Fleck, S.J. 1996. Muscle fiber hypertrophy, hyperplasia and capillary density in college men after resistance training. *J Appl Physiol* 81:2004-12

McCarger, L.J., Baracos, V.E., and Calandinin, M.T. 1989. Influence of dietary carbohydrate-to-fat ratio on whole body nitrogen retention and body composition in adult rates. *J Nutr* 199(9):1240-45.

McCusker, R.R., Fuehrlein, B., Goldberger, B.A., Gold, M.S., and Cone, E.J. 2006. Caffeine content of decaffeinated coffee. *J Anal Toxicol* 30(8):611-13.

McCusker, R.R., Goldberger, B.A., and Cone, E.J. 2003. Caffeine content of specialty coffees. *J Anal Toxicol* 27:520-22.

McNamara, D.J. 1992. Dietary fatty acids, lipoproteins, and cardiovascular disease. *Adv Food Nutr Res* 36:253-351.

McNaughton, L.R. 1986. The influence of caffeine ingestion on incremental treadmill running. *Br J Sports Med* 20(3):109-12.

Melo, G.L., and Cararelli, E. 1994-1995. Exercise physiology laboratory manual, 25.

Mendelson, J.H., Mello, N.K., Teoh, S.K., Ellingboe, J., and Cochin, J. 1989. Cocaine effects on pulsatile secretion of anterior pituitary, gonadal and adrenal hormones. *J Clin Endocrinol Metab* 69(6):1256-60.

Mensink, R.P., Zock, P.L., Katan, M.B., and Hornstra, G. 1992. Effect of dietary cis and trans fatty acids on serum lipoprotein[a] levels in humans. *J Lipid Res* 33(10):1493-501.

Metges, C.C., and Barth, C.A. 2000. Metabolic consequences of a high dietary-protein intake in adulthood: Assessment of the available evidence. *J Nutr* 130:886-89.

Miller, B.F. 2007. Human muscle protein synthesis after physical activity and feeding. *Exerc Sport Sci Rev* 35(2):50-55.

Miller, C.C., Park, Y., Pariza, M.W., and Cook, M.E. 1994. Feeding conjugated linoleic acid to animals partially overcomes catabolic responses due to endotoxin injection. *Biochem Biophysic Res Comm* 198(3):1107-12.

Millward, D.J. 1999. Optimal intakes of protein in the human diet. *Proc Nutr Soc* 58(2):403-13.

Morgan, R.E., and Adamson, G.T. 1959. *Circuit weight training*. London: Bell.

Morifuji, M., Sakai, K., Sanbongi, C., and Sugiura, K. 2005. Dietary whey protein increases liver and skeletal muscle glycogen levels in exercise-trained rats. *Br J Nutr* 93(4):439-45.

Moritani, T., and deVries, H.A. 1987. Re-examination of the relationship between the surface integrated electromyogram (IEMG) and force of isometric contraction. *Am J Physiol Med* 57:263-77.

Moritani, T., Muro, M., and Nagata, A. 1986. Intramuscular and surface electromyogram changes during muscle fatigue. *J Appl Physiol* 60:1179-85.

Mozaffarian, D., Katan, M.B., Ascherio, A., Stampfer, M.J., and Willett, W.C. 2006. Trans fatty acids and cardiovascular disease. *N Engl J Med* 354:1601-13.

Muthalib, M., Lee, H., Millet, G., Ferrari, M., and Nosaka, K. 2010. *J Appl Physiol* 109:710-20.

National Research Council. 1989. Protein and amino acids. In *Recommended dietary allowances*, 10th ed. Washington, DC: National Academy Press.

Nawrot, P., Jordan, S., Eastwood, J., Rotstein, J., Hugenholtz, A., and Feeley, M. 2003. Effects of caffeine on human health. *Food Addit Contam* 20(1):1-30.

Nelson, A.G., and Kokkonen, J. 2007. *Stretching anatomy.* Champaign, IL: Human Kinetics.

Newman, K.P., Neal, M.T., Roberts, M., Goodwin, K.D., Hatcher, E.A., and Bhattacharya, S.K. 2007. The importance of lost minerals in heart failure. *Cardiovasc Hematol Agents Med Chem* 5(4):295-99.

Ni, J.S., Wu, J.X., and Xiao, R.Q. 1994. The preventative and curative action of fish oil compound on early atherosclerotic lesions in the aortic of diabetic rats. *Chung-Hua Ping Li Hsueh Tsa Chih[Chinese Journal of Pathology]* 23(1):31-33.

Nielsen, F.H., and Lukaski, H.C. 2006. Update on the relationship between magnesium and exercise. *Magnes Res* 19(3):180-89.

Nielsen, O.B., de Paoli, F., and Overgaard, K. 2001. Protective effects of lactic acid on force production in rat skeletal muscle. *J Physiol* 536(Pt 1):161-66.

Nosaka, K., Newton, M., and Sacco P. 2002. Muscle damage and soreness after endurance exercise of the elbow flexors. *Med Sci Sports Exerc* 34(6):920-27.

Noth, R.H., and Walter, R.M. 1984. The effects of alcohol on the endocrine system. *Med Clin North Am* 68(1):133-46.

Nybo, L. 2008. Hyperthermia and fatigue. *J Appl Physiol* 104:871-78.

Nybo, L., and Nielsen, B. 2001. Hyperthermia and central fatigue during prolonged exercise in humans. *J Appl Physiol* 91:1055-60.

Obici, S., Feng, Z., Morgan, K., Stein, D., Karkanias, G., and Rossetti, L. 2002. Central administration of oleic acid inhibits glucose production and food intake. *Diabetes* 51(2):271-75.

Ohtsuka, A., Hayashi, K., Noda, T., and Tomita, Y. 1992. Reduction of corticosterone-induced muscle proteolysis and growth retardation by a combined treatment with insulin, testosterone and high protein-high-fat diets in rats. *J Nutr Sci Vitaminol* 38(1):83-92.

Opstad, P.K., and Asskvaag, A. 1983. The effect of sleep deprivation on the plasma levels of hormones during prolonged physical strain and calorie deficiency. *Eur J Appl Phys Occup Phys* 51(1):97-107.

O'Sullivan, U.P., Gluckman, D., Breier, B.H., et al. 1989. Insulin-like growth factor-1 (IGF-1) in mice reduces weight loss during starvation. *Endocrinology* 125:2793-95.

Oteiza, P.I., Olin, K.L., Fraga, C.G., and Keen, C.L. 1995. Zinc deficiency causes oxidative damage to proteins, lipids and DNA in rat testes. *J Nutr* 125(4):823-29.

Packer, L. 1997. Oxidants, antioxidant nutrients and the athlete. *J Sports Sci* 15(3):353-63.

Packer, L. 1998. Alpha lipoic acid: A metabolic antioxidant which regulates NF-kappaB signal transduction and protects against oxidative injury. *Drug Metab Rev* 30:245-75.

Packer, L., and Landvik, S.I. 1989. Vitamin E: Introduction to biochemistry and health benefits. *Ann NY Acad Sci* 570:1-6.

Packer, L., Tritschler, H.J., and Wessel, K. 1997. Neuroprotection by the metabolic antioxidant alpha-lipoic acid. *Free Radic Biol Med* 22(1-2):359-78.

Packer, L., Witt, E.H., and Tritschler, H.J. 1995. Alpha-lipoic acid as a biological antioxidant. *Free Radic Biol Med* 19:227-50.

Paffenbarger, R.S., Jr., Kampert, J.B., Lee, I.M., et al. 1994. Changes in physical activity and other lifeway patterns influencing longevity. *Med Sci Sports Exerc* 26(7):857-65.

Palaniappan, A.R., and Daim A. 2007. Mitochondrial ageing and the beneficial role of alpha-lipoic acid. *Neurochem Res* 32(9):1552-58.

Pariza, M.W., Ha, Y.L., Benjamin, H., et al. 1991. Formation and action of anti-carcinogenic fatty acids. *Adv Exper Med Biol* 289:269-72.

Parrish, C.C., Pathy, D.A., and Angel, A. 1990. Dietary fish oils limit adipose tissue hypertrophy in rats. *Metabolism: Clin Exp* 39(3):217-19.

Parrish, C.C., Pathy,D.A., Parkes, J.G., and Angel, A. 1991. Dietary fish oils modify adipocyte structure and function. *J Cell Phys* 148(3):493-502.

Patrick, L. 2002. Mercury toxicity and antioxidants: Part1: Role of glutathione and alpha-lipoic acid in the treatment of mercury toxicity. *Altern Med Rev* 7(6):456-71.

Pedersen, B.K., Steensberg, A., and Schjerling, P. 2001. Muscle-derived interleukin-6: Possible biological effects. *J Physiol* 536(Pt 2):329-37.

Philip, W., James, T., and Ralph, A. 1992. Dietary fats and cancer. *Nutr Res 12* (Suppl):S147-58.

Pitsiladis, Y.P., Smith, I., and Maughan, R.J. 1999. Increased fat availability enhances the capacity of trained individuals to perform prolonged exercise. *Med Sci Sports Exercise* 21(11):1570-79.

Podda, M., Tritschler, H.J., Ulrich, H., et al. 1994. Aplha-lipoic acid supplementation prevents symptoms of vitamin E deficiency. *Biochem Biophys Res Commun* 204:98-104.

Pogliaghi, S., and Veicstenias, A. 1999. Influence of low and high dietary fat on physical performance in untrained males. *Med Sci Sports Exerc* 31(1):149-55.

Posterino, G.S., Dutka, T.L., and Lamb, G.D. 2001. L(+)-lactate does not affect twitch and tetanic responses in mechanically skinned mammalian muscle fibres. *Pflugers Arch* 442(2):197-203.

Powers, M.*Guide to eating right when you have diabetes*. Hoboken, NJ: John Wiley & Sons. 2003: 130, 139.

Powers, S., and Howley, E. 2009. *Exercise physiology: Theory and application to fitness and performance*, 7th ed. New York: McGraw-Hill.

Prasad, A.S. 1996. Zinc deficiency in women, infants and children. *J Am Coll Nutr* 15(2):113-20.

Prentice, W.J. 1990. *Rehabilitation techniques in sports medicine.* Toronto: Times Mirror/Mosby College.

Proske, U., and Allen, T. 2005. Damage to skeletal muscle from eccentric exercise. *Exerc Sport Sci Rev* 33:98-104.

Rabast, U., Kasper, H., and Schonborn, J. 1978. Comparative studies in obese subjects fed carbohydrate-restricted and high carbohydrate 1,000-calorie formula diets. *Nutr Metab* 22(5):269-77.

Reid, M.B., Haack, K.E., Franchek, K.M., et al. 1992. Reactive oxygen in skeletal muscle. I. Intracellular oxidant kinetics and fatigue in vitro. *J Appl Physiol* 73(5):1797-804.

Ren, J.M., Semenkovich, C.F., Gulve, E.A., Gao, J., and Holloszy, J.O. 1994. Exercise induces rapid increases in GLUT4 expression glucose transport capacity and insulin-stimulated glycogen storage in muscle. *J Biol Chem* 269(20):14396-401.

Rennie, M.J., MacLennan, P.A., Hundal, H.S., et al. 1989. Skeletal muscle glutamine transport, intramuscular glutamine concentration, and muscle-protein turnover. *Metabolism* 38(Suppl 8):47-51.

Richardson, J.H., Palmerton, T., and Chenan, M. 1980. Effect of calcium on muscle fatigue. *J Sports Med Phys Fit* 20(2):149-51.

Rizza, R.A., Mandarino, L.J., and Gerich, J.E. 1982. Cortisol-induced insulin resistance in man: Impaired suppression of glucose production and stimulation of glucose utilization due to a postreceptor defect of insulin action. *J Clin Endocrinol Metab* 54:131-38.

Rose, D.P., Cannolly, J.M., Rayburn, J., and Coleman, M. 1995. Influence of diets containing eicosapentaenoic or docosahexaenoic acid on growth and metastasis of breast cancer cells in nude mice. *J Natl Cancer Inst* 87(8):587-92.

Rothman, R.L., Housam, R., Weiss, H., Davis, D., Gregory, R., Gebretsadi, T., Shintani, A., and Elasy, T.A. 2006. Patient understanding of food labels: The role of literacy and numeracy. *Am J Prev Med* 31(5):391-98.

Roy, B.D., and Tarnopolsky, M.A. 1998. Influence of differing macronutrient intakes on muscle glycogen resynthesis after resistance exercise. *J Appl Physiol* 84(3):890-96.

Ruegg, J. 1992. *Calcium in muscle activation.* Berlin: Springer-Verlag.

Ryschon, T.W., Fowler, M.D., Wysong, R.E., Anthony, A.R., and Balaban, R.S. 1997. Efficiency of human skeletal muscle in vivo: comparison of isometric, concentric, and eccentric muscle action. *J Appl Physiol* 83:867-74.

Sacheck, J., and Blumberg, J. 2001. Role of vitamin E and oxidative stress in exercise. *Nutrition* 17(10):809-814.

Sahlin, K. 1986. Metabolic changes limiting muscular performance. *Biochem Exerc* 16:22-31, 42-53.

Sallinen, J., Pakarinen, A., Ahtiainen, J., Kraemer, W.J., Volek, J.S., and Hakkinen, K. 2004. Relationship between diet and serum anabolic hormone responses to heavy resistance exercise in strength athletes and physically active males. *Int J Sports Med* 25:624-33.

Sallinen, J., Pakarinen, A., Fogelholm, M., Alen, M., Volek, J.S., Kraemer, W.J., and Hakkinen, K. 2007. Dietary intake, serum hormones, muscle mass and strength during strength training in 49-73 year old men. *Int J Sports Med* 28(12):1070-76.

Sanchez-Gomez, M., Malmlof, K., Mejia, W., Bermudez, A., Ochoa, M.T., Carrasco-Rodriguez, S., and Skottner, A. 1999. Insulin-like growth factor-I, but not growth hormone, is dependent on a high protein intake to increase nitrogen balance in the rat. *Br J Nutr* 81(2):145-52.

Sandretto, A.M., and Tsai, A.C. 1988. Effects of fat intake on body composition and hepatic lipogenic enzyme activities of hamsters shortly after exercise cessation. *Amer J Clin Nutr* 47(2):175-79.

Sangha, O., and Stucki, G. 1998. Vitamin E in therapy of rheumatic diseases. *Z Rheumatol* 57(4):207-14.

Saxton, J.M., and Donnelly, A.E. 1995. Light concentric exercise during recovery from exercise-induced muscle damage. *Int J Sports Med* 16(6):347-51.

Sayers, S.P., Clarkson, P.M., and Lee, J. 2000. Activity and immobilization after eccentric exercise: I. Recovery of muscle function. *Med Sci Sports Exerc* 32(9):1587-92.

Schoenle, E., Zapf, J., Humbrel, R.E., and Froesch, E.R. 1982. Insulin-like growth factor-1 stimulates growth in hypophysectomized rats. *Nature* 296:252-53.

Schurch, P.M., Hillen, M., Hock, A., Feinendengen, L.E., and Hollmann, W. 1979. Possibilities of calculating the fat-free body mass and its reaction to a carbohydrate-poor, fat-rich diet. *Infusionstherapie und Kinische Ernahrung* 6(5):311-14.

Schurch, P.M., Reinke, A., and Hollmann, W. 1979. Carbohydrate-reduced diet and metabolism: About the influence of a 4-week isocaloric, fat-rich, carbohydrate-reduced diet on body weight and metabolism. *Med Klin Munich* 74(36):1279-85.

Sebokova, E., Gar, M.L., Wierzbicki, A., et al. 1990. Alteration of the lipid composition of rat testicular plasma membranes by dietary (n-3) fatty acids changes the responsiveness of Leydig cells and testosterone synthesis. *J Nutr* 120(6):610-18.

Shamoon, H., Soman, V., and Sherwin, R.S. 1980. The influence of acute physiological increments of cortisol on fuel metabolism and insulin binding in monocytes in normal humans. *J Clin Endocrinol Metab* 50:495-501.

Sherwood, L. 1993. *Human physiology from cells to systems*, 2nd ed. St. Paul, MN: West.

Shultz, T.D., Chew, B.P., Seaman, W.R., and Luedecke, L.O. 1992. Inhibitory effect of conjugated dienoic derivatives of linoleic acid and beta-carotene on the in vitro growth of human cancer cells. *Cancer Letters* 63(2):125-33.

Sidery, M.B., Gallen, I.W., and Macdonald, I.A. 1990. The initial physiological responses to glucose ingestion in normal subjects are modified by a 3 day high-fat diet. *Br J Nutr* 64(3):705-13.

Sies, H., Stahl, W., and Sundquist, A.R. 1992. Antioxidant functions of vitamins. Vitamins E and C, beta-carotene, and other carotenoids. *Ann NY Acad Sci* 669:7-20.

Simmons, P.S., Miles, J.M., Gerich, J.E., et al. 1984. Increased proteolysis: An effect of increases in plasma cortisol within the physiological range. *J Clin Invest* 73:412-20.

Simopoulos, A.P. 1999. Essential fatty acids in health and chronic disease. *Amer J Clin Nutr* 70:S560-69.

Simopoulos, A.P. 2008. The importance of the omega-6/omega-3 fatty acid ratio in cardiovascular disease and other chronic diseases. *Exper Biol Med* 233:674-88.

Sjogren, K., Leung, K.C., Kaplan, W., Gardiner-Garden, M., Gibney, J., and Ho, K.Y. 2007. Growth hormone regulation of metabolic gene expression in muscle: A microarray study in hypopituitary men. *Am J Physiol Endocrinol Metab* 293:E364-71.

Soszynski, P.A., and Frohman, L.A. 1992. Inhibitory effects of ethanol on the growth hormone (GH)-releasing hormone-GH-insulin-like growth factor-I axis in the rat. *Endocrinology* 131(6):2603-8.

Starkey, D.B., Pollock, M.L., Ishida, Y., Welsh, M.A., Breshue, W.F., Graves, J.F., and Feigembaum, M.S. 1996. Effect of resistance training volume on strength and muscle thickness. *Med Sci Sports Exerc* 28:1311-20.

Staron, R.S., Karapondo, D.L., Kraemer, W.J., Fry, A.C., Gordon, S.E., Falkel, J.E., Hagerman, F.C., and Hikida, R.S. 1994. Skeletal muscle adaptations during early phase of heavy resistance training in men and women. *J Appl Physiol* 76:1247-55.

Steck, S.E., Chalecki, A.M., Miller, P., Conway, J., Austin, G.L., Hardin, J.W., Albright, C.D., and Thuillier, P. 2007. Conjugated linoleic acid supplementation for twelve weeks increases lean body mass in obese humans. *J Nutr* 137:1188-1193.

Swolin, D., Brantsing, C., Matejka, G., and Ohlsson, C. 1996. Cortisol decreases IGF-1 mRNA levels in human osteoblast-like cells. *J Endocrinol* 149(3):397-403.

Taouis, M., Dagou, C., Ster, C., Durand, G., Pinault, M., and Delarue, J. 2002. N-3 polyunsaturated fatty acids prevent the defect of insulin receptor signaling in muscle. *Am J Physiol Endocrinol Metab* 282(3):E664-71.

Terjung, R.L., and Hood, D.L. 1986. Biochemical adaptation in skeletal muscle induced by exercise training. *J Appl Physiol* 70:1021-28.

Tesch, P.A., Colliander, E.G., and Kaiser, P. 1986. Muscle metabolism during intense, heavy-resistance exercise. *Eur J Appl Physiol Occup Ther.* 55:362-366.

Thirunavukkarasu, V., Nandhini, A.T., and Anuradha, C.V. 2004. Fructose diet-induced skin collagen abnormalities are prevented by lipoic acid. *Exp Diabesity Res* 5(4):237-44.

Thompson, J.R., and Wu, G. 1991. The effect of ketone bodies on nitrogen metabolism in skeletal muscle. *Comp Biochem Physiol* 100(2):209-16.

Tipton, K.D., Ferrando, A.A., Phillips, S.M., Doyle, D., Jr., and Wolfe, R.R. 1999. Postexercise net protein synthesis in human muscle from orally administered amino acids. *Am J Physiol* 276:E628-34.

Tipton, K.D., Rasmussen, B.B., Miller, S.L., Wolf, S.E., Owens-Stovall, S.K., Petrini, B.E., and Wolfe, R.R. 2001. Timing of amino acid-carbohydrate ingestion alters anabolic response of muscle to resistance exercise. *Am J Physiol Endocrinol Metab* 281(2):E197-206.

Tomobe, Y.I., Morizawa, K., Tsuchida, M., Hibino, H., Nakano, Y., and Tanaka, Y. 2000. Dietary docosahexaenoic acid suppresses inflammation and immunoresponses in contact hypersensitivity reaction in mice. *Lipids* 35(1):61-69.

Tsai, A.C., and Gong, T.W. 1987. Modulation of the exercise and retirement effects by dietary fat intake in hamsters. *J Nut* 117(6):1149-53.

Tuohimaa, P., Keisala, T., Minasyan, A., Cachat, J., and Kalueff, A. 2009. Vitamin D, nervous system and aging. *Psychoneuroendocrino.* 1:S278-286.

Underwood, L.E., D'Ercole, A.J., Clemmons, D.R., and Van Wyk, J.J. 1986. Paracrine functions of somatomedins. *J Clin Endocrinol Metab* 15:5-77.

Urban, R.J., Bodenburg, Y.H., Gilkison, C., Foxworth, J., Coggan, A.R., Wolfe, R.R., and Ferrando, A. 1995. Testosterone administration to elderly men increases skeletal muscle strength and protein synthesis. *Am J Physiol Endocrinol Metab* 269:E820-26.

U.S. Food and Nutrition Board. 1989. *Recommended dietary allowances,* 10th ed. Washington, DC: National Academy Press.

Vincent, H.K., Bourguignon, C.M., Vincent, K.R., Weltman, A.L., Bryant, M., and Taylor A.G. 2006. Antioxidant supplementation lowers exercise-induced oxidative stress in young overweight adults. *Obesity* 14(12):2224-35.

Vissers, M.N., Zock, P.L., Roodenurg, A.J., Leenen, R., and Katan, M.B. 2002. Olive oil phenols are absorbed in humans. *J Nutr* 50(5):1290-97.

Von Schacky, C. 2000. N-3 fatty acids and the prevention of coronary atherosclerosis. *Am J Clin Nutr* 71(Suppl 1):S224-27.

Wahle, K.W., Caruso, D., Ochoa, J.J., and Quiles, J.L. 2004. Olive oil and modulation of cell signaling in disease prevention. *Lipids* 39(12):1223-31.

Wahrburg, U., Martin, H., Sandkamp, M., Schulte, H., and Assmann, G. 1992. Comparative effects of a recommended lipid-lowering diet vs a diet rich in monounsaturated fatty acids on serum lipid profiles in healthy young adults. *Am J Clin Nutr* 56(4):678-83.

Wang, C., Caitlin, D.H., Starcevic, B., et al. 2005. Low-fat high fiber diet decreased serum and urine androgens in men. *J Clin Endocrinol Metab* 90(6):3550-59.

Wardlaw, G.M., and Insel, P.M. 1990. *Perspectives in nutrition.* St. Louis: Times Mirror/Mosby.

Wells, G. 2007. *Speeding recovery from training.* http://www.drgregwells.com/task-6-recovery-regeneratio/

Westerblad, H., Allen, D.G., Bruton, J.D., Andrade, F.H., and Lannergren, J. 1998. Mechanisms underlying the reduction of isometric force in skeletal muscle fatigue. *Acta Physiol Scand* 162:253-60.

Westerblad, H., Bruton, J.D., Allen, D.G., and Lannergren, J. 2000. Functional significance of calcium in long-lasting fatigue of skeletal muscle. *Eur J Appl Physiol* 83:166-74.

Westman, E.C., Yancy, W.S., Edman, J.S., Tomlin, K.F., and Perkins, C.E. 2002. Effect of 6-month adherence to a very low carbohydrate diet program. *Am J Med* 112(1):30-36.

Whitney, E., and Rolfes, S.R. 2008. *Understanding nutrition,* 11th ed. Independence, KY: Thomson Wadsworth.

Williams, J.H. 1991. Caffeine, neuromuscular function and high-intensity exercise performance. *J Sports Med Phys Fitness* 31(3):481-89.

Willit, W.C., Stampfer, M.J., Manson, J.E., et al. 1993. Intake of trans fatty acids and risk of coronary heart disease among women. *Lancet* 341(8845):581-85.

Wilmore, J.H., and Costill, D.L. 1999. *Physiology of sports and exercise.* Champaign, IL: Human Kinetics.

Wolfe, R.R. 2000. Protein supplements and exercise. *Am J Clin Nutr* 72:S551-57.

Wozniak, A.C., Kong, J., Bock, E., Pilipowicz, O., and Anderson, J.E. 2005. Signaling satellite-cell activation in skeletal muscle: Markers, models, stretch, and potential alternative pathways. *Muscle Nerve* 31:283-300.

Yancy, W.S., Jr., Olsen, M.K., Guyton, J.R., Bakst, R.P., and Westman, E.C. 2004. A low-carbohydrate, ketogenic diet versus a low-fat diet to treat obesity and hyperlipidemia: A randomized, controlled trial. *Ann Intern Med* 140:769-77.

Yoshida, H., and Kajimoto, G. 1989. Effect of dietary vitamin E on the toxicity of autoxidized oil to rats. *Ann Nutr Metab* 33(3):153-61.

Zafarullah, M., Li, W.Q., Sylvester, J., and Ahmad, M. Molecular mechanisms of N-acetylcysteine actions. *Cell Mol Life Sci* 60(1):6-20.

Zapf, J.C., Schmid, H., and Froesch, E.R. 1984. Biological and immunological properties of insulin-like growth factors I and II. *Clin Endocrinol Metab* 13:3-30.

Zorzano, A., Palacin, M., and Guma, A. 2005. Mechanisms regulating GLUT4 glucose transporter expression and glucose transport in skeletal muscle. *Acta Physiol Scand* 183(1):43-58.

Index

Note: The italicized *f* and *t* following page numbers refer to figures and tables, respectively.

About the Authors

Tudor O. Bompa, PhD, revolutionized Western training methods when he introduced his groundbreaking theory of periodization in Romania in 1963. After adopting his training system, the Eastern Bloc countries dominated international sports through the 1970s and 1980s. In 1988, Dr. Bompa applied his principle of periodization to the sport of bodybuilding. He has personally trained 11 Olympic Games medalists (including four gold medalists) and has served as a consultant to coaches and athletes worldwide.

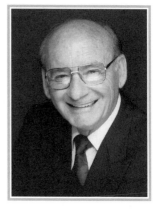

Dr. Bompa's books on training methods, including *Theory and Methodology of Training: The Key to Athletic Performance* and *Periodization of Training for Sports,* have been translated into 17 languages and used in more than 130 countries for training athletes and educating and certifying coaches. Bompa has been invited to speak about training in more than 30 countries and has been awarded certificates of honor and appreciation from such prestigious organizations as the Argentinean Ministry of Culture, the Australian Sports Council, the Spanish Olympic Committee, and the International Olympic Committee.

A member of the Canadian Olympic Association and the Romanian National Council of Sports, Dr. Bompa is professor emeritus at York University, where he has taught training theories since 1987. He and his wife, Tamara, live in Sharon, Ontario.

Mauro Di Pasquale, MD, a physician specializing in nutrition and sports medicine, spent 10 years at the University of Toronto teaching and researching nutritional supplements and drug use in sports. He wrote both *Bodybuilding Supplement Review* and *Amino Acids and Proteins for the Athlete* and has written hundreds of articles for *Muscle and Fitness, Flex, Men's Fitness, Shape, Muscle Media,* and *Ironman,* among many others. Di Pasquale was a powerlifter for over 20 years, winning the powerlifting world championships in 1976 and the World Games in 1981.

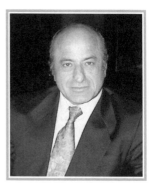

Di Pasquale received his medical degree from the University of Toronto and is a certified medical review officer. Currently the president of the International United Powerlifting Federation and the Pan American Powerlifting Federation, he lives in Ontario.

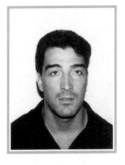

As a former professional wrestler for the National Wrestling Alliance (NWA), bodybuilder, and kinesiologist, **Lorenzo J. Cornacchia** has directed extensive electrical myographical (EMG) research to identity which exercises produce the greatest amount of muscular electrical stimulation. In 1992, he conducted a research study with Dr. Bompa and various colleagues to scientifically determine the results of bodybuilders' use of periodization training methods, bodybuilders' use of performance-enhancing agents and the typical bodybuilding training method, and bodybuilders' use of the periodization method coupled with performance-enhancing agents. *Ironman* magazine published the results in their May 1994 issue, "Periodization vs. Steroids." Cornacchia also published the results in Dr. Di Pasquale's international newsletters, *Drugs in Sports* and *Anabolic Research Review*. Cornacchia coauthored *Periodization of Strength*. His EMG research was published in *Ironman's Ultimate Guide to Arm Training* (2001), *Ironman's Ultimate Bodybuilding Encyclopedia* (2002), and *Ironman's Ultimate Guide to Building Muscle Mass* (2003).

Cornacchia became an editor and author for *Ironman* magazine, writing a monthly column called "EMG Analysis," and directed extensive research studies in electromyography to determine which exercises produced the greatest amount of muscular electrical activation. Currently he is working with Dr. Di Pasquale on research dealing with supplementation and the metabolic diet.

Cornacchia received his BA in physical education from York University. Currently he is co-owner of a fitness establishment called FFX and is the president and shareholder of Pyrotek Special Effects, Inc., where he spends most of his time designing special effects for shows such as the Grammy Awards, Academy Awards, and BET Awards and for artists such as Iron Maiden, Lady Gaga, Van Halen, Rihanna, Taylor Swift, and Lil Wayne. Cornacchia resides in Miami, Florida, and Las Vegas, Nevada. His favorite pastime is watching the NFL's Cincinnati Bengals.

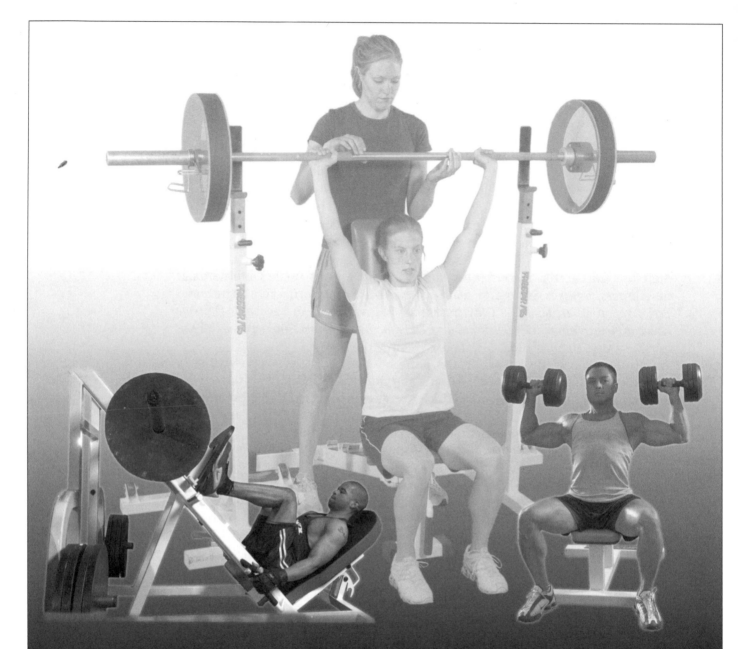